Celebrity Health
Narratives and the
Public Health

DATE DUE

Celebrity Health Narratives and the Public Health

CHRISTINA S. BECK, STELLINA M.A. CHAPMAN,
NATHANIEL SIMMONS, KELLY E. TENZEK
and STEPHANIE M. RUHL

McFarland & Company, Inc., Publishers
Jefferson, North Carolina

LIBRARY OF CONGRESS CATALOGUING-IN-PUBLICATION DATA

Beck, Christina S.
    Celebrity health narratives and the public health / Christina
S. Beck [and four others].
        p.   cm.
    Includes bibliographical references and index.

    ISBN 978-0-7864-7971-9 (softcover : acid free paper) ∞
    ISBN 978-1-4766-1907-1 (ebook)

    1. Mass media in health education.   2. Celebrities.
3. Health promotion.   4. Consumer education.   I. Title.

RA440.5.B43 2015
613.0285—dc23   2015019051

BRITISH LIBRARY CATALOGUING DATA ARE AVAILABLE

Front cover © 2015 Shutterstock

Printed in the United States of America

McFarland & Company, Inc., Publishers
    Box 611, Jefferson, North Carolina 28640
    www.mcfarlandpub.com

Table of Contents

Acknowledgments

Christie: I am very grateful to my co-authors, Stellina, Nathaniel, Kelly, and Stephanie for collaborating with me on this project (as well as to Tim McKenna for his contributions to our earlier article about celebrity health narratives). Work on this book has spanned several years, overlapping with other professional and personal adventures, but, especially given that celebrity health narratives have become even more prominent and intimate (with the advent of social media), I'm glad that it has taken some time to finish. I appreciate the continued support of the faculty in the School of Communication Studies at Ohio University and the many conversations that I have had with colleagues and students about this endeavor. Feedback from reviews of our article in *Health Communication* and conference presentation at the Central States Communication Association conference has enriched and advanced this book. On a personal note, my husband, Roger C. Aden, has, quite literally, made my role in this project possible. Thanks so much to Roger for everything that you do to make sure that everyone in our family has what they need, when they need it, including time for me to finish up a book only a few weeks after our oldest daughter got married. I am also so blessed for my daughters Ellie-Kate (age 6), Emmy (age 13), Chelsea Meagan (age 19), and Brittany (age 27) and grateful for their patience and sacrifice, especially during the last few weeks of the project. I'll work on our trip to DisneyWorld now ☺ Finally, I praise God for all of His many blessings!

Stellina: Just when you think you know who you are, something comes along and makes you a stronger, better person. May we all have the courage to tell *our* story and encourage as many people as possible to be proactive about *their* health. To everyone who made this book possible: Past teachers, professors, family and friends, especially my mom, dad, and husband Aaron, thank you for your ongoing support and encouragement throughout my educational and professional careers. To the coauthors of this book, Christie, Kelly, Nathaniel, and Stephanie: You are all brilliant scholars and I thank you for your valuable contributions, immense encouragement, and inspiration throughout this journey of crafting such a beautiful book.

Nathaniel: I would like to thank the various celebrities both within and beyond this book that shared their health experiences with the public. Although this may not have always been their choice or desire, their stories continue to make a difference. I would also like to thank my coauthors for all of their feedback and hard work throughout this entire process.

Kelly: I would like to acknowledge and thank my colleagues who provided support throughout the process and listened to ideas and challenges during the writing process. I would like to thank the local coffee shop who provided the space for creative thought and a full cup to keep moving forward. I would also like to thank my family, who never stopped providing encouragement and support even when trips home were cancelled, travel plans changed, and I needed extra help with Maggie, our dog's, care. I hope that with this book and the difficult health conversations that are brought up, if the readers are experiencing similar situations or need help, they find the courage to seek support to find physical and spiritual peace.

Stephanie: I dedicate this work to some of the most significant women in my life: my mother, my sisters, and my mentors, Lynn M. Harter, Mary Albert Darling, and Suzette Turpel—your lives, your work, and your love are beautiful examples that we do not need celebrity status to make extraordinary contributions to our world.

Preface

CHRISTINA S. BECK

I admit it. Every now and again, my eye drifts ... wanders away from my rather boring cart of groceries and up to the enticing racks of magazines that line the check-out aisle. Yes, I have an Inquiring Mind, and, sometimes (not always, though!), I skim headlines about the rich and famous, observe less than flattering photographs of celebrities, and note captions that question the health status of people whom I "know" but have never met—all while waiting to pay for my weekly shopping.

As I was working on my book *Communicating for Better Health: A Guide through the Medical Mazes* (Beck, 2000), I realized that I wanted to include a chapter on public dialogues about health. As I gathered material for that portion of the book, I recalled those images from the check-out aisle and started to think about other celebrities who chose to share their private health-related sagas with the public—Annette Funicello, Christopher Reeve, Tracey Gold, among others. I realized that their private-turned-public health narratives constitute important contributions to broader conversations about health, wellness, illness, and even death.

What began as the collection of a few examples for a small section of a chapter in another book has morphed into the development of a data set over the past 17 years that currently encompasses information on over 200 celebrities who have confided personal health details through television and print interviews and, increasingly, interactions with fans on various forms of social media. As time ensued, the stacks under my office desk grew. After obtaining and enlisting an apprentice from the Honors Tutorial College to pursue more leads and print transcripts from various news programs and talk shows, the mound under my desk expanded even more, especially given that this data collection dovetailed with the emergence of social media and reality television and proliferation of television outlets—a perfect storm, if you will, for intensified attention to the personal concerns of public figures, particularly with regard to health issues.

As I continued to clip, buy, and tape items that could be related to this research, my life continued to unfold. Since my work on this project began in 1997, I have welcomed two more daughters (for a total of four children), co-edited another book, and served as editor of *Communication Yearbook*, president of the Central States Communication Association, and first vice president of the National Communication Association. Although I never would have intended to drag the celebrity health narrative project out for so long, I am grateful that something always seemed to come up and distract me from getting back to it, given that these years have enabled me to gather data as this unique phenomenon in both pop culture and public health communication unfolded.

Moreover, delayed attention to these materials allowed me to amass just the right team of coauthors. In 2011, I invited four smart, talented, and eager individuals—Stellina Aubuchon, Timothy McKenna, Stephanie Ruhl, and Nathaniel Simmons—to join me on this project and to begin sifting through the files that overflowed from under my desk (yes, images from hoarding shows might be appropriate). We wrote a paper that earned a Top Paper Award in the Central States Communication Association's Health Communication Interest Group (and that subsequently became an article in *Health Communication*). During our CSCA top paper panel, attendees offered enthusiastic feedback on our findings and urged us to develop our work into a book-length project. Four members of the initial team elected to do so. (Tim McKenna opted to focus on other research more closely related to his program of research, including his dissertation, and we then added Kelly Tenzek, an accomplished health communication scholar, to the team.)

For the book project, we enhanced our data set by collecting additional material from online discussion boards, Twitter, and Facebook as we developed chapters. In all, data for this volume includes books that were authored by celebrities, Congressional records, television show transcripts, magazine and newspaper articles, Facebook and Twitter posts, and online discussion board comments, reactions to blogs or online articles, and, in the case of one of our chapters, survey research. Notably, throughout this book, we only include references to cases in which celebrities speak out about their own health condition or a health situation with an intimate personal connection (or where loved ones of a celebrity speak out, such as the family of former National Football League player Junior Seau regarding traumatic brain injury). This book does not focus on paid celebrity spokespeople because we consider those contributions to differ significantly from personal accounts (see related argument by Houston et al., 2011), with the exception of our chapter on Paula Deen (for reasons that we specify in chapter 5).

We appreciate McFarland's excitement about this project, and we marvel at the book that we have produced over the past 15 months since we obtained our contract. Concurrently, life certainly "happened" for all of us. All of my co-authors found new jobs, and three of them (Nate, Stephanie, and Stellina) finished their dissertations while writing chapters on this book. Stellina got married, and I rejoiced in the marriage of my oldest daughter just days before our book deadline (not to mention the various activities and accomplishments of my other three girls that demanded my attention over those months). I mention these other personal and professional details as a means of underscoring the postmodern blurring and interweaving of our lives. Instead of singular, simple, linear lives, we juggle, multitask, and manage as the varied and complicated threads of our personal and professional lives intertwine and reflexively flavor each other. As such, our life narratives are implicitly messy, complex, and entangled.

The lives of celebrities are perhaps even more so, especially when they wrestle with a health challenge. Usually such a challenge is a deeply personal and private matter; the intense glare of the public eye, amid the increasingly interactional and intimate enactment of life as a contemporary celebrity, can prompt a recasting of a "just private" health experience into a "private-yet-public" health narrative. As we detail throughout this book, emergent "private-yet-public" celebrity health narratives function rhetorically and relationally to inform and inspire onlookers, powerfully reframing conversations about potentially stigmatizing illnesses and drawing attention to relatively unknown ones. Further, as we elaborate, celebrity narratives continue to influence personal perspectives of fans as well as impact public policy on funding and health-related research. We argue that this work constitutes an important contribution to discussions of fandom and implications of popular culture for public health conversations.

We hope that you enjoy reading this book as much as we have had fun while writing it!

CHAPTER ONE

Personal Challenges, Public Struggles

An Overview of Celebrity Health Narratives and Implications for Public Health Conversations

Michael J. Fox energetically skateboarded into the hearts of big-screen audiences in the *Back to the Future* trilogy as Marty McFly. Thus, as an actor seeking to keep options open for future roles, Fox found himself in a difficult position as he subsequently navigated his career as a youthful actor amid his diagnosis of Parkinson's disease, traditionally envisioned as an "old person's" condition (see Beck, 2005; Fox, 2002). For a number of years, Fox tried to mask the symptoms. Ultimately, he realized that he could no longer do so, and he revealed his illness to Barbara Walters in a special interview, transitioning his private health issue into a public one. Indeed, as Fox noted in his book, *Lucky Man*, he changed from an individual who confided only in close family and friends to an activist for research about Parkinson's disease, creating a foundation to raise money and testifying before Congress in a quest for federal funding.

Notably, Fox's experience exemplifies an increasingly prevalent form of public dialogues about health and, concurrently, an intriguing artifact of contemporary popular culture (Beck, Aubuchon, McKenna, Ruhl, & Simmons, 2014). As we elaborate throughout this book, celebrities have long captivated public attention, and, with ever expanding and diversified mediated accessibility to public figures, those in the spotlight must implicitly wrestle with what to share, what to conceal, and why and how to do so. Especially in terms of health issues, such disclosures by prominent individuals hold the potential to influence health awareness, prevention, and responses, and, potentially, policy as others read or hear about a celebrity's illness and/or, perhaps, his/her appeal for action or aid.

Celebrity health narratives have certainly not gone unnoticed in the mainstream press. Recent examples include widespread coverage of Robin Roberts' return to *Good Morning America* in February 2013, after battling cancer; episodes of *Katie* (2013, January) and *The Doctors* (2013, February) that were both dedicated to the topic of celebrity health narratives, and Oprah's interviews in January 2013 with Lance Armstrong about his drug use and resulting implications for the foundation that he created for cancer research. As we detail in this book, when a celebrity decides to disclose a diagnosis to a reporter (or update a Facebook status, send a tweet, or post an Instagram photo about it), especially in this era of social media, s/he initiates a very public and multi-faceted communicative firestorm, instantly propelling a previously private situation into a public discussion about everything from medical alternatives to motivations for sharing.

In this introduction, we frame our exploration of celebrity health narratives in terms of private-public boundary management and narrative theorizing, and we situate celebrity health narratives as powerful, multilayered, sometimes controversial, contributions to broader interactions about health and health policy. We also contextualize celebrity health narratives as increasingly dynamic and interactive in light of social media and participatory fan cultures.

Blurred Narrative Boundaries

On May 14, 2013, Angelina Jolie, an acclaimed actress, humanitarian, and mother, shocked readers of the *New York Times* by revealing her "strong choice" to undergo a preventive double mastectomy in an editorial on the Op-Ed page. Jolie's mother passed away from ovarian cancer in 2007. After learning that she tested positive for BRCA1 gene, Jolie opted to reduce her risk of breast cancer through a series of preventive surgeries to remove and then reconstruct her breasts (see also Tauber, Cotliar, Dennis, Jordan, Green & Cedenheim, 2013, May 27). As one columnist noted, Jolie's decision could readily be considered "understandable. She watched her mother struggle with breast cancer, then die of ovarian cancer.... Her maternal grandmother also had ovarian cancer" (Abcarian, 2013, May 21, para. 3). Indeed, sadly, only 12 days after her stunning disclosure, Jolie's aunt (her mother's sister) also passed away from breast cancer on May 26, 2013 ("Angelina Jolie's aunt dies of breast cancer," 2013, May 27).

During the course of the surgeries, Jolie remained visible yet mum, continuing to fulfill commitments while shrouding her medical saga in secrecy (Dillon, 2013, May 22). According to Dillon, "Brad Pitt and Angelina Jolie have played spies and assassins on the big screen, and in real life they covered their tracks during Jolie's preventive mastectomy surgeries," reportedly employing "untraceable rental cars and early morning appointments to avoid discovery" (para. 1–2). As partner Brad Pitt revealed in an interview with *USA Today* (Puente, Freydkin, & Mandell, 2013, May 15, p. 2A), "She could have stayed absolutely private about it, and I don't think anyone would have been none the wiser with such good results."

Yet, on May 14, 2013, Jolie disclosed her story to the world, confiding, "On April 27, I finished the three months of medical procedures that the mastectomies involved. During that time I have been able to keep this private and to carry on with my work" (para. 6). However, as she explained in her Op-Ed column, she shattered her silence "because I hope that other women can benefit from my experience. Cancer is still a word that strikes fear in people's hearts, producing a deep sense of powerlessness. But today it is possible to find out through a blood test whether you are highly susceptible to breast and ovarian cancer, and then take action" (para. 7). As Pitt noted in his interview with *USA Today* (Puente et al., 2013, May 15, p. 2A), "It was really important to her to share the story and that others would understand it doesn't have to be a scary thing. In fact, it can be an empowering thing, and something that makes you stronger and us stronger."

In her Op-Ed piece, Jolie (2013, May 14) painted a portrait of a devoted mother, yearning to take all necessary steps to be with her children as long as possible, of a wife with a supportive partner (Brad Pitt), and of a woman with options. Jolie explained, "My doctors estimated that I had an 87 percent risk of breast cancer and a 50 percent risk of ovarian cancer" (para. 3). According to Jolie, "I wanted to write this to tell other women that the decision to have a mastectomy was not easy. But it is one I am very happy that I made.... I can tell my children that they don't need to fear they will lose me to breast cancer.... I feel empowered that I made a strong choice that in no way diminishes my femininity" (para. 11–12).

Jolie's decision to discuss her response has sparked both praise and controversy ("Controversy of the Week: Jolie: A Powerful Message about Breasts and Cancer," 2013, May 31; M. Roberts, 2013, May 14). Editorial boards for the *New York Times* and *USA Today*, fellow celebrity breast cancer survivors (such as Sheryl Crowe), and a wide range of columnists heralded Jolie's courage and transparency about such a personal matter. In her article titled, "Angelina Jolie's Courageous Act Will Save Women's Lives," *Los Angeles Times* columnist Abcarian (2013, May 21) hailed Jolie's willingness to shed light on this sensitive topic, noting that "[w]ith her star power and ability to stoke an insatiable public interest, Jolie, 37, has the potential to help save lives by raising awareness. With the stroke of a pen, she makes genetic testing seem less fearsome and helps destigmatize mastectomy" (para. 4). The front page head-line on the May 15, 2013, issue of *USA Today* boldly proclaimed: "Her mas-tectomy could change women's lives" (see Puente et al., 2013, May 15, p. 1A). Nearly a year later, Nolte (2014, March 4) reported that the vast majority of publications and commentary cast Jolie's decision and disclosure in a positive light, in spite of potentially problematic aspects of the story.

Critics cautioned against branding the disclosure as universally "good," with at least one linking her to owners of the genetic test. Alleging that Jolie could actually be "part of a clever corporate scheme to protect billions in BRCA gene patents" and "influence" the approaching "Supreme Court deci-sion," Adams (2013, May 16) contended that "[i]f you pull back the curtain on this one, you find far more than an innocent woman exercising a 'choice.' This is about protecting trillions in profits through the deployment of carefully-crafted public relations campaigns designed to manipulate the pub-lic opinion of women" (para. 2).

Even some practitioners who do not suspect such financially driven motivations acknowledged the controversial nature of Jolie's disclosure as well as potentially negative ramifications. Referring to the "Angelina Effect," Kruger et al. (2013, May 27) asserted in *Time* magazine that "the seeming straightforwardness of Jolie's case masks a much murkier reality, one that involves science, policy and probabilities, not to mention Americans'—indeed everyone's—tendency to observe what the famous do and then conclude that we should do the same" (para. 6). *The Week* noted: "Jolie deserves full credit for publicly explaining her decision, said Peggy Orenstein in NYTimes.com, but many doctors worry it will actually 'add fuel to a culture of fear' about breast cancer" ("Controversy of the Week," 2013, May 31, p. 4). Dr. H. Gilbert Welch (2013, May 18), a professor of medicine at the Dartmouth Institute for Health Policy and Clinical Practice and guest CNN contributor, commented that he read Jolie's editorial and, at first, "couldn't understand initially ... the concern expressed by others" (para. 5). However, Welch continued,

> As the day wore on, the story dominated the news. I didn't fully appreciate how much Ms. Jolie is admired and respected and had neglected to consider just how powerful a celebrity personal anecdote could be. If American women saw themselves in Angelina Jolie—then that would be a problem. Because the logical next question is: Should I get a preventive mastectomy? Then I realized some-thing was missing in her piece: something that should have been printed in big black letters: *NOTE: This story is not relevant to more than 99 percent of American women* [emphasis original] [para. 5–9].

Clearly, regardless of intentions or even influences on health practices, Jolie's piece in the *New York Times* instantly redefined her formerly private health issue into a topic ripe for public conversation. Puente et al. (2013, May 15, p. 2A) commented that "[i]n 2008, actress Christina Applegate was forced into discussing on TV her breast cancer and mastectomy because someone leaked her medical records to *The National Enquirer*.... Not Jolie. She took control of her own narrative." As we now explain, though, Jolie implicitly and inevitably yielded that control just as soon as the story surfaced in the public sphere, triggering not only a public onslaught of conversation about this important issue but also, by virtue of sharing her story with the world, providing an opening for others in the general public to comment, critique, congratulate, and, essentially, co-author her emergent health narrative.

Preserving Privacy

> It wasn't just that a supernova movie star had her breasts surgically removed to improve her chances of not getting breast cancer. It was how Angelina Jolie—a woman who is rarely without a paparazzi scrum in pursuit—was able to do it in secret, and then announce it on her own terms. This never happens. Until Tuesday. The next shock was how the news went over with people who love her, people who loathe her, or people who, up until yesterday, didn't give a fig about her [Puente et al., 2013, May 15, 1A].

Public figures (such as politicians, actors, musicians, prominent business officials) have long sought to manage their public images by carefully guarding what they consider to be private (and potentially damaging or face-threatening) information (for related arguments, see Petronio, 2000, 2002, 2004, 2007, 2010, 2013; Petronio & Kovach, 1997; Petronio & Reierson, 2009). In her theory of Communication Privacy Management, Petronio (2000, 2002) argues that, in interpersonal and family relationships, individuals must carefully navigate just how much (and what and when) to reveal otherwise private details to others as well as reflect on possible benefits and costs of disclosure. Confiding personal details can draw others near, yet, depending on the reaction of those others, that same information can drive them away.

Disclosure of potentially face-threatening details in the public sphere also comes with a similar risk of alienation due to stigma. In his classic work, Goffman (1963) situated stigma as the communicative co-construction of some feature (such as a disease or physical characteristic) as societally dispreferred. Revealing such an attribute involves risking adverse financial, emotional, physical, and/or relational consequences. Thus, individuals must wrestle with the potential benefits of disclosing something that others might treat as problematic versus concealing that condition or characteristic. Especially for a celebrity, reputation constitutes a significant factor in obtaining opportunities (such as acting jobs) and fostering desired relationships with fans and co-workers. Do the "pros" of disclosing (such as increased immediacy, potential to help others, some degree of control over one's own narrative) outweigh the "cons" (negative reactions by others, loss of ability to narrate one's own narrative in one's own time)?

However, protecting privacy boundaries can be particularly difficult for people in the public eye. The ever inquiring minds of fans (and readers of popular supermarket tabloids) want to know if an actress has an eating disorder or if an actor has an addiction. Photographers utilize advanced technology to capture images of celebrities at every turn, and reporters scrutinize video and photographs and scramble for tips to determine if an actor suffers from a serious affliction. Patrick Swayze expressed frustration with invasive media attention after his diagnosis with stage-four pancreatic cancer amid his preference for privacy. In his 2009 book, *The Time of My Life*, Swayze (with his wife, Lisa Niemi) wrote that he elected to delay telling his mother about his cancer diagnosis until after she went through her own eye surgery, but a reporter showed up at his mom's door and broke the news instead. According to Swayze, "Unfortunately, those morally bankrupt souls at the *National Enquirer* had other ideas.... Human decency is apparently an afterthought when there's money to be made selling tabloids" (p. 237).

Just as the decision to disclose such diagnoses is complicated and layered in our private lives when we don't happen to be celebrities, such choices become even more multi-faceted when individuals struggle with potential public revelations. Swayze obviously wanted to wait to disclose his condition to his mother out of concern for her health—very much mirroring considerations that even people out of the public eye must navigate. With celebrity status, though, comes the additional factor of managing public persona and perceptions.

Berger (1985, October 3) wrote, "For more than a decade, the name Rock Hudson was synonymous with masculine good looks" (para. 7). Yet, when Hudson appeared on the television show *Dynasty*, he looked tired and frail, and, according to costar Linda Evans, he seemed hesitant to share a scripted kiss (http://video.pbs.org/video/2326560754/). A short while later, Hudson shocked fans and the entertainment community with the news that he had AIDS. Not only had he concealed his homosexuality to "protect his macho image," he became "the first major U.S. celebrity to die of complications from AIDS" ("Hollywood icon Rock Hudson dies of AIDS," 1985, October 2, para. 1). Especially given the confusion and fear surrounding HIV/AIDS in the early 1980s, Hudson's reluctance to kiss Evans and to disclose his condition made sense. As Evans noted in the PBS documentary *Pioneers of Television*, she even subsequently experienced stigma, given that she had touched lips with Hudson during the scene, as dread of catching the misunderstood disease prompted other actors to avoid contact with her (http://video.pbs.org/video/2326560754/).

Although Hudson sought to preserve his privacy to avoid such reactions, the eventual disclosure resulted in "an outpouring of concern for him and for other victims of the disease" (Berger, 1985, October 3, para. 6). Berger noted,

> On Sept. 19 many well-known entertainers joined in a special performance to help raise money to find a cure for AIDS, and although Hudson, who bought $10,000 worth of tickets, was reported too ill to attend, he did send a telegram. It said in part: "I am not happy that I am sick. I am not happy that I have AIDS. But if that is helping others, I can at least know that my own misfortune has had some positive worth" [para. 24].

Private-Yet-Public Health Narratives

Over 40 years before Angelina Jolie made the "bold choice" to reveal her preventive double mastectomy, in the 1970s, former First Lady Betty Ford recognized the potential to transform her own personal health issues into very public teachable moments. At a time when few dared to utter words such as "breast" or "breast exams" (and spoke in hushed tones about problems with "the bottle"), Betty Ford earned widespread acclaim for candor about her bout with breast cancer and her struggles with alcohol. According to Stone (2011), Ford's openness saved lives by motivating many to obtain early detection through breast exams and then encouraged others to seek help after her own frank admission that she needed help to overcome alcoholism.

Notably, the very decision to disclose transforms something that might usually be intimate into a quite public matter. For example, while Jolie and Pitt were preserving their privacy, they controlled their own narrative—the ways in which they wanted to handle intricate medical details and decisions, how they told their children (and when), as well as related emotional and relational meanings, perspectives, and identities. They co-constructed how to talk about the health decision (and when) as well as the ways in which it impacted (or did not influence) their lives, perspectives, or responses. To borrow from Petronio (2000, 2002, 2004, 2010, 2013), they fervently managed their privacy boundaries in terms of this particular issue, and, as such, they carefully and artfully molded the emergent health narrative as partners and then as a family with their children.

With the publication of her editorial, though, Jolie automatically broadened those boundaries to include people quite literally around the world. Petronio and Caughlin explained,

> CPM proposes that people characterize private information as something they own. However, people often bestow various degrees of ownership to others when disclosure takes place, making them shareholders. Because of this communicative process, private information can move from being personal to collective as individuals disclose to others [2006, p. 37].

In the next section, we detail how transformations of personal health narratives into more public ones enable others who learn the news to become co-authors as they, in turn, spread and/or comment on the once private story. As Beck et al. (2014) noted, "Through such disclosures, people implicitly draw others into their emergent, fluid, life narratives and, in the case of health issues, involve those others in their health narratives" (p. 245).

Narrating Our Lives

In his beautifully written book, Arthur Bochner (2014) offered a thoughtful and comprehensive history of narrative theorizing, interwoven with his own journey as an academic. We recommend it as a resource on various strands of interdisciplinary work on the nature of narrative. In addition to illustrating how narrative permits rich insights into life experiences, through his own autoethnographic reflections, Bochner's volume traces traditions of narrative theorizing with a depth that extends beyond the scope of our work in this book. However, as a means of framing our investigation of celebrity health narratives, we highlight the following key issues.

In his description of the narrative paradigm, Fisher (1984, 1985a, 1985b, 1987a, 1987b, 1989, 1994) contended that narrative constitutes an inherent and essential feature of human life. According to Fisher (1984, p. 2), "By 'narration,' I refer to a theory of symbolic actions—words and/or deeds—that have sequence and meaning for those who live, create, or interpret them." Fisher (1984, p. 8) continued to assert that "[i]n theme, if not in every detail, narrative, then, is meaningful for persons in particular and in general, across time and place."

Through our physical actions, emotional reactions, and choices (including what to share with others and what to keep to ourselves), we craft our life (and illness) narratives as we chart the course of our existence (see, for example, Frank, 2010; Harter, 2013; Harter, Japp, & Beck, 2005). This potential freedom and flexibility can foster creative treatments (and expressions) of situations as individuals interpret, respond to, and, perhaps, challenge "the way things 'are,'" prevalent storylines, or "master" narratives (see, e.g., Bamberg & Andrews, 2004; Charon, 2009; Cole, 2010; Harter, 2009; Harter, Scott, Novak, Leeman, & Morris, 2006; Lalvani, 2011; O'Malley-Keighran & Coleman, 2013; Smith-Chandler & Swart, 2014). For example, Angelina Jolie resisted a more typical trajectory of waiting for disease before taking action, electing the double mastectomy as a preventive measure rather than treatment for an existing illness. She proactively sought the blood test, opted for surgery, and broke the news to the world on her own terms.

Notably, the co-construction of meaning involves not simply a "teller" but also others who experience or encounter that symbolic experience and make sense of it in their own ways, according to their own backgrounds, perspectives, and lived realities. As Fisher (1987a, p. 64) argued, "Rationality is determined by the nature of persons as narrative beings—their inherent awareness of *narrative probability*, what constitutes a coherent story, and their constant habit of testing *narrative fidelity*, whether or not the stories they experience ring true with the stories they know to be true in their lives."

By conceptualizing narrative as implicitly dialogic and temporal, we maintain that contributions to the narrative (by all co-tellers) reflexively impact identity construction (see, e.g., Bamberg, 2012; Pederson, 2013; Redman, 2005) as well as the emergent narrative. Thus, as individuals expand their privacy boundaries (such as Jolie writing the op-ed piece), they inherently (although not necessarily intentionally) permit and, indeed, invite commentary on and co-authorship of "their" respective stories. Stephens (2011, p. 66) emphasized that "the construction of narrative may be understood from performative and dialogical perspectives as always a joint enterprise with an active audience." Expanding privacy boundaries implicitly results in redefining "my" story as "our" story in that responses of others (and their respective retellings) reshape and flavor the ever emergent narrative (see also DeFina & Georgakopoulou, 2008; Seaton, 2008).

Reflecting on Fisher's (1984, 1985a, 1987a) claims regarding narrative, we realize the potential power of a narrative to impact others (see related arguments by De Graaf, Hoeken, Sanders, & Beentjes, 2012; Green & Brock, 2000; Kim, Bigman, Leader, Lerman, & Cappella, 2012; Lane, Miller, Brown, & Vilar, 2013; Lee, Hecht, Miller-Day, & Elek, 2011; S. T. Murphy, Frank, Catterjee, & Baezconde-Garbanati, 2013; Niederdeppe, Kim, Lundell, Fazili, & Frazier, 2012; Shaffer, Tomek, & Hulsey, 2014) if it makes sense, if it "rings true," to others.

When Jolie made the decision for the double mastectomy, she had to believe that it was the best course of action, based on available information, feedback from trusted confidantes, etc. No one else mattered beyond her closest family members. However, the disclosure of her surgical choice stretched the scope of her story beyond herself to encompass others who read about her medical saga, talked with others (in person and online), and reflected on the weight of Jolie's words for themselves and their own health (for related work on "witnessing," see Ong, 2014). People could (and did) add their perspectives (critical and complimentary) to Jolie's narrative as they crafted editorials or letters to the editor, conversed on talk shows, and chatted at the water cooler, essentially participating in a public co-narration of Jolie's ongoing health situation. Countless others could now play "Monday morning quarterback" about a decision that did not directly affect them but that *could* be relevant or inspirational if some aspect of the story resonated with them. Moreover, the shifting of a formerly private health narrative into public discourse transforms those "outsiders" into emergent co-stakeholders on the ever evolving story of one person's private health situation unfolding in a quite public arena.

EMERGENT CO-STAKEHOLDERS

For both Angelina Jolie and Betty Ford, revealing private health concerns constituted a choice made willingly. For Michael J. Fox and Rock Hudson, the decisions to disclose their respective diagnoses came much more grudgingly. For all in the public eye, navigating the balance of maintaining personal boundaries amid intense public scrutiny has become increasingly challenging and complicated, especially in this era of social media.

In 1985, Meyrowitz explained that the advent of television enabled viewers to develop parasocial relationships with people that they observed on screen. According to Meyrowitz, as viewers watch characters, news commentators, or political figures on television, they feel as if they come to know them. (For related work on parasocial relationships, see also Earnheardt & Haridakis, 2009; Hartmann & Goldhoorn, 2011; Kassing & Sanderson, 2009; E. Lee & Jang, 2013; Ramasubramanian & Kornfield, 2012; Savage & Spence, 2014; Sood & Rogers, 2001.) Nearly 30 years later, especially with the advent of social media, the "fourth wall" has continued to crack as public figures now routinely tweet about their daily activities and interact with fans on Facebook about some (but not usually all) aspects of their private lives (for related arguments, see Baym, 2010; Booth, 2010; W. J. Brown & Basil, 2010; Evans, 2011; Gauntlett, 2011; High, Oeldorf-Hirsch, & Bellur, 2014; H. Jenkins, 2006; H. Jenkins, Ford, & Green, 2013; Kackman, Binfield, Payne, Perlman, & Sebok, 2011; E. Lee & Jang, 2013; Marwick, 2013; Papacharissi, 2011; Thackeray, Burton, Giraud-Carrier, Rollins, & Draper, 2013; van Dijck, 2013;

Wheeler, 2013), blurring the space between "front" and "back" stages (see Goffman, 1959). Beck et al. (2014) noted that "[d]igital media has altered how people orient to media and others, transforming previously passive 'audience members'" into active co-participants (see, e.g., Baym, 2010; Booth, 2010; Evans, 2011)" (p. 247). Beck et al. noted that "[i]n this hyper-mediated environment, private and public 'boundaries' lack clear demarcations, even in the context of something as personal as a health condition when one happens to be a public figure" (p. 247).

Through those blurred boundaries, with a focus on an illness or injury as a mutual foe, some fans can identify with celebrities on a deeper (and more personal) level as fellow patients. According to K. Burke (1950/1969, p. 21), "two persons may be identified in terms of some principle they share in common, an 'identification' that does not deny their distinctness" (see also Brock, 1999; Wolin, 2001). The following passage from a mother of a fan of then 15-year-old Nick Jonas exemplifies the intimate connection triggered by a shared diagnosis:

> Nick, I am not familiar with your music, but my six-year-old daughter just loves your band. We found out last week that she is type 1 diabetes. When she discovered that you also had this terrible condition it actually bought [sic] a smile to her face. It made her realize that life will go on. We are now just members of a club that no one wants to be a part of. Give your mom a big hug because as a parent that has a child with diabetes this is one of the hardest things to go through. Our prayers are with you. Courtney's Mom ["Diabetes has not slowed down 15-year-old Nick Jonas," 2008, April–May, Comments section].

For Fox, Hudson, and Ford, as well as for the nearly 200 other celebrities in our data set, interactions with fans and admirers as well as opportunities for activism contributed mightily to their own health journeys as well as to public dialogues about health and wellness. In her 1999 book, *Care Packages: Letters to Christopher Reeve from Strangers and Other Friends*, Dana Reeve, wife of the actor best known for his role as Superman, heralded fans for their love, support, and messages of encouragement after Christopher fell from his horse and became paralyzed. In his foreword to the book, Christopher noted,

> When I broke my neck on May 27, 1995, it was like entering a dark tunnel. I couldn't go in alone. My family and my closest friends would have to come with me. As we began to inch our way forward in the dark, suddenly there was light. It came from the thousands of letters that were sent to us from all around the world. Many were from old friends and people I had worked with in the past. But most of them were from complete strangers who felt compelled to write out of pure empathy and compassion. Every day during my stay in intensive care, Dana or one of our family would read handfuls of letters to me. And as I listened,

I soon understood something new: that these letters were not from strangers, just people I had never met. For the first time I realized that all six billion of us on this tiny blue marble are essentially the same—in fact, it is not so hard to understand and see ourselves in others. We are only strangers if we choose to look away [pp. ix–x].

CELEBRITY HEALTH ACTIVISM

Notably, Christopher Reeve did not just benefit from outpourings of support. After his condition stabilized, he worked on behalf of others with spinal cord injuries, establishing the Christopher and Dana Reeve Foundation (to raise money for spinal cord research) and representing the community in testimony before Congress, lobbying for additional funding and advocating for stem cell research (see Gerosa, 1999; Reeve, 1999; Smolowe et al., 2006).

Farrah Fawcett, best known as a beautiful star of the hit 1970s television show, *Charlie's Angels*, originally hoped to capture a "story of survival" (Rutenberg, 2011, May 27, para. 20) by documenting her own cancer journey. Rutenberg recounted,

> When a recurrence of her anal cancer was diagnosed in 2007 she began filming her doctor visits and then decided to make a documentary. She said she wanted to highlight what she saw as the slow process of drug approvals in the United States and treatment advances in countries like Germany, where she was seeking a cure [para. 20].

According to Rutenberg, Fawcett's raw and riveting video diary, as she sought (and struggled with) treatments (and as her body began to fail), became "a seminal moment in television history when it was broadcast in May 2009—making Ms. Fawcett 'the first American celebrity to film herself dying,' the *New York Post* wrote" (para. 4). Rutenberg noted that the Emmy-nominated documentary aired on NBC just six weeks before Fawcett passed away on June 25, 2009. By all accounts, Fawcett hoped to depict cancer realistically and, in so doing, reveal the ravages of the disease and promote options beyond the United States.

> Much of "Farrah's Story" includes real-life footage of Farrah (taped by her good friend, Alana Stewart) visiting doctors & going through treatments, surgery, & recovery. Alana, at one point, had suggested that they needn't tape all of it; but Farrah told her that this was "what cancer is" (kudos, Farrah) ... so, fair warning: there's footage of her throwing up, in there (sick from anesthesia ... she counted herself vomiting 76 times, total, once), & going through the pain & hair loss & good news & bad ... *all* of the real stuff that cancer brings ["'Farrah's Story'— Video of Cancer Documentary Now Available Online," 2009, May 16, para. 3].

The documentary was never intended as a sensational bid for attention or sympathy; instead, Fawcett hoped to use her celebrity status and personal experience as a means by which to "address shortcomings she saw in American cancer treatment and to present it in art-house style" (Rutenberg, 2011, May 27, para. 10) as her video diary intimately exposed and illuminated the harsh realities of a disease that most prefer not to even acknowledge—anal cancer. In memory of her fight for survival and quest for alternatives, the Farrah Fawcett Foundation continues to raise awareness and money for HPV-related cancer research and patient assistance programs (http://www.thefar-rahfawcettfoundation.org/mission).

As we elaborate throughout this book, celebrity health narratives prompt involvement with fans and others who care about a particular disease or condition, prompting the co-narrators/co-stakeholders turned fellow activists to spread information about a health situation, encourage early detection and prevention efforts, perhaps support a celebrity's foundation, and, on some occasions, lobby Congress for research funding. With Congress, celebrities find sympathetic (and, perhaps, star-struck) legislators, willing to become co-stakeholders as well in that they devote precious time on the House or Senate floor to personal narratives about particular health issues.

In her article in *Quarterly Journal of Speech*, Lisa Gring-Pemble (2001) repeated the question: "Are we going to now govern by anecdote?" (p. 341). Although her analysis pertained to congressional hearings about welfare recipients, the question could easily be posed about celebrity health advocates who offer testimony regarding various illnesses and appeals to fund research. Although we do not debate the merit of such research or desirability of attention to diseases or conditions, even some of the celebrities that are featured in this book have wondered aloud about access and decisions seemingly based on case-by-case publicity (i.e., "disease of the week") rather than a more systematic approach.

Regardless of perspectives on equity or access, instances of celebrity health activism continue to spark public dialogues about issues related to a particular illness or injury such as preventive care, testing, diagnosis, research, and/or general awareness (see W. J. Brown & Basil, 2010; Darman & Teslik, 2006; Gerosa, 1999; Kalb, Wingert, & Foote, 2000; Mann, 2007, July 31; Nocera, 2009, January 15; Nolte, 2014, March 4; Smolowe et al., 2006; Wujcik, 2009, March; see also related work by Espejo, 2009). For example, Hilton and Hunt (2010) considered the potential "missed opportunity" of coverage of Jade Goody's public battle with (and death from) cervical cancer (p. 368), referring to the "Goody Effect," yet, Elliott (2009, March 22) argued, based on Goody's willingness to disclose and discuss her illness, that "[c]ancer screening experts are reporting a massive surge in the number of young women coming forward for screening—some for their very first test" (para.

4). Hollander (1993) noted Magic Johnson's influence on individuals to seek HIV testing (as did W. J. Brown & Basil, 1995; B. Brown & Baranowski, 1996; Casey et al., 2003). Cram et al. (2003) found a significant increase in colono-scopies after Katie Couric's awareness campaign (see also Malkin, 2000, March 12). As we detail throughout this book, celebrities who share infor-mation about their illnesses generate "buzz" that translates into awareness, action, and activism.

Preview of Coming Attractions...

As we concluded in our earlier article (Beck et al., 2014), celebrity health discourse extends prior work in the communication discipline on public-private boundaries (for related work, see Petronio, 2000, 2002) as well as on narrative theorizing (DeFina & Georgakopoulou, 2008; Harter et al., 2005; Sharf, Harter, Yamasaki, & Haidet, 2011; Stephens, 2011). This book enables us to explore implications of decisions about privacy and disclosures in terms of the personal health journeys of public figures as well as to analyze rami-fications of such decisions for emergent public narratives about issues of pre-vention, screening, stigma, body image, illness, physical challenges, and even death and dying.

Although earlier works have concentrated on individual celebrities, this book offers two unique dimensions. First, drawing from our extensive data set, we highlight core themes and trends across this important form of health communication and intriguing aspect of contemporary popular culture. Second, unlike any other account of celebrity health narratives, this book embraces a uniquely dialogic approach. We envision narratives as col-laborative and co-constructed, and, as such, we integrate voices from indi-viduals who respond publicly to celebrity health narratives through Twitter, Facebook, discussion boards, and letters to editors of publications. Building from DeFina and Georgakopoulou (2008) and Seaton (2008), as we argued earlier, with personal disclosures, individual journeys necessarily evolve into shared stories, co-authored through discourse, discovery, and mutual deliberation as they unfold dynamically and temporally (see Beck et al., 2014). Especially in this era of Twitter and other social media opportunities, we affirm that such an approach is vital to grasping the complexities of these narratives.

As such, this book contributes to important conversations about health, popular culture, fandom, media, and narrative theorizing. As the following chapters detail, these narratives foster dynamic, increasingly mediated public conversations about varied relational and medical aspects of health and wellness, and this book provides an excellent foundation for understanding the dimensions and implications of that discourse, especially in terms of awareness about conditions and inspiration for seeking preventive measures and/or care. Further, given the amount of activism that results in raising money and/or lobbying before Congress, we assert that communication scholars should examine the ethical, political, and logistical consequences of celebrity involvement in public health policy and health research. This book offers an excellent start to those critical scholarly conversations.

Originally, we had envisioned dividing the book into two core areas—implications of celebrity health narratives for celebrity and fan health journeys and celebrity health narratives as forms of public health activism. However, after researching and reflecting on our varied cases, we realized that those functions of celebrity health narratives are inherently intertwined. Disclosures by celebrities and comments by others in the general public and mainstream media both work reflexively to construct, shape, and direct the ever emergent public-yet-private narrative—and that narrative implicitly contributes to broader discussions about the particular disease, health, wellness, and, sometimes, even death and dying.

As we begin the book, we concentrate on the ways in which celebrities and others co-narrate (and, on occasion, challenge and contest) the story as they join it "in progress." In some cases, the story unfolds with a spirit of support and admiration, as we exemplify in chapters with a focus on Brooke Burke-Charvet and Kim Kardashian. These chapters illuminate and underscore the dynamic, evolving nature of these celebrity health narratives. Through ongoing dialogue, these private-yet-public narratives can also enhance perceived common ground and foster a sense of community and social support with other co-stakeholders, opening virtual doors for dialogue about related issues, including the need for testing and treatment.

However, as we have hinted in this introduction, not all celebrities welcome the intense glare of media attention, and, certainly, the revelation of (or speculation about) a health issue can result in public debate over what would otherwise be construed as private matters. As such, we draw in work on contested narratives as well as Fisher's narrative theorizing as we seek to understand controversy that ensues when some aspects of certain narratives fail to "ring true" with various co-stakeholders (see especially chapters on Catherine Zeta-Jones, Paula Deen, and Keira Knightly, and a broader chapter on instances of celebrity death due to drug or alcohol abuse). As we tackle those chapters, we reflect on issues of identity, social responsibility, and preferences for privacy and personal control.

In the second portion of the book, we transition to the challenges of and opportunities for celebrity health activism amid concurrent desires to frame desired individual identities, beginning with the complex world of sports. We continue that conversation by spotlighting examples of blurred boundaries between "reel" and "real" life for a host of actors on daytime drama, and we complete the volume with powerful chapters on the tireless advocacy of Giuliana Rancic, Robin Roberts, and Mary Tyler Moore.

Notably, this book encompasses a wide range of health-related conditions, including various forms of cancer, psoriasis, mental illness, type 1 diabetes, body image (and potential eating disorders), traumatic brain injury, infertility, type 2 diabetes, and reflections on substance abuse. We spotlight intense struggles for survival and reactions to tragic celebrity deaths.

As we bring the book to a close, we herald the recent examples of Amy Robach, Hugh Jackman, and others, and we ponder the implications of this form of health-related discourse, both in terms of setting an agenda for (increasingly virtual) water-cooler interactions as well as public policy decisions. Indeed, many of us do "have an inquiring mind" (to paraphrase the long-time ad for the *National Inquirer*), and, to borrow from an E. F. Hutton commercial, when a celebrity talks, "people listen." However, as we hope that you will note from this book, they also consider, respond, and contribute to the emergent discourse. To that end, as the following chapters detail, celebrity health narratives serve the powerful function of starting public dialogues about extremely important issues related to health and wellness, and those public conversations work to advance awareness about preventing, living with, and, sometimes, dying from illnesses and injuries through compelling personal life journeys.

CHAPTER TWO

From Actress to Cancer Patient

Brooke Burke-Charvet Dances through Thyroid Cancer

Mom, co-host (*Dancing with the Stars*), author (*The Naked Mom*), and CEO of her own fitness line (Brooke Burke Body), Brooke Burke-Charvet now adds cancer survivor to her list of successes. Brooke travels the nation, sharing her story and spreading the message about the importance of routine physical examinations, stemming from her scare with thyroid cancer. This chapter reviews Brooke's story, including her diagnosis and recovery from thyroid cancer. Analyzing both news interviews and video posts on Brooke's personal blog, this chapter examines viewers' reactions and discussions as the public makes sense of and identifies with this celebrity and her illness.

Brooke Burke-Charvet—Actress, Television Personality and Cancer Patient

Television host and co-host, actress, author, CEO, dancer, and spokesperson are all roles that can be found on Brooke Burke-Charvet's resume. Her career began when she was known as Brooke Burke, the host of E! Network's *Wild On!* (1999–2002)—a show that followed Brooke around the world, as she experienced food, culture, and nightlife in sexy places around the world (e.g., Casablanca, Rio, Miami, etc.; IMDB, 2014a). Brooke Burke married actor David Charvet (*Baywatch* hunk) in 2006, and she took his name, Brooke Burke-Charvet. Brooke is most commonly known as both the Season Seven mirror ball trophy winner on ABC's *Dancing with the Stars* (2008) and, shortly after her victory, the co-host of ABC's *Dancing with the Stars* (eight seasons—

21

2010–2013). Additional accomplishments for Brooke include CEO of her companies, Baboosh Baby and Brooke Burke Body, as well as her blog, ModernMom.com (Twitter.com, 2014). Brooke has also been the spokeswoman for Sketchers and contracted commercials with major companies such as Coca-Cola, Discover, and Anheuser Bush. In 2011, she added author to her resume as she published her first book, *The Naked Mom: A Modern Mom's Fearless Revelations, Savvy Advice and Soulful Reflections*. In this book, she documented her experiences as a mother, wife, and career woman, sharing her writing as a testament to women about life's realities—accepting that nothing in life is perfect and encouraging women to celebrate their abilities and limitations, guilt-free.

Brooke Burke-Charvet has led an exciting life from the big screen to wife and mother of four beautiful children. In addition to television host and co-host, actress, author, CEO, dancer, and spokesperson, Brooke Burke-Charvet now includes cancer survivor as part of her life story. In this chapter, we provide a brief description of thyroid cancer, acknowledge other celebrities who have been affected by this disease, and highlight how Brooke Burke-Charvet overcame her disease in the spotlight.

The Thyroid Gland: An Overview

We might not think about our endocrine system and all of the tiny cells, nerves, and glands that function to regulate our bodies each and every day. The thyroid gland, or the butterfly-shaped gland located in the base of the neck, plays an important role in overall health and wellness. Weighing less than one ounce, the thyroid gland controls how fast our bodies convert vital nutrients into energy. It helps to keep the body in check by using iodine to produce hormones that are responsible for regulating a person's energy and emotional balance, blood pressure, heart rate, body weight, and body temperature (Mayo Clinic, 2014a).

Health problems associated with the thyroid gland are classified as structural problems resulting in a kind of thyroid disease (Cleveland Clinic, 2014). The most common forms of thyroid disease include hyperthyroidism, hypothyroidism, and thyroid cancer (Mayo Clinic, 2014a). If the body produces too much hormone and the thyroid gland cannot keep up, the body uses energy more quickly, resulting in hyperthyroidism. On the flip side, hypothyroidism occurs when the thyroid gland produces an inadequate amount of hormones and the body uses its energy more slowly (clevelandclinic.org, 2014). The thyroid gland is made up of two types of cells, follicular cells and C cells, or parafollicular cells. Cancer of the follicular cells is called Follicular thyroid cancer and cancer of the parafollicular cells is called Papillary thyroid cancer (American Cancer Society, 2014b). Thyroid cancer occurs in the cells of the thyroid, and, if left untreated, those cells can expand into nearby tissues in the human body (Cleveland Clinic, 2014; see also Mayo Clinic, 2014a).

According to the American Cancer Society (2014b), thyroid cancer is the "most rapidly increasing cancer in the U.S." (para. 5), with an estimated likely diagnosis of some 63,000 new cases in 2014. Between 1973 and 2002, researchers and doctors have observed instances of thyroid cancer increase by 140 percent (Davies & Welch, 2006). Women are three times more likely to develop thyroid cancer than their male counterparts. Women also develop thyroid cancer at a younger age (their 40s and 50s) than men (their 60s and 70s). Although the rates seem to be accelerating in the United States, the Mayo Clinic (2014a) credited advances in new technologies for detecting these cancers in their earliest stages.

The survival rate for thyroid cancer is quite magnificent. If caught early, the five-year survival rate for thyroid cancer is nearly 100 percent; people who live five years without a reoccurrence (growing, spreading, or return) of the thyroid cancer are typically considered cured. Treatment options include two or more of the following: removal of the thyroid gland, radioactive iodine treatment, thyroid hormone therapy, beam radiation therapy, or chemotherapy (American Cancer Society, 2014b). The aftermath of thyroid cancer treatments often includes the inability to have children later in life and daily medication (a synthetic hormone that helps regulate the thyroid) for the remainder of the survivor's life (American Cancer Society, 2014b; Cleveland Clinic, 2014).

THYROID DISEASES IN THE LIMELIGHT

Although the thyroid is small, disorders such as thyroid cancer affect thousands of people each year, and celebrities have certainly brought attention to this disease. According to FoxNews.com (2014), many celebrities have shared their diagnosis of a thyroid disorder with the public. Graves' disease has affected hip-hop star Missy Elliott. In an interview with *People Magazine*'s Debra Lewis-Boothman and Dahvi Shira (2011, June 23), Missy reported, "I feel great" (para. 7), and she noted, "Under my doctor's supervision, I've been off medication for about a year and I'm completely managing the condition thru diet and exercise" (para 7). Graves' disease has also impacted former first couple, George H. W. Bush and Barbara Bush. Actress Kim Cattrall suffers from Hashimoto's disease, a disorder where the immune system attacks the thyroid gland, causing hypothyroidism.

The queen of daytime television, Oprah Winfrey, suffers from both hypothyroidism and hyperthyroidism and required thyroid medication until her thyroid became regulated. In the January 2009 edition of *O, The Oprah Magazine*, author John Hastings wrote that Oprah's thyroid problems have balanced to control and that she no longer takes medication. In that article, Oprah uses her diagnosis as an opportunity to educate the public about the thyroid gland and potential related diseases. Hyperthyroidism also affects reality television star Kelly Osbourne and fitness expert Jillian Michaels. Film critic Roger Ebert, and actresses Angie Everhart, Brooke Burke-Charvet, and Sofia Vergara have all battled thyroid cancer.

Of these celebrities, Brooke Burke-Charvet has been the most vocal advocate about thyroid disorders. Since Brooke's public announcement, Sofia Vergara (known for her presence on the hit television show on ABC, *Modern Family*) has also used her celebrity status as a platform for raising awareness for early detection of thyroid cancer as well as supporting those already diagnosed with thyroid cancer. Through her campaign, "Follow the Script," Vergara has informed others about the importance of consistent treatment of thyroid-related issues while recalling her experience with thyroid cancer over a decade earlier ("Follow the Script," 2014). Although compelling, Vergara's campaign efforts began well after she was already in remission. We devote the remainder of this chapter to Brooke Burke-Charvet's journey through thyroid cancer and why she chose to share her story with the world through various forms of social media from shortly after her diagnosis.

Brooke Burke-Charvet's Personal Home Video Announcement

On November 8, 2012, at only 41 years old, Brooke went public with her diagnosis of thyroid cancer, alerting fans on her blog, ModernMom.com, about her pending surgery. Burke-Charvet posted a video to her fans and fellow mothers, letting them know what was going on directly from her:

> I need to have thyroid surgery and a thyroidectomy, which means I'm going to have a nice big scar right here across my neck. [Brooke points to her neck, drawing a line with her finger along where the scar will be after the surgery.] I don't get to just walk around and pretend like nothing happened or not follow up or not share it, because it's going to be pretty much dead center. [Brooke gestures to the same spot on her neck.] I don't want anybody to read about it and get

the wrong idea, or think that I'm sick, because I'm not. I feel really good. I've actually never felt better. That's what's so crazy about this whole thing, and you never ever think that some tiny nodule, something that I didn't even know was going on inside my body—I went for a regular physical, and that's how I discovered this [2012, November 8, para. 12].

Brooke explained in her video that, of all cancers, "doctors say this is a good kind of cancer to have. Good cancer [with air quotes added by Brooke]—that sounds so crazy! But my doctor did tell me that this is a happily-ever-after kind of thing." She exuded a warm and encouraging attitude in her public address, and she noted on her blog that she aimed to share a message of hope and strength with her fans:

> Here's the way I see it: I'm just going to make a positive out of this negative thing. I'm going to be a really good patient and do everything I need to do.... I'm ready to deal with it, and I'm going to be fine. I feel really, really strong.... I'm going to fight through this, and as crazy as it is, my head is in the right place. It's going to be good [Burke-Charvet, 2012, November 8, para. 13].

In her video message, Brooke revealed a different side to her fans—in her house, on what looks like a sofa or bed, wearing sweatpants, a T-shirt, and no make-up (as opposed to displaying a spray-tanned body or wearing a fancy gown as she might during a television appearance), she exhibited a raw, vulnerable persona and became perhaps even more relatable to her fans.

In response to Brooke's public message about her cancer, support poured in from her ModernMom.com community and Facebook and Twitter fans. Some offered words of encouragement and support or confided their own cancer experiences. Based on an analysis of Facebook, Twitter, and blog responses, three themes emerged from her posts and followers' feedback. As we detail in the remainder of this chapter, the first theme, *Fans Relate to Brooke*, discusses how people share their stories with Brooke and even take this gesture one step further by encouraging her to contact them. The second theme, *Surgical Badge of Honor*, focuses on how Brooke's fans both disclose their personal scars and also provide Brooke with words of wisdom and hope. In the third theme, *Wild On! Prevention*, we detail how Brooke uses her story as a means of encouraging early detection of cancers through prevention efforts.

Fans Relate to Brooke

On November 8, 2012, Brooke shared her vulnerable home video with Facebook friends, announcing her diagnosis of thyroid cancer. In her Facebook post to her fans, she commented, "Today is as good as any to share my diagnosis. Here is a vulnerable home video. I wanted you to hear it straight from me" (2012, November 8). Shortly after Brooke posted her story, she received a flood of responses from her fans, with a total of 179 likes of her post; 33 people shared her story with others on Facebook, and 181 fans left her with words of support. Also on November 8, 2012, Brooke posted another message on Facebook, taking ownership of her health saga, noting, "Here's the story, from me to you … it's all over the internet now, but this is my home video message." A response of 315 likes, 79 shares, and 304 messages continued to flood her inbox. Both Facebook posts included a home video message that linked back to Brooke's ModernMom.com blog. Throughout the Facebook and blog posts, fans uploaded personal details about their own cancer journeys as a means of commiserating with Brooke, as a fellow cancer patient (and, hopefully, survivor), and invited her into their personal spaces for advice and comfort.

Fans Related to Brooke through Shared Cancer Experiences

Brooke's fans envision her journey as a reflection of their own, empowering her with the strength to survive. In an article posted on Brooke's ModernMom blog, titled "Brooke Burke Inspires Others to Share Their Cancer Stories," an anonymous fan wrote:

This was me exactly two years ago … found at a routine physical, with no symptoms or family history. I was the healthiest I had ever been in my life and to hear the word cancer is scary to say the least. Especially when you have four kids as I do. Thyroid cancer is cancer, whether it's the best one to have or not. Be grateful that it's the best to have but don't allow anyone to discount your feelings [2012, November 8, Comments Section].

On Facebook, Brooke's fan, Mireya, explained:

Brooke, I hear your story and it's like I'm hearing my own story about thyroid cancer. I'm a thryroid [thyroid] cancer survivor also. I got diagnosed three years ago and it simply changed my life. My best advice to you is to have lots of faith and let your loved ones be there for you. That will be the key to your recovery. I definitely understand what you are going through! I went ahead and joined "Thyca" which is a thyroid cancer survivor group. You will get to meet other people who are going through the same thing. May God bless you and help you through this. Xoxo [2012, November 8].

Also on Facebook, Harriett explained,

Brooke, your story is so similar to mine. It has been 7 years since I went for an annual physical and it was the Nurse Practicner [Practitioner] that found the nodule. Of course, they are not malignant but the endocrinologist did the needle biopsy and I ended up having 3 nodules and 1 was malignant. I had a great surgeon in Marietta, GA and did such a great job on my incision that it is barely noticeable and a necklace covers the scar. All that said, if you have to have cancer this is the type to have. My prayers are with you as you have surgery and recover … [fan continues about her Facebook photo] [2012, November 8].

Finally, Kristina, a Facebook fan explained,

Same story here … routine gyn checkup found a lump … biopsy, had full thyroidectomy due to the cancer … that was 12 years and 3 kids ago! I had to have a second surgery 4 years ago because I had it come back (even after the radioactive iodine) … your doc said the same thing mine did "if you are going to get cancer, this is the one you want" … while I still didn't want it, it has given me new views on life and how I live each day! [2012, November 8].

In all four of these examples, Brooke's fans positioned their own stories as like looking into a mirror and seeing their own reflections in that their respective cancer narratives resemble Brooke's path. At the time of these posts, Brooke had only found out that she had thyroid cancer, thus no treatment had occurred, yet, her fans provided rich insight to her future and what to expect in terms of a successful recovery. They verified her assertion that thyroid cancer is the best cancer to have and that she can and will overcome this small bump in her life. In a post on Facebook on February 6, 2013, Brooke thanked her fans: "Thank you to everyone for sharing your stories, thoughts and words of inspiration. It really means the world to me. I send you all of my love and more." Just two months after her December 5, 2012, surgery, Brooke again expressed gratitude to her fans for their continued support and encouragement through their respective life stories. Their survival narratives inspired Brooke during her darkest days.

Fans Related to Brooke and Invited Her into Their Personal Space

As people shared their very similar cancer experiences with Brooke, they began to cross over from the public space to private corners. These fans reached out to Brooke in public spaces by commenting on her open Facebook wall, Twitter, and video message on YouTube.com, and some then invited her to enter a private space for the two of them to talk on an even more personal level.

The following examples occurred in response to the posts listed above from Brooke's announcement about her diagnosis on her Facebook page and YouTube post (2012, November 8). Timothy stated, "I survived … 5 years cancer-free … if I can help in any way, don't hesitate to contact me … hugs" (2012, November, 8). Tonya said, "Brooke, I have had the same diagnosis, gone through a Thyroidectomy and all is GREAT! You will do just fine and live with this "Good" Cancer. Please private message me if you have any questions" (2012, November 8). Traci explained to Brooke, "You will be in my prayers! My Thyroid was removed last year, I understand. Please inbox me if you'd like to speak pvt [privately]. May God Bless You & Keep You" (2012, November 8). Cheryl Z. took the public to private conversation a step further, offering her personal email account to Brooke, "I had the same cancer 4 yrs ago. If you want to chat about this … you can reach me at xxxxx@hotmail. com. It is always good to have someone to ask questions … [email edited to preserve confidentiality]" (2012, November 8).

In addition to these four messages from fans, Cheryl K. provided Brooke with a message of support on Facebook:

> If you want any help or have any questions about how I got through it all, surgery, after surgery, my surgeon, how I feel now, anything, I am on Facebook and please feel free to message me. I would be happy to help you. Sincerely Cheryl [2012, November 8].

David posted the following information on Brooke's Facebook wall:

> Sounds like Hurtle Cell Neoplasm—the type I had. Get a good surgeon and he will place the cut line in the natural fold of your neck. You will see it if you stretch your neck but otherwise it will be practically invisible. I can tell you in detail how my surgery went and the post-op testing and the follow up care. The U.S. Army treated it very aggres[s]ively once they determined the type of thyroid problem and I am still here 22 plus years later. If you want to know any more— just let me know. Best of luck to you [2012, November 8].

On YouTube, Sharon extended her support to Brooke as well:

> Thank you for sharing your story! My 19-year-old daughter was diagnosed with thyroid cancer 2 years ago and started a foundation 5 months later called Bite Me Cancer (see it online). She raises research dollars and awareness for thyroid cancer (the fastest growing cancer in the U.S.) as well as help other teens with cancer. We would be honored to stay in touch with you. She'd love to talk to you sometime. She's an active sophomore in college trying to helps others [https://www.youtube.com/all_comments?v=6yvZuWuSIHU].

As these examples attest, Brooke's fans trust her enough to invite her into their personal, private space. One fan even publically offered her personal email address to her celebrity idol just in case she wants to chat with her about cancer. We do not know if Brooke took any of these fans up on their offer to have a private conversation with her about thyroid cancer and their experiences, off-screen (i.e., in a more private arena, such as private Facebook messages, email, etc.), but it is interesting to see how an open, raw celebrity video prompted fans to put themselves in a vulnerable state by uploading personal contact information and private health-related details (see related arguments by Petronio, 2002, 2004).

The exemplars also indicate that Brooke's fans employ media (e.g., Facebook) as a space and a place for parasocial relationships to unfold. Baek, Bae, and Jang (2013) defined parasocial relationships as unilateral bonds between performers (i.e., celebrity) and their respective audience members/fans. These fans use media portals like Facebook as outlets where they can engage in supportive communication, including advice and emotions from performers, thus strengthening their connection with and closeness to the celebrity (see High et al., 2014; see also E. Lee & Jang, 2013; Meyrowitz, 1985; Ramasubramanian & Kornfield, 2012; Savage & Spence, 2014; Sood & Rogers, 2001). These spaces allow fans and celebrities to co-define their roles (see Baym, 2010; W. J. Brown & Basil, 2010) as cancer patient and survivor, not merely "fan" and "celebrity" by virtue of Brooke's heavy presence on the television screen throughout the last 20 years (*Wild On!*, *Dancing with the Stars*, etc.). As they assert a relationship with Brooke and identify with her as fellow thyroid cancer patients/survivors (see related argument by K. Burke (1950/1969), some situate themselves as more than just "fans" (see related work by Meyrowitz, 1985). By extending the parasocial relationship through the shared health experience, some fans felt comfortable enough to invite Brooke into their personal space. Thus, in addition to offering a platform for users to share their likes, desires, and experiences (Antheunis, Tates, & Neiboer, 2013; High et al., 2014), these reactions affirm the use of social media for expressions of mutual social support, even between people who will likely never meet face to face.

Surgical Badge of Honor

In her video announcement on her Facebook page and ModernMom.com blog, Brooke discussed with her fans that she will have a scar on her body after her surgery to remove the cancerous nodule on her thyroid gland. Brooke explained, "I need to have thyroid surgery and a thyroidectomy, which means I'm going to have a nice, big scar right here across my neck" (2012, November 8). In her message to her fans, she admitted,

> I don't get to just walk around and pretend like nothing happened or not follow up or not share it, because it's going to be pretty much dead center [referencing the future scar that will be on her neck]. I don't want anybody to read about it and get the wrong idea, or think that I'm sick, because I'm not [2012, November 8].

Instead of her fans seeing her with a scar across her neck without a personal explanation from her, she opted to announce in advance what will be happening to her. She concluded by commenting, "Here's the way I see it: I'm just going to make a positive out of this negative thing. I'm going to be a really good patient and do everything I need to do."

As responses to her video messages poured in, fans voiced support and encouragement to Brooke as she approached her surgery. They attempted to alleviate the possible stigma surrounding a scar on the neck, and they referenced scars on their own necks due to their personal experiences with thyroid cancer, identifying with Brooke's self-proclaimed surgical badge of honor.

Fans pointed to Brooke's enduring beauty and noted that a scar would not change that quality. Others gave her a different perspective on how to view such reminder of a scary time in her life. Both functioned as forms of support.

Jen wrote on Brooke's Facebook wall that "[w]hen I see your scar I'm going to think, that's the exit door the cancer took when it left your body. Sending prayers for your upcoming return to health!" (2012, November 8). James added that "[s]cars are just signs of living life ... you have a lot of people supporting you ... wishing you a speedy recovery" (2012, November 8). Debbie told Brooke that "[t]he scar will only show how soon they found it and [how] STRONG you are.... You will still be beautiful" (2012, November 8). Even the Thyroid Cancer Awareness page (2012, November 8) weighed in on Brooke's conversation, asserting, "You can do this! Your scar will be your badge. Wear it proudly! Blessings to you" (https://www.facebook.com/pages/Thykidz-Thyroid-Cancer-Awareness/90237802618). Last, Jimmy expressed his admiration for Brooke, saying, "I have admired you for so long. You have an inner beauty that no scar can disfigure. hugs and kisses to you!" (2012, November 8).

In all, Brooke's fans and supporters upheld her characterization of the scar as a surgical medal of honor, signifying her future status as a survivor of thyroid cancer. Their words of wisdom and encouragement underscored that she would remain beautiful with the scar and that no scar could take away who she is.

Brooke's video message revealing her recent diagnosis of thyroid cancer triggered especially strong reactions from others who had walked the same trail. Fans emptied their hearts out in support to her upcoming battle with cancer. On Facebook, Nena explained how her scars are signs of victory and Brooke's scar can be one too:

> Prayers for you. i have two beautiful scars on my body one is on the left side of my neck and one on the stomach from a feeding tube. i am going to tell you i remember asking the doctor are you sure the scar won't be that bad and he tells me don't worry. i was upset that i have scars on my body but you know what i love my scars it lets me know that cancer did not beat me and it's now 11 yrs

and i am more beautiful now than ever and i am 47 yrs old I am like a bottle of wine the older the better. brooke i am here for you if you ever need someone to talk to. girl you are going to be more beautiful than you are now I am jealous [2012, November 8].

Nena referred to her scars as beautiful and a reminder that cancer did not beat her. She offered herself to Brooke as a support system and reassured her that she would be even more beautiful even after she beats cancer. Cheryl K. acknowledged the scar but downplayed it by suggesting ways to minimize it:

Hi Brooke ... 2½ years ago at age 45 I also was diagnosed with thyroid cancer. It also was found by my internist at my annual physical. It was terrifying, but everything is ok. I take synthroid every day, follow up blood tests every few months and an ultra sound every year. Re the scar, I choose not to piton [have] any scar treatments so I have a scar, but it looks like it's part of my neck. If you are worried about it, you can put scar cream on and I think thy [that] eventually you won't even see it at all [2012, November 8].

Cheryl K. noted that creams will help reduce the appearance of scars and that she should not worry about it too much. Likewise, Vickie, another fan of Brooke's, discussed her thyroid disorder and heralded the potential symbolism of the scar on Brooke's Facebook page:

Brooke, I had my thyroid destroyed with radioactive iodine when I was younger at 18, so it didnt develop into cancer. I am now 49 and still taking my hormones and feeling great. You are a beautiful woman and a scar is worth saving your life. I may need possible neck surgery in the very near future so we can have matching scars.... I have an MRI tomorrow.... Best of luck and stay positive.... Love u [2012, November 8].

Vickie mentioned that she might potentially resemble Brooke in the near future if her MRI reveals that her thyroid disorder has turned into full-blown cancer, but she reminded Brooke that, regardless of what happens, concern about a scar is not worth dying for. Kristina brushed Brooke's comment about scars off in a very concise, yet assuring way, noting on Facebook that "the scar is really nothing!!! no one even notices mine" (2012, November 8). Kristina, just like the other fans listed above, connected with Brooke and her soon to be "surgical badge of honor," but she crafted her response differently, simply telling Brooke that people do not seem to notice hers, implying that it might be the same for her.

On February 4, 2013, nearly two months after her thyroidectomy, Brooke posted an entry and photo of her scar on her ModernMom.com blog. She did so in honor of World Cancer Day and wanted her fans to know how she felt this morning in relationship to her scar. She explained that, while she prepared for such an important day, the scar that aligns her neck became ever so apparent to her. She reflected:

> For the first time, I allowed my battle wound to stop me. I began to wonder ... how I was going to cover it? Should I cover it? Will it be a focal point for audiences as I start my season back on TV? Will it be the first thing that people see when they are speaking to me? Those moments that I lost focusing on something that is now part of my journey, were not only moments for myself, but moments for everyone else today, on World Cancer Day [2013, February 4].

Her scar now serves as a reminder of her battle with cancer and her good fortune in surviving. She now has a surgical badge of honor forever present on her neck, in a prominent location that she and others can easily observe. She wrote in her blog, "I was incredibly lucky, but I am painfully aware of the number of people who are not as fortunate as me." The World Health Organization (WHO) reveals that worldwide, cancer is the leading cause of death, accounting for 8.2 million deaths in 2012 alone (World Health Organization, 2014). Having survived something that kills so many people each year is surely remarkable and, as we detail in the next section, inspiring.

WILD ON! PREVENTION

In her post titled, *Cancer. Me?* (2012, November 8), Brooke started off by writing, "Today is my day to share.... I'm sorry I left you hanging for the past few months regarding my thyroid results [Brooke links to a page on her blog where she posted about the thyroid test]. It's been a crazy experience. Here's my story: [the blog entry continues with a personal testimony and a video announcement to her fan]" (http://www.modernmom.com/98795a8a-3b3e-11e3-be8a-bc764e04a41e.html).

Even pre-cancer diagnosis, Brooke Burke-Charvet has been at the forefront of public service. She uses her fitness company, Brooke Burke Body, her public blog forum, ModernMom.com, as well as various social media as platforms for disseminating messages and providing a place for public discussion on various women's health topics (e.g., pregnancy, conception, parenting, etc.). Post-cancer diagnosis, she began to focus more on prevention in light of what happened to her regarding the early detection and treatment of her cancer. In an analysis of both social media posts by Brooke and messages from her fans and followers (e.g., Facebook and Twitter), as well as Brooke's blog, ModernMom.com, the theme of *Wild On! Prevention*, emerged. As we elaborate in this section, Brooke has dared to share her story with others in an effort to inspire them to be proactive in terms of their health and health care.

In a successful attempt to share her story with her fans and the world, Brooke linked her story from ModernMom.com to her Facebook page in two separate posts on November 8, 2012. On the same day, she also published her video on YouTube; to date, YouTube has recorded 535,444 views of her home video message (see https://www.youtube.com/watch?v=6yvZuWuSIHU). As a response to her story, a total of 1,151 people liked her posts on Facebook (n = 494) and YouTube (n = 657). A total of 1,067 people left Brooke a message on her Facebook wall (n = 485), YouTube stream (n = 574), or ModernMom.com blog (n= 8). Furthermore, 112 people shared her story on their Facebook news feed. In addition to these posts, Brooke also used World Cancer Day on February 4, 2013, as another opportunity to share her story again as well as promote cancer awareness. In her post on Facebook (also linked to her ModernMom.com blog), she included a picture of herself holding a "Stand ↑ 2C" sign which stands for Stand up to Cancer. Brooke's sign says "I stand up to 41 Million[;] Stephanie[;] Jerry" and her message said:

> It is World Cancer Day. I'm blown away by a new awareness of how many people in my life have cancer and, since my diagnosis, how many I have met that are still fighting the fight. If sharing my personal experience has helped even just one person, I can't tell you how happy that makes me. Thank you everyone for sharing your stories with me. How many people do you know who have been affected by cancer? I share my thoughts on today and what it means to me on my ModernMom blog [2013, February 4].

A flood of responses filled Brooke's Facebook page in the form of likes (n = 992), shares (n = 52), and messages (n = 82). Combining her messages from Facebook, YouTube, and ModernMom.com, a total of 1,149 messages include emotional responses to Brooke's raw, thoughtful personal home-video message in which she confided her cancer news to her fans and evidence of how her story has helped to encourage and promote early detection of cancer.

Brooke has utilized her celebrity status as leverage to communicate about cancer prevention and early detection and treatment. Her large fan base and followers on social media confirm that she has the ability to reach many people with her health messages. Fans have responded to her efforts to raise awareness of this fast-growing disease through details of her personal brush with cancer. One fan, MsAAJ, responded to Brooke's video on YouTube,

> I commend you for sharing your story. Each person that shares their story raises more awareness about these issues! You don't know how many women will reach out to their doctors because they see this! Please know that you (and your family) are continuously in my prayers!" [n.d.].

On Facebook, Melissa confided,

Glad you're okay! You look wonderful and healthy. I am also on this interesting "journey" just being diagnosed in October. I'm recovering from the thyroidectomy and lymph node removal. Now it's on to the RAI soon. TC awareness is so important, since it's easy to go undetected for a long time. Happy Holidays and Best wishes to you! [2013, December 5].

Bruce also weighed in on the Facebook conversation, adding,

I applaud your superlative activism and efforts to raise awareness. You are one very special lady! Cancer affects us all. It's unlikely that there are many people who haven't been affected, or at the very least, know someone diagnosed with cancer. My dad was only 53 yrs. Old when he died after a long hard battle with renal cancer [2013, February 4].

Kelly posted on Facebook,

What a positive attitude u have which is inspirational, u will be fine and bounce back stronger than u ever thought was possible, your family will get u through this rough patch in your life, but your a very motivated women with strength, my thoughts r with u at this difficult time [2012, November 8].

Marisol echoed the other comments on Facebook, stating,

Brooke your words have brought to life my thoughts and emotions. Being a thyroid cancer survivor, I thank you for bringing awareness today and many days. Thank you for writing on your blog and so eloquently describing what many people feel and have gone through [2013, February 4].

In addition to the messages above, Dana, from YouTube, explained, "Best wishes for good health Brooke. You will save many lives by sharing your story" (n.d.). Michele added, "I want to thank you for sharing—gives us all pause to stop and think. Life moves so fast we forget to slow down and be aware and so forth—god bless" (2012, November 8).

Brooke's fans commend her on re-framing the dark time in her life as one that has provided her with the opportunity to help others through awareness and education. By sharing her story with the world, she is advancing awareness of thyroid cancer (even thyroid diseases) and preventive efforts to catch them in their early stages. Through their posts, fellow cancer survivors, in particular, have praised Brooke for inspiring other women and men to get checked.

Beyond helping others be more aware of thyroid cancer and prevention efforts, Brooke's story has also functioned as a form of support for her fans and followers. Bree posted on Facebook:

Thank you for your story. You have also helped me through mine. I am not upset that I got this disease. I'm proud of my scars. I feel that we have been chosen for a special reason to help others. Xoxo [2013, February 4].

Building on the post above, Carrie extended, "Thank you for sharing your story. I will be 2 years post op in February and it is nice to hear stories of other moms going through the same thing as me. Stay strong and beautiful!" (2013, December 5). Likewise, Donna responded on ModernMom.com, saying, "Hi Brooke ... thanks for sharing your story. I can definitely relate. [Fan goes on to share her story.] You are truly an inspiration. I've been following your journey.... It's such a beautiful thing you're doing. Thanks again for sharing! Love from Toronto.—Donna" (2012, November 8).

These quotations affirm that Brooke's story has provided some with a sense of hope and inspiration as they continue on with their battle. Debbie posted on Brooke's Facebook wall about how she wished that she had had her to look up to as support when she battled thyroid disease many years ago:

> Brooke, I did not have cancer but had my thyroid out in April 2010. [Fan shares her medical journey with Brooke.] My pray[er]s are with you, and your family. Please keep us all informed. Thank you for sharing your story with us. I read many of the posts and have learned much more about this. I sat up night after night reading and reading about the surgery. [Referencing her medical journey 25 years earlier.] Wish I had some where to hear all these stories and not be as scared. Love and God bless you [2012, November 8].

This post confirms that even someone who battled thyroid problems in earlier years recognizes how Brooke is shaping the future of thyroid health by informing others through ongoing awareness. Her fans applaud her for "not allowing the tabloids to exploit" her (Facebook friend, Donna, 2012, November 8). They thank her for not keeping this matter private and for sharing her news in a public way. Shelli explained,

> Brooke, what a lovely, inspiring, honest video that was. Thank you for giving up some of your privacy in order to share the news; you will undoubtedly bring hope and strength to many people affected by cancer. You're in my thoughts and my Buddhist-equivalent-of-prayers and I know you'll pull through this with health and aplomb! [2012, November 8].

Cindi also wrote:

> Praying for a successful surgery and speedy recovery Brooke. As someone told me when I was diagnosed with cancer, God gave you the microphone, how you use the stage or what you choose to sing is up to you. Hugs and prayers [2012, November 8].

Brooke has used her celebrity status as a service, rather than prioritizing privacy. She continues to offer support and encouragement as she educates others on the importance of early detection of cancers. Post-cancer diagnosis, she has begun to focus more on prevention in light of what had happened to her. She admits in her 2014 post on ModernMom.com titled *Ultrasound, Biopsy and Fear*,

> Being a woman devoted to living a healthy lifestyle with no health concerns other than chronic fatigue and Hashimoto's, I casually blew off my doctor's recommendation to get a thyroid ultrasound after he felt a lump in my neck during my routine physical.

She recognized that she carelessly disregarded her doctor's wishes for her to have a routine scan to see if her thyroid disease had developed into full-blown cancer. We are unsure as to when the doctor made such recommendation, but, nonetheless, Brooke did receive an ultrasound that revealed she had thyroid cancer. Ever since this experience, Brooke has devoted much of her time to informing others of the importance of prevention and early detection of cancer through routine doctor visits, yearly mammograms, and yearly gynecological exams.

Her posts on Facebook and Twitter encourage people to get checked, screening early for cancers of all kinds. In December 2013, one year after her thyroid cancer surgery, she tweeted and posted multiple messages on Facebook about taking the initiative to get checked. She invited others to get examined too, asserting, "It's all about preventative medicine, early diagnosis & being responsible 4 our health. Get your regulate [regular] check ups, it can save lives" (2013, December 5). Fans like @Brian32223 on Twitter responded saying "I go tomorrow and next week." Also on December 5, 2013, Brooke tweeted and posted on Facebook, "Getting ready 4 a three hour check up. Yearly physical. Gotta do it." Fans poured in support, verifying the need to have yearly physicals as a way to take control of your health. Maria agreed with Brooke, saying, "That's how my Dr found the lump on my thyroid that ended up being cancerous, got to do it!!!" Judy echoed, "Being responsible for your own well being … awesome!" Other fans disclosed more, even sharing when their upcoming preventive visits will be. John wrote, "I have mine on Jan 2," and Matt claimed that "I am going to mine at 3:30 today." These fans affirmed their opinions and support for early detection through preventive measures like routine check-ups with your doctor. Later, on February 26, 2014, Brooke tweeted, "'Our health always seems much more valuable after we lose it.' I refuse to NOT b[e] healthy! Scheduling my yearly mammogram today @goodhealth."

These examples illustrate Brooke's active choice to self-disclose (Derlega, Winstead, & Greene, 2008) her personal and private thoughts and feelings related to her health with the public. In doing so, she has prompted other men and women to self-disclose by confiding their stories with the world, too. Her fans also demonstrate a sense of co-ownership of Brooke's public message, as demonstrated through the 164 people who shared her story on *their* respective Facebook walls. Petronio (2002) explained this co-ownership of personal information that requires the discloser of the information and the receiver to negotiate rules or parameters for disclosing this information. Since Brooke revealed this information on a public forum, she initiated opportunities for information to be leaked and shared. Furthermore, according to High et al. (2014), "Facebook users monitor the disclosures displayed in their friends' profiles, perceiving some disclosures as a request for support, and this attention to others' disclosure makes Facebook an active venue for supportive communication" (p. 79; see also Bender, Jimenez-Marroquin, & Jadad, 2011).

Together, Brooke and her followers construct a supportive environment, online in a public space (i.e., Brooke's Facebook page and blog, ModernMom.com), where people can go and learn more about, share their experiences with, and receive support for thyroid cancer. Although Brooke willingly used her celebrity status by confiding to the public, she has also taken the time to thank her fans who also choose to self-disclose as well, noting in a public Facebook post, "Thank you to everyone for sharing your stories, thoughts and words of inspiration. It really means the world to me. I send you all of my love and more" (2013, February 6).

Discussion

Through the innovative media platforms of Facebook, Twitter, and YouTube, celebrities like Brooke Burke-Charvet can share their stories of cancer diagnosis, treatment, and survival with their friends, family, biggest fans, and casual onlookers. While self-disclosing in such a public arena may be daunting to some, as we illustrate throughout this book, celebrities and their fans can co-construct social media as a supportive environment for disclosing and sharing personal health experiences (Bender et al., 2011; High et al., 2014). Revealing personal information on these digital platforms fosters parasocial relationships (Baek et al., 2013), implicitly broadening circles of intimacy in terms of disclosing and discussing personal information (Petronio, 2002). Together, celebrity and fans/followers co-own the emergent private-yet-public health narrative, as they support each other in light of the same or similar health problem.

In this chapter, we described how Brooke's fans responded and continue to respond to her cancer story, helping Brooke to cope with her new diagnosis and facilitating more intimate conversations about personal issues, blurring the lines even further between public and private conversations. These interactions through social media, in particular, extend perceptions of co-ownership of a celebrity's story, especially when fan and celebrity have experienced a similar health situation.

Notably, of the hundreds of social media posts and messages by Brooke's fans (n = 1,067), not one of them erred on the side of somewhat telling her to maybe reassess her priorities or think about this situation from a more rational point of view. When faced with the recent diagnosis of cancer, do many people automatically think about scars left on their body? Or do they think about survival so that they (i.e., celebrities) can continue the fame and fortune that their life has to offer? We see that the online environment truly was a supportive environment for Brooke and her fans to have an honest-to-goodness conversation about their fears, all while gaining the confidence that they need to tackle their disease.

Moreover, through her fitness company, Brooke Burke Body, and her personal struggles of cancer, Brooke promotes cancer prevention by permitting her fans even deeper into her private world. She allows her fans to know when she is scheduling and going to doctor's appointments. Through tweets and Facebook posts, she lets her fans follow her through her day, inviting them into her life; these efforts bring "outsiders" closer into her "private" life, strengthening and reinforcing that parasocial relationship. Extending from that relationship, Brooke then has the ability to reinforce messages of prevention and early detection because the fan identifies with Brooke as a friend, someone they should and can trust. Through her personal health experiences, her passion to educate people about the importance of a healthy lifestyle coupled with preventive efforts coming out on social media, and the help of her supporters, Brooke's public-yet-private health narrative has unfolded as a mutually supportive (and, likely, quite persuasive) form of health communication.

CHAPTER THREE

Just Like Kim

Fan Responses to Kim Kardashian's Battle with Psoriasis

A wise man once said, "The public eye never blinks."—Kourtney Kardashian (Seacrest, Bunim, & Murray, 2011)

The Kardashians have taken the public by storm. The "undisputed royal family of reality TV" boasts a number-one hit reality TV show, 30 products from perfumes to clothing lines, and even a nail polish collection (*Oprah's Next Chapter*, 2012, June 17). After the Kardashian family made Barbara Walters' 10 most fascinating people of 2011 list, Walters commented, "I have never heard more anger or dismay than [when] we announced that the people you are about to see were on our list…" (ForeverLoyaltyMgmt, 2011, December 17). Often referred to as "famous for being famous," the Kardashians have one member, in particular, who has propelled this family into the public's eye: Kim Kardashian.

Kim Kardashian is a "reality TV Star, businesswoman, socialite, spokeswoman, and cover model whose image and brand seem to be everywhere" (*Oprah's Next Chapter*, 2012, June 17). As of May 2014, Kim has over 21 million Twitter followers and has been named as "one of the biggest names in pop culture" (*ABCNews*, 2011, August 8). However, Kim's career has not been all glitz and glam. Kim, like most celebrities, must continually navigate public-private boundaries. For instance, Kim has received scrutiny from the public's gaze for her 72-day marriage to NBA star Chris Humphrey. However, nothing perhaps has caused more controversy than the one private matter that sparked public attention about her life.

A former member of Paris Hilton's entourage, Kim Kardashian first came to public attention in 2007 with a sex tape (ForeverLoyaltyMgmt, 2011, December 17). The tape propelled Kim to fame. This tape (intended to be private between Kim and her long-time singer, songwriter, record producer and actor boyfriend, Ray J) soon became a public phenomenon (ForeverLoyaltyMgmt, 2011, December 17). Oprah referred to this tape as "the notorious sex-tape that started it all" (*Oprah's Next Chapter*, 2012, June 17). As Walters put it, "Something private, became public, and before you knew it they had their own reality show, 'Keeping up with the Kardashians'" (ForeverLoyaltyMgmt, 2011, December 17), featuring the modern day "Brady Bunch" of the Kardashians and Jenner family (Forever-LoyaltyMgmt, 2011, December 17). This show encompasses part of Kris Jenner's (Kim Kardashian's mother) vision for her daughters, Kourtney, Kim, and Khloe, "based on the idea that there is no line between what is private and what is performance, what's real, and what's for the cameras" (ForeverLoyaltyMgmt, 2011, December 17). With this philosophy, not surprisingly, family members even actively discuss personal health information on the family's reality show.

Kardashian health, like most families', includes some painful history. In 2003, Kim lost her father, Robert Kardashian, to cancer, just eight weeks after he was diagnosed (*Oprah's Next Chapter*, 2012, June 24). The Kardashian family has discussed Robert's death (as well as numerous health topics) on *Keeping up with the Kardashians*—cancer, laser hair removal, plastic surgery, birthing alternatives, and even ways to make one's vagina smell/taste sweeter. Perhaps most prominently, Kim has openly shared reactions to and information about her psoriasis diagnosis on the show upon media speculation about splotchy legs captured in paparazzi photographs. Within the initial episode about her condition, Kim's dermatologist diagnosed her with psoriasis and explained that it is genetic and controllable, not curable. Reflecting upon her diagnosis, Kim said, "People don't understand the pressure on me to look perfect. When I gain a pound, it's in the headlines. Imagine what the tabloids would do to me if they saw all these spots?" (Allin, 2011, July 25, para. 3). The episode inspired a slew of video blogs on YouTube and comments on popular press articles and back street celeb gossip sites, as well as tweets on Twitter. Kim later even posted a photo of a heart-shaped psoriasis spot on her Twitter account. Kim wrote, "Kinda funny & gross but look at my heart shaped psoriasis! LOL Had to share!" ("Kim Kardashian Shows Off Her Heart Shaped Psoriasis," 2011, August 15, para. 4). Thus, in this chapter, we examine "follower" responses to Kim Kardashian's psoriasis as a case study in which to better understand ways in which perceived relationships with celebrities via technology influence health communication.

Health, Parasocial Relationships, Technology and Celebrities

As we have mentioned throughout our book thus far, the past few decades have included increased focus on celebrities' roles in promoting health from health practitioners and communication scholars (Beck, 2005; Beck et al., 2014; Bell, 2011; W. J. Brown & Basil, 1995; W. J. Brown, Basil, & Bocarnea, 2003a, 2003b; W. J. Brown & deMatviuk, 2010; Lerner, 2006). W. J. Brown and Basil (1995) discovered that "[c]elebrities may be very helpful in promoting disease prevention" (p. 361). Beck et al. added that "decisions to reveal intimate developments (such as a potentially embarrassing condition or a face-challenging disease) beyond close social circles are even more complicated, in light of parasocial relationships and, more recently, social media" (p. 245). Kim Kardashian offers an especially useful example, given that she consistently references her love for Instagram and Twitter within her reality TV shows, *Keeping Up with the Kardashians, Kourtney & Kim Take Miami*, and *Kourtney & Kim Take New York*.

Kim's heart-shaped psoriasis tweet received an array of responses ("Kim Kardashian Shows Off Her Heart Shaped Psoriasis," 2011, August 15). From love to hate, Twitter functions as a technological medium for the enactment of a parasocial relationship with Kim (for related arguments, see Hartmann & Goldhoorn, 2011; Kassing & Sanderson, 2009; E. Lee & Jang, 2013; Meyrowitz, 1985; Ramasubramanian & Kornfield, 2012; Thackeray et al., 2013). With the ability to reply, re-tweet and favorite posts, followers on Twitter are able to interact with celebrities. Research demonstrates that noncelebrities develop close emotional and psychological bonds with famous people whom they admire and then seek to role model their lives (W. J. Brown & Basil, 2010). In fact, W. J. Brown and Basil stated that "[m]illions of people have donated corneas, put on seatbelts, had cancer screenings, reduced risky sexual behavior, and made healthy lifestyle changes through their parasocial interaction and identification with celebrities" (p. 602).

As we have mentioned thus far in the book, through social networking sites such as Twitter and Facebook, celebrities can reveal aspects of their personal lives in the public sphere and, in so doing allow their lives to intersect with others, even noncelebrities (for related arguments, see Beck, 2012; Goffman, 1976). Through this dialectical relationship, both celebrity and "follower" are powerful and powerless. In related work, Žižek (1992) referred to this phenomenon as the "dialectic of the gaze" (p. 72). From this perspective, a fan or "follower" of a celebrity may experience the dialectic of the gaze simultaneously by holding a position of control (i.e., by contributing to the fame of the celebrity) while also remaining impotent, given that they remain passive witnesses of a celebrity's actions.

Nocera (2009, January 15) argued that some celebrities, such as the late Steve Jobs, implicitly yield privacy rights due to their celebrity status. As Nocera explained, "There are certain people who simply don't have the same privacy rights as others, whether they like it or not. Celebrities. Sports figures. And, at least in terms of his health, Steve Jobs" (para. 9). Nocera called for Jobs to resign from Apple if he desired health privacy, but he characterized information on Jobs' health status as vital for Apple's shareholders. This story illustrates modern-day expectations of those within the public gaze, especially individuals with whom the audience holds vested financial or emotional interest, such as a celebrity/businesswoman like Kim Kardashian. Thus, in this chapter, we sought to understand how identification with celebrity illness influenced public perception of health, ways in which celebrity illness and disclosures impact parasocial relationships (especially as enacted online), and fan identification with celebrity health, employing Kim Kardashian as an exemplar.

"Konnecting" with Kim

Just Like Kim: Identifying with Celebrity Illness

As we detail, numerous followers identified with Kim's struggle with psoriasis. They communicated a strong sense of identification with the celebrity due to her illness. Tweets mentioned a perceived friendship and/or identifying with Kim, citing psoriasis as a personal link or "one step closer" to being like Kim. Followers claimed to be like her, discussed feeling closer to her, and used words such as "twin" or "twinsies" and even "sisters" to describe their perceived and desired relationship.

Some fans claimed to be closer to Kim due to the onset or outbreak of psoriasis. For instance, Connor (2013, August 14) tweeted to Kim, "my severe psoriasis breakout has brought me even closer to my girl @kimkardashian." Similarly, Kate (2013, August 14) commented that "[t]he doctor claims I have psoriasis, which means that I'm one step closer to being like Kim Kardashian #kardashainatheart [sic]." One follower questioned her identification with Kim due to her possible psoriasis development on her arm. Katherine Anna (2013, February 13) posted [sic] "I also found a tiny spot of what possible psoriasis on my arm. Sad that my fist thought was now I'm closer to Kim Kardashian?"

In addition to being "closer" to Kim, some fans went one step further within their perceived relationship. Some commented that they were "twins" of Kim Kardashian because they both have psoriasis. Paigey ☼ (2013, August 12) tweeted that "Kim Kardashian has psoriasis and so do I so we're basically twins." Barbie Bitch (2012, November 12) noted that "[m]e and my twin Kim

Kardashian have psoriasis." Similarly, Ashley (2013, January 28) asserted that "me and @KimKardashian are psoriasis twins." NACHO (2013, January 28) also claimed, "OMG. @KimKardashian were twinses!! We both have Psoriasis. Lol." One fan questioned if she was a twin with Kim due to her psoriasis occurring in similar locations to Kim. Brooke (2013, April 7) said, "So if me and Kim Kardashian have psoriasis in the same spots does this mean were [sic] twins????" Such discourses not only equated the tweeter's identity with Kim but also worked to elevate the poster's status to a celebritized position.

Not everyone claimed to be a twin or identical to Kim, but many identified with Kardashian because of their common psoriasis battle. As Burke (1950/1969) argued in his classic book, *A Rhetoric of Motives*, "In being identified with B, A is 'substantially one' with a person other than himself. Yet at the same time he remains unique, an individual locus of motives. Thus he is both joined and separate, at once a distinct substance and consubstantial with another" (p. 21). The following tweets illustrate this sense of solidarity by some fans.

Michelle (2013, March 31) asserted that "I have psoriasis. Kim Kardashian has psoriasis. Therefore I am Kim Kardashian." Similarly, FrejaHopwood 🥀 (2012, November 13) maintained that "Kim kardashian has psoriasis I have psoriasis, therefore I am Kim kardashian #yeahhh." Brett (2013, 5 Apr), said, "im kim kardashian with this psoriasis on my leg." Samantha (2013, May 10) invited others to "[j]ust call me the Kim Kardashian of Psoriasis. Damn xxxx genes ... #itchyitchyitchy." These tweets attempted to position the tweeter as one with Kim by connecting the psoriasis dots between Kim and themselves.

Some followers claimed to be "sisters" with Kardashian due to their (perceived) shared psoriasis. REEM (2013, June, 18) said, "If I find out I have psoriasis then I am officially @KimKardashian long lost sister." Even though this follower did not have psoriasis, she suggested that, if she were to be diagnosed with it, she would, in fact, be a long lost Kardashian. Kat (2013, June 13) posted that "Kim Kardashian has psoriasis and I have psoriasis so pretty much were [sic] sisters." Such tweeters underscored common attributes in their efforts to identify with the celebrity, stressing that a shared diagnosis of psoriasis (although certainly undesirable on a personal level) afforded yet another means through which fans could achieve (at least perceived) consubstantiality with the celebrity (see related works by Brock, 1999; Burke 1950/1969; Wolin, 2001).

Indeed, for some fans, having psoriasis, like Kim, constructed positive connotations. For instance, lana (2013, December 12) noted that "me and kim kardashian both have psoriasis, cute x x." This follower perceived it "cute" to share psoriasis with Kim. Hannah (2013, May 10) wrote, "Been diagnosed with psoriasis. Ah well, if you're going to have a disease, you want it to be one that kim kardashian has as well #brightside." In addition to being "cute" and desirable, these fans described sharing a diagnosis with Kim something to be celebrated, in spite of personal discomfort. babel (2012, December 11) commented that "having psoriasis in common with @KimKardashian woo." Such tweets reveal that those followers value their psoriasis diagnosis as a means to align or identify with Kim. Celebrity publicity in this case prompted construction of an illness as "cute" (as opposed to other more potentially stigmatizing descriptors), which fans might find acceptable in order to "be like Kim."

As we detail, followers specified other attributes, characteristics, or possessions, in addition to psoriasis, that made them "just like Kim." For example, numerous followers commented that they had the same area of psoriasis outbreaks on their body, as well as shared taste in men and bedding. Samantha (2013, January 8) asserted that "Me and Kim kardashian both have psoriasis and big butts. We are officially twins." Laura (2013, January 27) claimed, "Me and kim kardashian: giant boobs, and psoriasis. We could totally be bff' S. In a sexy way." Keith (2013, March 7) argued, "I'm like @KimKardashian. I date black guys AND I have psoriasis!" Joey (2013, March 1) tweeted that "[n]ot only do @kimkardashian and I both have psoriasis but we also have the same bedding!!" Lauren (2013, February 17) posted, "[s]ince Kim Kardashian has Psoriasis does that make it sexy? 👀 " Similarly, Jocelyn (2013, February 17) wrote, "Kim Kardashian makes psoriasis fabulous." Kathryn (2013, February 16) commented that "Kim Kardashian has psoriasis, I feel so cool!!!" These tweets "go the extra step" by identifying not only with Kim's psoriasis, but also with another physical characteristic or asset that this particular Kardashian sister possesses. Moreover, these tweets affirm that, for some reason(s), connecting with this particular celebrity mattered and that they clearly associate Kim's diagnosis as now an integral dimension of her image.

Kim = Psoriasis

As we will detail throughout this chapter via examples of Twitter activity, publicity about her psoriasis has linked the image of Kim Kardashian to the disease. This perception constructed Kim as an unofficial, yet "official" spokesperson, and, therefore, expert on psoriasis. Indeed, fans noted that references to psoriasis prompted thoughts of Kim Kardashian. For instance, Ashlee (2013, March 20) tweeted to Kim "@KimKardashian I am sitting here watching a show called The Food Hospital they are talking about foods to help with psoriasis. I thought of u." Tremecia (2012, November 27) said, "I remember when my brother thought I had psoriasis and was like 'omg you have the Kim kardashian disease' smh." Kidrauhl † (2012, November 1) asked "Is it bad that when I saw a psoriasis commercial, I thought of Kim Kardashian?" Ciara (2013, February 14) responded, "Ahahahaha whenever I see a commercial about psoriasis I automatically think of Kim Kardashian #crazyfanprobs #hatemyself" In many ways, these comments demonstrate that Kim's public discussion of psoriasis provides context or a "more real" way of knowing and understanding what it means to have psoriasis. Through Kim's willingness to expose the "back stage" of psoriasis (see Goffman, 1959), Kim advances dialogue about this otherwise potentially stigmatizing condition, by merging fact and values, reason and emotion (Fisher, 1984, 1987a) and identifying with others who struggle to manage this health issue (see related work by Burke, 1950/1969).

Learning about Psoriasis

When celebrities make their private health matters public, they educate the public and increase public understanding of the illness/disease. Numerous tweets revealed that Kim's discussions of psoriasis led them to be educated about the autoimmune disorder. For instance, Elena (2012, November 9) tweeted to "@KimKardashian you taught me all of the symptoms of psoriasis. #lifesaver." Adeelah (2012, November 15) noted that "I don't think I'd know what's Psoriasis if it wasn't for Kim Kardashian." Nicola (2012, October 30) offered her diagnosis to another person on Twitter, tweeting that "@MrsNicolaMcLean looks like psoriasis hun, Kim kardashian recently showed pics of her with it, google and see if looks similar x."

Upon learning about possible treatments from Kim, fans treated recommendations as legitimate and viable. For example, in one episode of her reality TV show, Kim Kardashian stole her sister's breast milk in order to put it on her psoriasis after reading online that it was a cure-all liquid. Afterwards, fans reported learning about this remedy. For example, Kendra (2013, February 12) wrote, "Thanks to @KimKardashian I now know that breast milk is good for my psoriasis lmao." Sydney (2013, March 4) shared that "Jack just told me to rub breast milk on my psoriasis because Kim Kardashian did it. #TooMuchTv #ThanksFoTheAdviceFlack." Summer (2013, March 20) mentioned that "I'm only trying breast milk to cure my eczema because it worked for @KimKardashian and her psoriasis. Hopefully it works just as well!" valll (2013, July 16) suggested, "So many people have it and it hurts so baddd ☺ maybe I should try breast milk like Kim Kardashian #psoriasis pic.twitter.com/FJ8vifeFOQ."

We are concerned that fans would employ recommended cure-alls, given that Kim has no medical education. When celebrities, such as Kim, discuss illness and treatments (even without overtly endorsing possibilities for other people), they resemble the white-coat actors in pharmaceutical commercials.

INSPIRATIONAL

Followers find Kim's revelation to be inspiring. Akter (2012, November 27) wrote, "@KimKardashian @leannrimes both of you are inspirational in your support and awareness of Psoriasis :)" J U N A ♥ ⋛ (2013, April 26) said, "@KimKardashian's heart-shaped #psoriasis. She's been my inspiration in fighting psor. She's preggy&Godbless her baby!" каяєи ᨔ (2013, January 28) boasted that "if @KimKardashian isn't ashamed of her skin condition Psoriasis then I shouldn't either bout my Psoriasis." Beary (2013, January 29) confided that "knowing someone as perfect as @KimKardashian has psoriasis makes me feel better about having it hHa." Jasmin (2013, January 30) wrote [sic], "I actually look up to @KimKardashian. me and her both have psoriasis and she handles it like its nothing. I need to start doing that, too." J E S S (2012, November 13) asserted that "[t]he fact that Kim Kardashian has psoriasis makes me feel 100x better." Vanessa (2013, April 5) wrote, "Knowing how open Cara Delevingne and Kim Kardashian are about their psoriasis is making me feel a bit, well … more normal, and confident." Katie (2013, April 5) wrote, "@KimKardashian I just found out today I got psoriasis but it make [sic] me feel more confident in myself that someone like you can deal with it :)" Rachel (2013, February 7) shared that "[s]eeing beautiful women like @CariDeeEnglish and @KimKardashian battle psoriasis w/ such empowerment makes me feel like I'm still beautiful ♥ " bambino—(2013, February 8) revealed that "the fact @KimKardashian has psoriasis makes me feel better when I have out breaks of it." Angela (2012, December 16) mentioned that "every time I freak out about having psoriasis my mom reminds me that @KimKardashian has it too and I instantly feel better. #loveher." Alex (2013, March 26) wrote, "if this is Psoriasis at least I can tell myself @KimKardashian rocks it and is fabulous #itsakardashianlife."

Additionally, followers expressed encouragement that someone as beautiful and talented as Kim had a "flaw" or "imperfection." Behind the glitz and glam, having psoriasis showcased her humanity, which increased her attraction and fans' desire to identify with her. Some delighted in Kim's "imperfection." Valerie (2013. January 28) commented that "@KimKardashian has Psoriasis. Hmm she's not so perfect after all. But breast milk is sure to be the cure!! #KKTM." Meghan (2013, January 28) said, "I bet none of you knew

Kim Kardashian has psoriasis. We all have flaws." Meghan Nelson (2013, January 28) tweeted that "I think it's great how open @KimKardashian is about her psoriasis. It just goes to show no one is perfect ❤ " Jess (2013, January 30) wrote, "why did I just find out that Kim Kardashian has psoriasis? guess that perfect bitch really couldn't have it all. HA." MuchLoveJaimie (2013, January 29) revealed, "I forgot Kim kardashian has psoriasis! She's not perfect!!! How wrong is it tho that it makes me feel better about my self hahaha." Beneé (2013, November 7) confided that "[i]t makes me happy that Kim K gets psoriasis from time to time." Jade (2012, December 30) recalled a conversation: "Me: 'When you're feeling down, just remember you're the sperm that won.' Bestfriend: 'Or remember that Kim kardashian has psoriasis.'" Olivia (2013, February 10) shared that "Kim Kardashian has psoriasis. I am a terrible person for saying this but that kind of makes me happy."

Kim's revelation inspired research projects and presentations for school coursework as well as career choices. Brianna (2013, January 29) wrote, "I love how Kim Kardashian has inspired the topic for my advanced biology project #psoriasis." Sarah (2013, January 9) wrote, "Learning about psoriasis in biology so I can become a doctor and cure @KimKardashian." Kamikazee (2013, February 14) wrote, "doing my first immunology paper on psoriasis bc @KimKardashian has it. perfect reason to learn, and keep up with kim. :) lol." Such educational inspiration revealed ways in which celebrity health disclosures and public discussion can create disease-curing interest and awareness. In addition to being inspired by Kim, fans demarcated her as an expert as evidenced throughout numerous solicitations for advice.

SOLICITING ADVICE

As someone who has openly discussed her private health matter, Kim became an expert in the eyes of her followers. Yazeed (2013, January 30) queried, "@KimKardashian my brother referred me to your show when he was diagnosed with psoriasis. Any tips btw? :(" Shivam (2013, February 1) asked, "@KimKardashian how did you fix your psoriasis? I got it too, would like to be able to make it go away, thanks!" Sam (2013, January 18) wrote, "@KimKardashian hi Kim, My names Sam from the UK, my brother suffers from psoriasis and i heard you do too, pls can you recommend a cream?" Angie (2013, February 11) inquired, "@KimKardashian what do you use for your psoriasis? I have it on my elbows, so irritating!" Jessica (2013, February 9) questioned, "@KimKardashian what do u use for psoriasis as I am a sufferer.?" Maria (2013, June 16) wrote, "@KimKardashian I have psoriasis just like you, can you recommend me a treatment? Any lotions that you've used that worked?" In addition to soliciting advice, fans demonstrated their parasocial relational concern for Kim as they suggested cures to her for her psoriasis.

SUGGESTING CURES

Throughout the tweets collected, numerous followers offered caring comments for Kim Kardashian in terms of suggesting cures and treatments to help alleviate her psoriasis outbreaks. For instance, Rikki (2013, February 14) suggested, "@KimKardashian you should try acupuncture and Chinese herbs for psoriasis they really work!!" Arielle (2013, April 6) commented, "@KimKardashian you should stop using @KourtneyKardash's breast milk and go to the Dead Sea for your psoriasis." Rhonda (2013, February 1) asserted, "@KimKardashian You should try going gluten free to help w/psoriasis. #glutenfree #celiac @Glutenfreeworks." Anna (2013, February 15) claimed, "@KimKardashian—Hey Kim! You should read wheat belly! It may significantly help with your Psoriasis :)" p3g88 (2013, February 1) shared, "@KimKardashian wanted to let you know of something for your psoriasis to use is olive oil. its all natural and good for your skin." Selenatoя (2012, November 27) suggested, "@kimkardashian I know you have psoriasis and I had and put ice on the area and helped a lot. Why don't you try? It might work." Harlee ♡ (2012, November 11) recommended, "@KimKardashian watching your episode about psoriasis, I have it too, try Psoriasin gel from Walgreens, its magic!" MARGOT (2013, February 8) encouraged, "@KimKardashian used crest toothpaste with crystals and added a little water. Leave for 5 min. and in a month it was gone." Raerae (2013, March 20) wrote, "@KimKardashian use the cream that farmers use on cows utters for ur Psoriasis. It's works. Xx." In addition to suggesting cures to Kim, which demonstrated a caring behavior from her fans, fans tweeted pleas of help with their own psoriasis relief.

PLEAS FOR HELP

Kim also fulfills the parasocial role of a "Good Samaritan." We do not know whether Kim obliged or not through these tweets, but the tweets do reveal "pleas for help" on Twitter. Daniel (2012, November 27) asked, "@KimKardashian Your #psoriasis won't magically go away. Use your fame to help find a cure. There are great doctors looking for a cure." Aliza (2013, November 28) inquired, "@KimKardashian I need your help. Who treated your psoriasis? My beautiful 9-year-old has it. Any help would be great." Kristie (2013, January 10) wrote, "@KimKardashian what's the best medication you used for psoriasis? Plz plz help. Xoxo." Donnamarie (2013, March 22) inquired, "@KimKardashian I have psoriasis too. Any natural trtmnts u think wk best? I was laidoff n my selfestm is super low during the intervwing [*sic*]." Farrah (2013, May 25) begged, "I need breast milk for my psoriasis, I get the same thing as Kim kardashian occasionally and nothing else works!!!!" By pleading for help, fans demonstrated their parasocial expectation of Kim. Through their tweets, fans underscore a parasocial relationship in that they oriented to her as a celebrity and "friend," with implied expectations for helping her supporters when they demonstrate need or ask for help (see related work by Meyrowitz, 1985).

Discussion and Conclusion

This chapter expands health and mass communication research by analyzing ways in which followers of Kim Kardashian's Twitter account enact parasocial relationships via identification with the celebrity and her disorder. First, identification with Kim influenced public perception of psoriasis in a myriad of ways. Followers exhibited a strong desire to obtain the "sexy illness" in order to be more like the celebrity. In this instance, followers attempted to exonerate their own illness and likelihood to that of Kim Kardashian, compelling followers to not only state their similarity with Kim's psoriasis, but also to list multiple characteristics that make them just like Kim. Additionally, Kim's continual discussion of psoriasis increased knowledge, advanced awareness, and even spurred students to research medical topics in reports. As this case indicated, celebrities can become illness experts, with fans seeking information and even help from someone who has little (or no) medical expertise other than personal experience with the illness.

Second, this study revealed that celebrity illness disclosure and dialogue solicited parasocial relationship interactions in terms of identification with the celebrity and illness. For example, followers communicated their parasocial relationship by identifying with the celebrity by claiming one is "just like Kim," one step closer, or that they are, in fact, Kim's long lost sister. Additionally, these relationships offered social support for the celebrity, who may or may not engage by responding to tweets, as demonstrated through caring behaviors where followers offered cures and advice on how to eliminate the celebrity's ailment.

Finally, the comments reveal three dominant rhetorical strategies that individuals employed in order to identify with celebrity illness: Claiming "twinsies," caretaking behaviors as evidenced through offering advice to Kim, and pleas for help, which demonstrated a relational expectation that Kim will help them in their time of need. Claiming "twinsies" in this study referred to instances where individuals ascribe celebrity-like status and traits to themselves by pointing out a similarity that existed between said speaker and the celebrity target. Caretaking behaviors involved measures in which followers suggested medical remedies or suggestions on some type of action Kim should perform in order to alleviate her psoriasis suffering. Through "pleas for help," followers demonstrated their parasocial relational expectation of Kim. When solicited for help, Kim was expected to reciprocate the same caretaking behaviors others have offered to her, which demonstrates the perceived dyadic relationship between the two parties.

As we will detail at the end of the book, this chapter affirms that social media comprise an increasingly prevalent way that fans and celebrities exchange information and that expanding privacy borders between fan and celebrity influences parasocial interactions in a new way that created instant expectations and relational reciprocity. For example, instead of just sharing information with Kim, fans also expected Kim to share information with them. This perceived reciprocity expectation influenced the celebrity-fan relationship. As such, fans treated Kim as a valued source of information about psoriasis as an "expert" and as a "friend."

CHAPTER FOUR

"I never wanted to be the poster child for this"

Catherine Zeta-Jones and Bipolar II Disorder

Michael Douglas and Catherine Zeta-Jones, a prominent Hollywood super couple, attract attention on the red carpet as well as in the tabloids, and Michael's bout with throat cancer and Catherine Zeta-Jones' reluctant public conversation about her diagnosis of bipolar II disorder have certainly launched this celebrity pair into the spotlight. In this chapter, we begin our discussion of celebrity health narratives that are not nearly as tidy and positive as the ones that have been enacted by Brooke Burke-Charvet and Kim Kardashian. As we note in this focus on Catherine Zeta-Jones' personal response to her bipolar II disorder in addition to online comments, not all celebrities necessarily desire for their respective identities to be linked with a particular illness, and they do not all wish to serve as "experts" or "advocates." Yet, as reactions to Catherine Zeta-Jones' protest that "I never wanted to be the poster child for this [bipolar II disorder]" suggest, some onlookers contest a more private story, arguing that the price of fame equates not only disclosures of personal information but also efforts on behalf of the "greater good" (Dillon, 2012). After discussing CZJ's celebrity status and bipolar II disorder and reviewing the theoretical framework for this chapter, we consider mixed reactions to Catherine Zeta-Jones' quest to shift her public health narrative back to a private matter.

Catherine Zeta-Jones' Stardom

This mother of two is no stranger to the spotlight. Catherine Zeta-Jones came to fame in the 1990s for her role in a TV drama series entitled *The Darling*

Buds of May. CZJ also received an "Oscar [for best supporting actress] and Bafta award in 2003 for her role in the film adaptation of the musical *Chicago*" (Fallon, 2011, April 13, para. 5). Throughout the '90s, CZJ consistently held supporting actress roles in films and miniseries such as *Christopher Columbus: The Discovery, Catherine the Great, The Phantom, Titanic,* and *The Mask of Zorro* (IMBD, 2014b). According to the IMDB, her performance in *The Mask of Zorro* propelled her stardom into roles such as *Entrapment, Traffic, Ocean's Twelve,* and *The Haunting,* and, in 2009, CZJ's first Broadway role in *A Little Night Music* earned her a Tony award. However, her fame intensified when she became part of a Hollywood super couple.

First Came Love, Then Came the "Private" Health Concerns

In 2000, CZJ and fellow actor Michael Douglas tied the knot in what has been referred to as a fairy-tale wedding (Malkin, 2014, January 12). CZJ and Michael Douglas have constantly been in the spotlight for their fame, marriage, and health. Despite marital troubles in 2013 which involved a brief separation, this Hollywood celebrity couple seemingly exemplifies the adage that true love does conquer all, and they walked on the red carpet together again in April 2014 (E. Lee, 2014, April 16). However, their very public careers and marriage have also put them in the spotlight as they wrestled with personal health issues very much in the public eye. First, Michael Douglas was diagnosed with throat cancer in 2010, but, in January 2011, he announced that he was cancer-free after six months of treatment (Hass, 2012, December).

CATHERINE'S BIPOLAR II DISORDER.

CZJ sought treatment for a challenging year of dealing with multiple stressors including Michael's cancer as well as his former wife's suing him for a portion of royalties from his movie, *Wall Street: Money Never Sleeps* (Salahi, 2011, April 14). She spent five days at the Silver Hill Hospital in Connecticut for treatment for bipolar II disorder (Fallon, 2011, April 13, para. 7). CZJ's "surprise admission came the same day [as] a *National Enquirer* cover story" on the event (Dillon, 2012, December 7). In an interview with *Oprah*, Michael mentioned that CZJ never wanted this diagnosis to become public, but she reluctantly confirmed her illness after someone within the hospital reportedly sold the story to the press (Reeves & Clarke, 2011, April 26). A family friend told *Star* magazine that life stressors exhausted CZJ, confiding that "[s]he had to go into treatment because she hadn't been taking her bipolar medication—she was the last thing on her mind [because she put others first]" (Schwartz, 2013, September 16, p. 36). CZJ sought a second round of inpatient treatment in April 2013. However, soon afterward, Michael commented that his throat cancer had been caused by oral sex. The family friend claimed that "Catherine went absolutely berserk.... What he was trying to say was that throat cancer wasn't just due to his smoking, that there were loads of other causes, including oral sex. But it came out wrong. Catherine was horrified" (Schwartz, 2013, September 16, p. 36).

During an interview with *InStyle* magazine, CZJ explained, "I'm not the kind of person who likes to shout out my personal issues from the rooftops, but with my bipolar becoming public, I hope fellow sufferers will know it's completely controllable. I hope I can help remove any stigma attached to it" (Puente, 2012, November 13, para. 4). Additionally, she expressed optimism that "those who don't have it [bipolar II disorder] under control will seek help with all that is available to treat it" (*Huffpost Celebrity*, 2012, December 12, para. 2).

CZJ's actions prompted praise and support from medical professionals and fans alike. Mark Davies, from Rethink Mental Illness, observed that "[w]hen people such as Catherine Zeta-Jones speak out it makes a big difference to the millions of other people facing mental illness. It shows them that they are not alone and that mental illness can affect anyone, rich or poor, famous or otherwise" (Fallon, 2011, April 13, para. 11). Former *Today* show and *Dateline NBC* host Jane Pauley, who also has bipolar II disorder, asserted that "[i]t's not an exaggeration to say she has made the world a safer place for people who have the diagnosis, are afraid of being diagnosed or will one day be diagnosed. Her impact in the world of the arts has been considerable. But this might be bigger" (Baker, 2011, April 21, para. 2).

In an interview with *People*, a close friend of CZJ said, "If this were something else—pills, drugs, whatever—it would have been an easy out. There is some weird taboo about this. But she's like, 'If I had diabetes, I would say I had diabetes and I would get treatment for it.' She didn't ask for this disorder" (Cotliar & Tauber, 2011, May 2, p. 54).

Notably, CZJ joins other famous actresses, such as Carrie Fisher (*Star Wars*) and Patty Duke (*The Miracle Worker*) who have acknowledged their battles with mental illness. Duke (1987, 1992) wrote two books, chronicling her experiences with manic depression, and Fisher has openly discussed her struggles with bipolar disorder and addiction (see E. Johnson, 2013, April 20). However, CZJ's openness about her bipolar II disorder has not necessarily been willingly transparent. During an interview on *Good Morning America*, cohost Elizabeth Vargas spoke with the actress about her up-and-coming film, *Playing for Keeps*. When asked about her bipolar II disorder, CZJ said,

> You know what? I'm sick of talking about it, because I never wanted to be the poster child for this. And I never wanted this to come out publicly. It came out. And so I dealt with it in the best way I could. And that was just saying that look, "Hey, I'm bipolar." Everyone has things going on and we deal with them the best we can. We can't jump from the rooftop shouting, you know about "I have this, look at me, victim." *No.* we all have issues in life. And I'm really happy that I have great friends, great support and that's all you can do [*Good Morning America*, 2012, December 7, para. 7].

CZJ's attempt to negotiate her privacy boundaries in this public eye, as illustrated through this excerpt, serves as the focal point for this chapter. As Wheeler (2013) detailed, celebrities have increasingly leveraged their fame as springboards for activism, and, as scholars have argued, the internet has afforded individuals (even those who might not have otherwise risen to some degree of fame) with ever increasing opportunities for connecting with and influencing others (E. Lee & Jang, 2013; Marwick, 2013). However, CZJ's expressed desire to reclaim her "own" narrative has been challenged by others who assert that "celebrity status" comes at the cost of privacy.

In this chapter, we explore this issue of "owning" a narrative. If we accept that narratives constitute fluid, emergent, collaboratively co-constructed stories (e.g., Bamberg, 2012; Bamberg & Andrews, 2004; Harter, 2009; Harter et al., 2005, 2006), what happens when disputes occur that involve an individual's privacy, preferences, and perspectives (see related work by Lalvani, 2011; Redman, 2005) amid challenging and very intimate life situations (see Pederson, 2013)? As we detail in this chapter, CZJ's personal illness narrative has become contested by some fans and onlookers as they herald an implied master narrative of "the greater good" over CZJ's desire to step aside as "poster child."

In an article entitled, *Catherine Zeta-Jones, Please Don't Stop Talking About Bipolar Disorder!*, Kaufman (2012, December 10) wrote, "People love hearing that celebrities have the same problems they do. Zeta-Jones has become *more* relatable, not less, since she came out" (para. 9). Kaufman argued that, "[b]y removing mental illness from the conversation, Zeta-Jones risks alienating fans, not winning them over" (para. 9). He proceeded to assert that "[h]er lack of shame will speak volumes, and set an example for other people with mental illness to stop blaming themselves and start getting the treatment they need. That's the opposite of being a 'victim' or an empty 'poster child'; that's showing true strength" (para. 11).

Managing "Private" Turned "Public" Narratives

Communication Privacy Management (CPM) theory proposes individuals "consider private information something they own, and over which they desire control" (Petronio, 2002, p. 9). CPM employs a boundary metaphor to discuss levels of permeability for disclosure. A person's culture, gender, perceived risk/benefits, motivations, and context influence privacy rules that govern discloser decisions. When an individual chooses to disclose personal information, others become "co-owners" of that information. Bute and Vik (2010) referred to CPM as an ongoing, unfinished practice that requires constant attention and management. As we have noted thus far, celebrities are no exception, and, in fact, their boundaries become more problematic as their popularity grows and/or accessibility to fans expands through means such as social media, even when a celebrity decides that s/he no longer enjoys the focus on a very personal concern, such as a mental illness.

CZJ: Reluctant "Poster Child"

REDUCING STIGMA

Goffman (1963) defined stigma as "an attribute that is deeply discrediting" (p. 3). According to Goffman, stigma may be an individual or group attribute that renders a person to be inferior, tainted, discounted, and/or unworthy of association. Goffman defined three classifications of stigma: (a) physical abnormalities, (b) imperfections of character, and (c) tribal/racial stigma. Physical abnormalities and tribal/racial stigmas are generally visible; whereas imperfections or character flaws may be invisible to the naked eye. The act of self-disclosure, or when people are outed, bring such "flaws" into the spotlight. Stigmas may be face-threatening. Agne, Thompson, and Cusella (2000) described imperfections of character as discreditable and, once disclosed, may result someone in being discredited, which renders a loss of face. Within interpersonal relationships, the threat of losing face exists since perceptions of what is a "stigma" may differ person to person. Scrambler and Hopkins (1986, p. 33) referred to fears of stigmatization as "felt stigma" and prejudice against stigmatized individuals as "enacted stigma."

Goffman (1963) asserted that stigma is socially constructed and, therefore, located within social interaction, which may be changed. On *Good Morning America*, Dan Harris said, "Anytime you have a high profile case like this it really is an opportunity to educate people about mental illness which, as you know, is so often stigmatized" (Salahi, 2011, April 14, para. 2). Similarly, in response to an online press article regarding CZJ's disorder, one reader, Jim, wrote, "It helps to de-stigmatize the disorder or any mental disorder for that matter when celebrities go public with their having it" (Gicas, 2012, December 7, Comments Section). Similarly, JAD expressed, "I'm glad she spoke out about her condition. It makes others with mental illnesses feel normal" (C. Johnson, 2012, December 7, Comments Section). These comments reinforce the destigmatization process that occurs when celebrities go public with their health narratives.

Lipp (2011) suggested that stigma is best alleviated on policy, local, and individual levels. Past research on celebrity health disclosures revealed that each of these levels can be influenced when celebrities' public and private lines blur as a result of their personal health information being shared with the public (Beck et al., 2014). Link and Phelan (2006) argued that "stigma places people at a substantial social disadvantage with respect to these resources, it increased their exposure to risks and limits access to protective factors, potentially adding to their burden of disease or disability" (p. 529). Reeders (2008) described narratives as one way in which to overcome public health stigmas. Therefore, CZJ's narrative holds the power to assist in destigmatizing bipolar II disorder. For instance, one fan, Terri, commented, "Thank you Catherine for speaking out about the disorder and showing it can affect anyone regardless of wealth and status. Perhaps chipping away at the stigma" (Kirkova, 2013, July 21, Comments Section). Similarly, MannyHM wrote on April 15, 2011,

> Of all the beautiful faces in the world I'm glad Catherine Zeta-Jones has decided to associate hers with bipolar 2 disorder. Stigma and shame having to do with mental illness is completely unnecessary and has gone on way too long. This wonderful actress is doing a lot of good educating the public. For all of us living with this disorder, I thank her for her courage! [Health Media Ventures, 2014, Comments Section].

Stigma is not only associated with producing stress for its recipient (Gibbs & Fuery, 1994; Link & Phelan, 2006), but it also serves as a trigger for bipolar II disorder (International Bipolar Foundation, 2014). Therefore, CZJ's revelation held the potential to not only contribute to the destigmatization of this illness, but also to lower stress triggers for individuals suffering from bipolar II disorder. Online comments on news articles reflected that CZJ's disclosure helped reduce stigma against bipolar II disorder on individual levels. In fact, responders contended that celebrity health disclosures are needed for destigmatization of mental illness. Lauren praised CZJ's disclosure, noting, "Well done to her for being open about her condition and not letting it define or rule her life in anyway—this is what we need to remove certain stigmas and help others with mental illnesses to understand that they are not alone and they are not to be ashamed of it" (C. Johnson, 2012, December 7, Comments Section).

Lauren not only commended CZJ for her bravery, but she characterized CZJ's actions as essential for helping stigmatized individuals to not be ashamed. Similarly, Brenda m expressed, "I wish more people spoke candidly about their mental health challenges. The stigma needs to disappear so those who haven't been seeking proper attention for their challenges will not be so afraid to do so" (Blacklow, 2013, July 22, Comments Section). Jennifer wrote, "I too have been diagnosed with bipolar disorder. I commend Catherine Zeta-Jones in her willingness to come forward about her own experience. The more we talk about mental illness, the greater the understanding becomes and the less stigma is associated with it" (Macatee, 2012, November 14, Comments Section). Brenda, Lauren, and Jennifer's comments revealed that individuals may find strength through celebrity health disclosures, which ultimately combat the stigma attached to their illness. Destigmatization is not only a plausible reality when celebrities disclose but, increasingly, an expected or assumed role.

'Tis a Celebrity's Role

Clearly, some individuals contended that celebrities, such as CZJ, are expected to "give back" to the public and to use their position for the greater good. Therefore, they oriented to CZJ's disclosure and candor about her bipolar II disorder as positive for the "greater good" and, further, a now required expectation. In other words, fans and onlookers generally anticipated co-owning CZJ's personal health information. This anticipation extended Petronio's (2002) co-ownership discussions to public personalities, such as CZJ and other celebrities. Reactions to CZJ prompt us to coin the term *detached co-owners* to highlight the interplay between the observer and the observed. Such a term enhances understanding into the dialectic of controlling and being controlled. This construct extends from prior work on parasocial relationships between fans and celebrities in that fans feel a sense of connection with people in the public eye (W. J. Brown & Basil, 2010; Earnheardt & Haridakis, 2009; Hartmann & Goldhoorn, 2011; Kassing & Sanderson, 2009; Meyrowitz, 1985; Ramasubramanian & Kornfield, 2012; Savage & Spence, 2014; for related work on fandom, see, e.g., Gray, Sandvoss, & Harrington, 2007; Hills, 2002; Jenkins, 2006).

"Detached co-owners," once vested, expect to be kept "in the loop" on their investment. Since CZJ could not actually develop and maintain intimate personal relationships with her fans and followers, *detached co-owners* refers to relationships that are largely one-sided but may refer to individuals who supported CZJ in some way such as by paying to see one of her movies, etc.

Online comments to popular press articles revealed assumptions regarding the celebrity's role as well as their anticipation and expectation that they have a right to CZJ's privacy, due to their vested interest in her celebrity status. For instance, Tightwad wrote, "Sorry, but if you're going to use people to make you rich and famous, you've established a relationship with the public. You are going to have to answer questions in bad times as well as good. It comes with the territory" (Daily Dish, 2012, December 7, Comments Section). Tightwad demarcated not only a relationship with the public, but the expectation that questions will be answered. In other words, CZJ must share truthfully and fully personal information because this information isn't just "hers," but is perceived to be "ours." CZJ's bipolar II disorder does not belong to her. It belongs to each of "us" who made CZJ a celebrity. Similarly, Shall wrote, "If you're in the public eye ... it's the publics business to ask" (Daily Dish, 2012, December 7, Comments Section). This quote too demonstrates that CZJ's business is "our" business. Popnfresh argued, "Sorry, Cathy, but you're a celebrity. If you want reporters to stop asking you these questions, stop putting yourself in front of reporters. You made the choice to stand in the spotlight and reap the financial rewards of stardom. If the spotlight is getting a little too hot for you, step out of it. Don't whine about it" (Daily Dish, 2012, December 7, Comments Section).

Popnfresh characterizes "whining" when she sought to reinforce her privacy boundaries, which speaks to the anticipated role of CZJ as celebrity. In the perspective of such fans, celebrities should share without restraint; thus, they implicitly affirm that celebrities' privacy rights are not like those of non-celebrities (see related work by Nocera, 2009, January 15). Popnfresh's use of "Cathy" demonstrates a familiar relationship with CZJ, which speaks to the detached co-owner relationship that Popnfresh implies. Similarly, Denise acknowledged, "I understand her wanting that to not be a topic but she knows that being a celeb the good and the bad are going to be out there and talked about" ("Catherine Zeta-Jones: I Don't Want," 2012, December 8, Comments Section). Although sympathetic, Denise demarcates the celebrity role as including disclosing personal health information. Denise's use of "the good and the bad" may be replaced with "knowing your personal health information."

SOCIAL RESPONSIBILITY

Some commenters believed not disclosing or continuing to talk about her bipolar II disorder made CZJ selfish. In other words, it was her social responsibility and obligation to continue talking about her disorder. Through such comments, fans/onlookers contend that part of a celebrity's role is to "give back" to the public, in this case, through providing personal health information to the public. Such an expectation revealed the anticipatory collaborative story-building process. CZJ, as celebrity, is intertwined with life narratives of fans and onlookers, and, as such, she ought to mesh her pages with people in the public in their respective storybooks (see, e.g., related argument by Beck, 2012).

For instance, Misty asserted that "[w]hether they like it or not people look at and up to celebrities. Yes, there is the 'It's my life, leave me alone' path, but, at the same time, she really made so many people with bi-polar disorder feel not so 'weird' or alone. It's a shame with all her influence she'd rather stay on the selfish path" ("Catherine Zeta-Jones: I Don't Want," 2012, December 8, Comments Section). Similarly, Elsa said, "instead of moaning and groaning she should embrace the sickness and educate the public" ("Catherine Zeta-Jones: I Don't Want," 2012, December 8, Comments Section).

More vocal fans argued that CZJ's social responsibility included using her voice to share her story, educate the public, and contribute to destigma-tizing mental illness. For instance, Guest reprimanded CZJ: "Shame on her. She has the blessed opportunity to help SO MANY PEOPLE, as someone who sufers [sic] from Bipolar Disorder i do not have a voice. It is a disease that no one takes seriously. So I have nothing but sadness for someone with SO much, that wants to give so little back" ("Catherine Zeta-Jones: I Don't Want," 2012, December 8).

In this excerpt, Guest refers to CZJ as someone who has much but shares little. Such an action discredited CZJ from fulfilling her perceived social responsibility to the public. Guest voiced disappointment and sadness that CZJ did not embrace the opportunity to improve the lives of individuals with bipolar II disorder. Guest's use of "no one takes it seriously" speaks to the stigma that exists, which may be lessened through CZJ's vocal efforts. Similarly, Serina argued,

> Sure Michael J Fox will forever be the actor with Parkinson's, but because of that, and the work, and attention he has brought to the disease has raised so much aware4ness and money for a cure of this disease. He chooses not to stop using his voice about Parkinson's. Way to go Michael! Come on Catherine … it was you who I thought of when I was diagnosed with bipolar recently, and it was you who gave a more positive outlook on this disease. Build awareness of Bipolar, Catherine…. Keep talking about it! ["Catherine Zeta-Jones: I Don't Want," 2012, December 8, Comments Section].

Serina compared and contrasted CZJ with Michael J. Fox, an actor and a well-known spokesperson for Parkinson's disease. This commenter not only encouraged Catherine to keep talking about it but indicated that people already associate her name with bipolar. When celebrities do, such as MJF, they are praised, but, when they do not meet public expectations, others chastise them for failing to keep the issue in the public arena. Blah_Blaher_Blahest wrote, "Instead of crying crocodile tears, that you think that you are the poster child for an affliction, that you proclaimed to the media, and that most people have to suffer with on a much bigger scale, why don't you reach out and try to help others?" ("Catherine Zeta-Jones: I Don't Want," 2012, December 8, Comments Section).

Similarly, Wendy asserted that "[i]t's too bad she doesn't want to be a 'poster child' for being bipolar. She could accomplish so much more good than just being an actress" ("Catherine Zeta-Jones: I Don't Want," 2012, December 8, Comments Section). Wendy's comment revealed that speaking out not only benefits others and allows CZJ to fulfill her social responsibility but that she could actually achieve a higher level of "doing good." In spite of the potential "greater good" of personal disclosure, notably, not everyone perceives CZJ's social responsibility to be a voice and face for bipolar II disorder.

Supporting Privacy Boundaries

Comments extended CZJ's co-ownership to include "public defenders." In this chapter, we coin *public defenders* to refer to individuals who have become aware of another's privacy via mass media that speaks to defend an individual's, usually a celebrity's, right to privacy. For instance, Joe wrote, "Give her a fracking break. She is an absolute beautiful woman who has been caught in the Holyweird idiots and she deserves some privacy" (C. Johnson, 2012, December 7, Comments Section). Joe not only demanded CZJ to be given a break but also noted that she deserved privacy. Similarly, Geomancer contended that "Ms. Jones has now made it clear that she has no desire to be a poster child (spokesperson) for the disease, so let's respect her wishes" (Daily Dish, 2012, December 7, Comments Section). Geomancer respected CZJ's wish not to be the "poster child" for bipolar II and requests for others to respect her wishes. These two commenters illustrated that public defenders stand up and "defend" the privacy boundaries of others, even celebrities. Although also detached co-owners, due to their understanding of CZJ's health information, public defenders seek to help the target reinforce and strengthen their privacy boundaries. In other words, public defenders helped their target reinforce their privacy boundaries by fending off attacks or potential intrusions from another.

Some public defenders affirmed CZJ's right to privacy as a tactic to reinforce her privacy boundaries. Missylalawhite emphasized,

She shouldn't be the poster child for this, the media made it that way. Let the woman talk about what she wants to talk about in an interview. I agree with her, it gets tiring to have them talk about her being bipolar during almost every interview. She's had enough and has every right to be tired of it [Gossipcop, 2012, December 7, Comments Section].

Missylalawhite blamed the media for making CZJ the poster child for bipolar II. In other words, Missylalawhite envisioned the media as a culprit that sought to intrude upon CZJ's privacy boundaries. Missylalawhite reinforced CZJ's belief that "it gets tiring" by aligning her own view with CZJ. Additionally, she stressed to others that "she's had enough" and has "every right to be tired." Similarly, another sought to bolster CZJ's privacy boundaries by questioning the expected role of CZJ to share her health narrative. ignorancereigns suggested that "[h]er personal life is just that, personal. Why should she have to be the one to be the poster child for something she struggles with" ("Catherine Zeta-Jones: I Don't Want," 2012, December 8, Comments Section)? ignorancereigns not only reinforced that personal life should be kept personal to only CZJ but also asked why CZJ must be the poster child, encouraging others to critically examine why they anticipate such a role for her.

One commenter disputed the notion that it was CZJ's social responsibility to share her personal health experiences. Dani explained,

Your illness is your business ... no one else's ... if you do not wish to discuss it then you have every right not to ... it is not Catherine zeta Jones job to make any one feel better about their own illness ... if you are bipolar that is your cross to bear ... not up to anyone else to make you cope with it or feel better about it ... illness for some people is a very personal issue ... that is the reason for HIPPA laws [Gossipcop, 2012, December 7, Comments Section].

This statement highlights divergent perspectives on the perceived role and performance of celebrities in the public and private sphere as well as legal ramification and protection as the ultimate public defense for privacy boundaries. Dani explained that HIPPA laws exist to protect an individual's personal health information.

One commenter believed that CZJ should be awarded privacy due to her talent. Lagoon Crow noted, "This woman is spectacularly beautiful, AND she happens to be extremely talented. Leave her alone on anything she doesn't want to discuss" (Daily Dish, 2012, December 7, Comments Section). Lagoon Crow echoed the call for individuals to "leave her alone on anything she doesn't want to discuss." This statement reinforces and publicly defends CZJ's privacy boundaries by directly informing others that their action is not appropriate. Similarly, Felicia objected to the expectation that discussing her illness constitutes CZJ's social responsibility. She wrote,

> Actor are not super humans. Beneath the surface they are like us all. Some of them choose to take up causes and discuss them and some of us do not. It is not fair to say she an obligation because she has been in movies to discuss in every interview her personal battles with mental health [Gossipcop, 2012, December 7, Comments Section].

Felicia commented that actors are not super humans but, instead, are like "us." "Us" within this instance refers to all "noncelebrities." Felicia explained that CZJ should not be under the social obligation, or responsibility, to discuss her personal mental health battles in every interview. This statement defends CZJ and urges fairness and a sense of humanity to be extended to individuals within the spotlight.

Conclusion

The public's reaction to CZJ's claim that she did not want to be the "poster child" for bipolar II disorder prompted mixed reactions regarding public orientation to a celebrity's role with public dialogues about health. On one hand, numerous commenters perceived CZJ's story to be not just hers, but ours. In fact, such individuals affirmed that her role as a celebrity required her to "pay-it-forward" by forfeiting her right to privacy. In other words, they characterized speaking about experiences with bipolar II disorder as her social responsibility. Due to ways in which they envisioned CZJ's voice to help reduce stigma related to mental health illnesses, and, in particular, bipolar II disorder, some fans and onlookers treated this form of advocacy as her social responsibility. However, others have publicly defended CZJ's right to privacy. Our discussion of these varied roles work to extend and enhance understanding of Petronio's (2002) Communication Privacy Management Theory related to co-owner relationships.

In this chapter, we coined the term *detached co-owners* to highlight the interplay between the observer and the observed. This term extended Petronio's (2002) definition of co-owners to highlight the dialectic of controlling and being controlled. Alternatively, and similar to female performers' observations (A. G. Murphy, 2003), celebrities experience a dialectic of agency and constraint, simultaneously objectifying an observed subject via attention and inquiry. In other words, celebrities have agency to do as they like, but, at the same time, they are implicitly constrained by those that observe their performance and come with their own expectations about social responsibility and preferences for degrees of disclosure regarding personal health information. Detached co-owners police this dialectic as a means to compel celebrities to perform preferred public tasks and roles. Such an active, vocal role with the celebrity's privacy boundaries highlighted a perceived stakeholder claim in the celebrity's performance, role, and status as celebrity. Detached co-owners largely experienced their role from a one-sided perspective, but may attempt to interact with celebrities via online forums and social media sites.

Additionally, this chapter extended Petronio's (2002) conceptions of co-owners to include "public defenders." This chapter coined "public defenders" as individuals that attempt to defend another individual's right to privacy. Public defenders, in this instance, are made aware of CZJ's health narrative via mass media. Public defenders enacted various rhetorical strategies to reinforce and, therefore, make their target's privacy boundaries less permeable. As demonstrated in this chapter, such strategies may include: (a) calls for fairness and a sense of humanity to be extended to perceived violated individuals, (b) directly informing others of inappropriate demands or actions, (c) reminding perceived intruders of legal ramifications, and (d) asking the perceived intruder to critically examine why they anticipate and/or seek out such information from their target. We noted these strategies within this chapter, but they do not comprise an exhaustive list of ways in which public defenders may attempt to reinforce another's privacy boundaries.

This chapter illustrates the complexities of multiple co-stakeholders working to collaboratively shape and refine the emergent narrative, actively voicing preferences for participation and expectations of action. Through comments, onlookers implicitly co-negotiated and affirmed the "rights" to "her" story and even contested its future direction by disputing CZJ's own attempts to reframe the narrative as "private," not "public." As such, this case reveals conundrums with regard to privacy management in the public sphere and raises questions about ethical and moral responsibilities of individuals who hold the potential to raise awareness or engage in activism by virtue of their own personal stories and struggles.

CHAPTER FIVE

"I get diabetes just watching Paula Deen"

Public Responses to Paula Deen's Type 2 Diabetes Diagnosis

In a land where restaurants such as the *Heart Attack Grill*, famous for triple-bypass burgers, and *Man vs. Food* exist, the United States is no stranger to extreme, and dare we say *unhealthy* cuisine. Ozerky (2012, January 3) asserted that "[t]he U.S. is a strange and conflicted country when it comes to food [see related works by Harris & Bargh, 2009; Phillipov, 2013; Stefanik-Sidener, 2013]. We love our tacos, hate our scales, and live in a state of perpetual shame" (p. 56). Interest in cooking and food has prompted entire television shows and networks devoted to regional cuisine (see Buscemi, 2014) and treatment of food preparation as both empowerment and enactment of unique personalities (see S. Holland & Novak, 2013). As these endeavors attest, food can facilitate the accomplishment of particular cultures and cultural identities (Atkins-Sayre & Stokes, 2014; Buscemi, 2014; Goncalves, 2013), complicating critique based on "merely" nutritional or health information.

This chapter focuses on Paula Deen, a continual limit-pusher and chef specializing in traditional U.S. Southern cooking (and former star of two shows on the Food Network). Paula is credited with creating her own heart attack—the Krispy Kreme Burger. This burger includes "a half-pound beef patty topped with bacon and egg fried in butter, served *with glazed donuts in lieu of a bun*" ("The Krispy Kreme Burger," 2008, June 9).

Paula, the "self-crowned queen of Southern cuisine" (Moskin, 2012, January 17), stirred up a big batch of controversy when she confided to the world that she had type 2 diabetes (and acknowledged that she had known for three years). As fans expressed concern, critics slammed her ethics for continuing to promote high-calorie, high-fat, and often deep-fried, Southern cooking for so long after her diagnosis, without uttering a word to fans and viewers about potential consequences (see Conley, 2012, January 18; Holland, 2013; Kisken, 2012, January 21; Ledger-Enquirer, 2012, January 17; Ozersky, 2012, January 3).

> Thousands of Ms. Deen's fans tweeted their support and posted messages of sympathy on her Facebook wall Tuesday. But many others questioned her motives in concealing the condition for so long, or said they spotted hypocrisy in her decision to profit from an illness that they believe she had abetted [Moskin, 2012, January 17, para. 8].

In this chapter, we consider the complicated and controversial case of Paula Deen. As Moskin (2012, January 17, para. 7) noted, Deen's dilemma (as a particular type of chef wrestling with a diagnosis that, perhaps, stemmed, at least in part, from her cuisine) "adds a fresh story line to a rolling national debate about obesity, with elements of celebrity, schadenfreude and the current popular class warfare." Deen's decision to stay silent for three years, all while continuing "to educate the nation on how to prepare her signature sugar and saturated fat-heavy delights" (Le Miere, 2012, February 24, para. 5), opened the floodgates for personal and professional criticism. One dietitian, Kendall Dyer, argued that "it's disappointing that, as a celebrity, she is not using her announcement as a 'teachable moment'" (Macmillan, 2012, February 5, para. 14). Responding to critics, Deen offered up some resistance to that implied duty: "Like I told Oprah a few years ago, honey, I'm your cook, not your doctor. You are going to have to be responsible for yourself" (Nash, 2013, January 17). Pastry chef Kate Dunbar concurred, arguing that "[t]his is her own personal medical information. What she cooks and what she has are two very different things" (Kisken, 2012, January 21, para. 21).

Ironically, Deen made matters even more messy by disclosing her personal health situation at the same time that she announced a partnership (and financial agreement) with Novo Nordisk, a pharmaceutical company that markets products for individuals with diabetes, and proclaimed that she *did* want to help people with diabetes. Notably, Deen is the only person that we feature in this volume to receive financial benefits for discussing her health issue. We opted to include her for two key reasons. First, Deen's personal health saga has contributed greatly to larger public conversations about nutritional choices, obesity, and diabetes well beyond the efforts for which she was compensated, and we believe that reactions online (especially through Twitter) exemplify a contested narrative in which followers actively and openly disputed and mocked Deen's personal health situation by means of participating in the larger public forum. Second, even though Deen's financial arrangement ended with Novo Nordisk due to another scandal, she has continued to engage in advocacy and awareness efforts about type 2 diabetes.

After we share background information about Deen's empire, we discuss her disclosure, alliance with Novo Nordisk, and Twitter responses to the news of Deen's diagnosis.

The Paula Deen Empire

Paula began her career selling bagged lunches to office workers in Savannah, Georgia (Kisken, 2012, January 21). However, what began from humble means grew to an empire rich with partners, endorsers, and numerous possibilities. At the time of her health disclosure, Paula had two shows which aired on the Food Network, *Paula's Best Dishes* and *Paula's Home Cooking*. Additionally, Paula developed a number of Deen-branded products, which include "everything from cookbooks and eyeglasses to hams and mattresses" (Ozersky, 2012, January 3, p. 56). Deen even created a butter-flavored lip balm with the tag line, "Put a little South on your mouth," which is available for purchase in her retail store next to her *The Lady & Sons* restaurant in Savannah, Georgia. Deen also produces a bimonthly magazine, *Cooking with Paula Deen*, and has published over a dozen cookbooks, which, collectively, have sold more than 10 million copies (Underwood, 2012, May).

The Diagnosis, the Disclosure
and the Drug Company

Initially struck by denial, Paula Deen had to be convinced that she really suffers from type 2 diabetes. Once persuaded, Paula reportedly still "didn't feel ready to go public because she was still 'absorbing it'" (Satran, 2012, October 15, para. 5). Waiting on God to send her a message when it was time to reveal her secret, she noted, "To say I'm a very religious person, I can't say that, because I don't go to church. But I'm a very spiritual person. I knew that the opportunity to share would present itself" (Satran, 2012, October 15, para. 7). Additionally, Deen claimed that "[s]he was waiting to come forward until she could offer her 'friends' some 'hope'" (Ozersky, 2012, January 3, p. 56). With an estimated 25.8 million people with diabetes in the United States, costing roughly $245 billion in 2012 (American Diabetes Association, 2014) in addition to the physical toll on patients and their families, Paula's "hope" held the potential to impact millions affected by diabetes.

‗ Novo Nordisk

When contacted by pharmaceutical company Novo Nordisk to partner for a diabetes campaign, Deen said that they "fell out of their chairs" when she told them that she, too, had type 2 diabetes (Satran, 2012, October 15, para. 8), in spite of rumors on the Internet and even speculation in the *National Inquirer* on May 2, 2011, about her health. On January 17, 2012, Deen appeared on the *Today* show, telling Al Roker, "I'm here today to let the world know, that it is not a death sentence" (Nash, 2013, January 17). Deen reiterated that she waited to disclose her diagnosis because she wanted "to bring something to the table when I came forward and I've always been one to think that I bring hope because I've had lots of obstacles in my life y'all" (Nash, 2013, January 17).

The timing of Deen's disclosure on the same day that she announced her partnership with Novo Nordisk fueled public criticism. Novo Nordisk, the world leader in diabetes care, manufactures the drug that Deen reportedly takes for her diabetes. Paula Deen and her sons, Bobby and Jamie, joined Novo Nordisk on its national "Diabetes in a New Light" initiative, which (perhaps not so coincidentally) launched the same day as Paula came forward with her diagnosis. This educational and awareness campaign offers adults with type 2 diabetes management strategies, such as healthier versions of Paula Deen's famous recipes (Deen, n.d.), increasing physical activity (Moskin, 2012, January 17), and managing stress. The campaign also spotlighted the Deens at diabetic cooking events throughout the United States (Clarke, 2012, January 17). Through this campaign, Paula indicated: "I want to encourage those of you with type 2 diabetes to walk in my footsteps and make one small change to better control your disease" (SFGate, 2013, March 6, para. 3).

Paula commented, "I had been given lemons and I had to try and make lemonade—without sugar" (Hamm, 2012, July 9, para. 4)! As Paula asserted, "I could not come out and say, 'Hey, y'all, I'm type 2 diabetic,' and turn around and walk off. I had to have solutions" (Underwood, 2012, May). Paula presented Novo Nordisk as part of that solution. According to Paula, "They gave me the power to reach masses of people and to bring information" (Underwood, 2012, May). As a paid spokesperson, Deen proclaimed, "I'm giving a percentage to the American Diabetes Association" (Underwood, 2012, May). Deen acknowledged, "We have a financial agreement, but I'm doing this program because I want to inspire people" (Hamm, Chiu, Fogle, Mascia, & Prabhakar, 2012, January 30, para. 5). A representative for Novo Nordisk emphasized that "Paula Deen is someone people can relate to. We applaud her bravery for helping people the best way she knows how and are proud to call ourselves her partner" (R. Roberts & Elliott, 2012, January 19). Deen served as a paid spokesperson until her later racism scandal resulted in a loss of endorsements and business deals, including her arrangement with Novo Nordisk, in 2013 (http://www.huffingtonpost.com/2013/06/27/paula-deen-novo-nordisk_n_ 3509855.html).

Continuing the Conversation

In addition to public appearances through the Novo Nordisk campaign, Deen has commented widely on her journey with type 2 diabetes, crediting moderation, increased exercise, and smaller portions, as well as cutting back on sweet tea, with helping her to lose more than 30 pounds (Carlyle, 2012, July 18). In an interview with *Prevention*, Paula said, "There are so many people out there that need hope and encouragement. And I could help bring that" (Underwood, 2012, May). Deen urged people to "[g]o to their doctor and ask to be tested for diabetes and then get on a program that works for you" (Nash, 2013, January 17). Deen has continued to raise awareness for diabetes, especially during National Diabetes Awareness Month. As she claimed, "To celebrate National Diabetes Month, I'm going to be posting daily tips and facts to my Twitter and Facebook so that we can fight this disease together" (http://www.pauladeen.com/blogs/blog_view/paula_celebrates_ national_diabetes_awareness_month, para. 3). Deen noted: "When my life is over and you hear my name, I hope you associate the word 'hope' with it" (Roberts & Elliott, 2012, January 19). As she commented, "I'm a big believer that sharing your story can not only motivate yourself, but also inspire others to take care of their health" (SFGate, 2013, March 6, para. 14).

A Contested Private-Yet-Public Health Narrative

Throughout her career, Deen's cooking has constantly come under fire, forcing her to deal with considerable "heat in the kitchen," so to speak. Her use of butter, cream, and the deep-fryer rallied critics and supporters to her side. Ozersky (2012, January 3) claimed her Food Network success was largely based on her "personal élan and a freewheeling indifference to health concerns that in today's climate seemed in some weird way heroic" (p. 56). When Deen revealed her diagnosis, not many expressed surprise. Ozersky quoted a diabetes cookbook co-author, Chef Franklin Becker, as asserting that "Paula Deen was going to have some kind of health problem. It might not have been diabetes, but it would have been something. If you cook that way, if you eat that way, you're going to get issues" (p. 56). Similarly, Anthony Bourdain, a New York–based chef, voiced outspoken criticism of Paula Deen. Bourdain labeled Paula as the "worst, most dangerous person in America" due to her cooking (Conley, 2012, January 18, para. 5). Upon Deen's disclosure, Bourdain said, "When your signature dish is hamburger in between a doughnut, and you've been cheerfully selling this stuff knowing all along that you've got Type 2 Diabetes…. It's in bad taste if nothing else" (Conley, 2012, January 18, para. 6).

Deen reported being shocked by the negative responses that she received to her disclosure. She said, "I couldn't understand the haters" (Satran, 2012, October 15). Yet, upon sharing her news with the general public and media, she has not been able to "put a lid on" ensuing discourse, commentary, or, in the case of Bourdain, outright scorn (for related work on contested narratives, see, for example, Harter, 2009). Although Paula tried to tell a story of concern and compassion for others, unlike most patients with diabetes, Paula has endured "an epic public scolding because of her cooking and eating habits" (Moskin, 2012, January 17, para. 12). To borrow from Fisher (1984, 1985a, 1985b, 1987a), for many, key parts of her narrative didn't fit together or ring true—the delay in disclosure, the partnership with Novo Nordisk, the continued commitment to cooking that could contribute to health problems. The clash of varied ethical, moral, and ideological perspectives ensued, "boiling over" on the Internet as fans, followers, and individuals with diabetes offered their own reactions and accounts by writing to Paula, posting numerous posts online, such as on popular press articles, and interacting with Deen on social media sites such as Twitter. As we detail in this section, we certainly found mixed responses to Deen, with some linking her to diabetes, others blaming her for the disease, still others connecting diabetes to a "good time," and some calling her an "inspiration."

Paula Deen Is Diabetes

Goffman (1976) claimed that celebrities not only "link their own private lives to the public domain, but also link the lives of private persons to it" (p. 11). We recognized such a linkage in terms of Paula Deen and type 2 diabetes through the ways in which various people on Twitter not only discussed and interacted with Paula but also through tweets in which the public associated Paula Deen with the disease. In fact, seeing Paula, or products/people that reminded them of Paula, prompted some to think of type 2 diabetes, and vice-versa. For example, John wrote, "I think Paula Deen is just diabetes that grew around a person (2012, November 2). Paula's brand of cooking, so central to her public persona, certainly fits with possible perceptions of food that might contribute to diabetes. The Cuban Prometheus tweeted, "[i]f Hippocrates is the father of medicine, that makes Paula Deen is the mother of Diabetes right?" (2013, January 31). Deen as the mother of diabetes bears a symbolic image of womanhood and birthright. By being the "mother" to diabetes, at least this particular fan cast her as someone to foster, care for, and ensure its longevity.

Some connected Deen so much with type 2 diabetes that even seeing someone who resembled Paula purportedly prompted a craving for buttery food, and, as some even noted, diabetes. HalfPastAwesome tweeted, "Coulda sworn I just saw Paula Deen in Springfield. I now have a craving for butter & some mild diabetes" (2012, October 30). On the surface, this tweet implicitly treats diabetes as something that could be desirable. Even if HalfPastAwesome was most likely joking, this flip reference to a serious health issue also exemplifies a disturbing aspect of the emergent narrative that we address later within this chapter.

Products associated with Paula ignited not only the conflation with Deen to diabetes, but expressions of fear that her products may circulate and infect individuals with diabetes. Mad Dan commented, "I'm scared to death the Paula Deen cookware will give me diabetes" (2012, December 24). Similarly, Alicia Marie claimed, "Buying a 'diabetes cookbook' from @Paula Deen is like buying a detox kit from your friendly neighborhood drug dealer" (2013, June 21). Through these tweets, individuals stigmatized those products, regardless of potential attempts at humor, by implying that people could become "infected" with diabetes by using and even smelling Deen's merchandise. For example, 24601 remarked, "I discovered that Paula Deen makes candles that smell like her food, meaning I could literally INHALE the diabetes" (2013, March 21). These tweets marked Paula Deen products by insinuating that they could somehow be "contaminated" with diabetes and worked to mock Deen's illness and, therefore, type 2 diabetes.

Further, some fans and followers observed that Paula Deen's cooking shows exposed viewers to high-fat, butter-induced, deep-fried, Southern cooking—or at least a very stereotypical version of Southern soul food and, essentially, promoted type 2 diabetes. In fact, Jordan suggested, "If someone offers you food and says, 'It's from a Paula Deen recipe,' they're offering you diabetes" (2013, February 12). BreBre tweeted, "Paula Deen sends up the diabetes bat signal every time she turns her stove on" (2013, April 16). Even the perception of Deen's cooking screamed diabetes to some viewers. Lauren claimed, "Everything Paula Deen makes looks like heaven and diabetes all wrapped in one" (2013,

January 30). Additionally, Elliott argued, "Give a man a fish, and you feed him for a day. Give Paula Deen a stick of butter and she'll give that man diabetes" (2012, November 30). Such tweets suggest that Deen's cooking doesn't result in food, but rather in diabetes. Steph said, "Paula Deen doesn't cook.... She whips up a batch of diabetes on a daily basis!" (2012, December 6).

As demonstrated through various tweets, some posted that even watching her show could spread diabetes. In fact, Erin tweeted, "I get diabetes just watching paula deen" (2012, November 24). Relatedly, Nikki asked, "Did you know that you can contract Type 2 diabetes if you watch two consecutive episodes of Paula Deen's cooking show?" Further, Laura asserted that "[w]atching Paula Deen make beer batter deep-fried cupcakes is giving me diabetes" (2012, December 27). On the most surface level, these tweets advanced the idea that, by watching television, viewers could "catch" type 2 diabetes.

On a deeper (or perhaps more ironic) level, these participants may very well have been sarcastic in their tweets, but they most certainly still spread misperceptions and inaccuracies through the ongoing public discussion about and depiction of type 2 diabetes. Furthermore, although we certainly caught ourselves chuckling at some of the tweets too, we argue that such attempts at humor regarding such a serious disease are problematic. Would someone likely believe that merely watching an episode of television could cause diabetes? Possibly not. However, making fun of diabetes undermines not only Paula Deen—such comments interject a levity into the public discourse that could not only confuse but also add a layer to the emergent narrative that could work to stigmatize individuals who suffer from and wrestle with complications on a daily basis. Such contributions to the public discourse went beyond bashing Paula Deen and her private health situation; they inherently treated type 2 diabetes as an appropriate topic for humor.

Notably, some challenged Paula's cooking ethics and then engaged in questionable ethical participation in the emergent narrative themselves by tweeting misinformation or attacks. One tweeter named austyb wrote, "Paula Deen's bread pudding WILL give you diabetes, and she seems pretty unremorseful about it" (2013, January 8). Additionally, Daniel asserted that "Paula Deen is hellbent on giving the world type II diabetes" (2012, December 4). These tweets not only raised concerns about Paula's cooking ethics but also went further by blaming Paula for type 2 diabetes.

BLAMING PAULA

Being a celebrity in our contemporary age is marked with ascribed credibility (Tolson, 2001). However, Paula's decision not to disclose her diagnosis earlier than later diminished her credibility with onlookers. Janae D said, "da bish [*sic*] lied about it for 2 years. I'm never eating a deep fried chicken wing covered in donut glaze and bacon again!!" (2012, December 13). In response to her nondisclosure, TLH claimed, "paula deen get on my nerves. She help fatten us all but not say shit when she got diabetes" (2013, January 10). Even organizations associated with Deen endured scrutiny based on affiliation. Barclay noted, "There's an aspect of running a food channel where it's a public trust. It's irresponsible to keep her on air" (2012, December 24). He later tweeted, "When Paula Deen finally admitted that she had diabetes, she marketed it. This person should not be allowed to cook publicly" (2012, December 24). Lawrence also challenged her ethics, claiming that "Paula Deen works both sides of the street, pushing diabetes-inducing food, and then pushing drugs to treat it" (2013, May 6).

Many tweeters challenged Paula's intentions. Elizabeth asked, "Does anyone else have a problem w/ this woman 1st helping to make America even fatter, then capitalizing on her own diabetes?" (2013, February 1). Such questioning led tweeters to make judgments regarding Paula's personal ethics. Cziriak claimed, "Paula deen got diabetes so she could endorse it" (2013, February 22), perhaps indirectly referencing her partnership with Novo Nordisk or her implied advocacy of the type of food that she cooks. Josh addressed that issue even more pointedly, asking "Paula Deen endorsed diabetes medicine? Attn South: We've come full circle. That's a conflict of interest if I ever saw one" (2013, June 14).

Many tweets blamed Paula for increasing type 2 diabetes. Kay questioned, "Wonder how many people Paula Deen took 'down the diabetes lane' teaching Southern cooking?" (2013, February 11). Badri said, "The irony of paula deen releasing a video on diabetes, does this bitch not realize she's the cause of diabetes in god knows how many people?" (2012, December 16). Similarly, Brooke tweeted, "Paula Deen raising awareness about diabetes…. She's the reason I'm going to have diabetes" (2013, April 8). Such tweets wonder if Deen has a moral obligation to protect others as a celebrity chef. Guttman (2000) cautioned individuals to carefully weigh potential harm and risks "against possible benefits to be gained from the intervention" (p. 43). As a celebrity chef, the solution is not necessarily clear. Should Paula Deen have been responsible for issuing cautions about eating too many of her recipes?

"Excited" about Getting Diabetes

However, as we have indicated, not everyone blamed Paula at all. Derk responded to an online article about Deen's health announcement:

People, lay off Paula. Her food is old school and the way most Americans used to eat and many still do. Her style isn't probably as much a culprit in obsessity and other diseases in this country as is all the processed junk, high fructose corn syrup and partially hydrogenated corn oil laden diets many live on. I get so tired of sanctimonious health freaks who analyze every freakin morsel they put in their body. It's obsessive and in the end, their diet often turns out not so healthy after all. Would I eat Paula's recopies on a daily basis, no. But I do throw caution to the wind now and then and make equally glutinous dishes. Life's too short. My grandmother cooked and ate like Paula and lived a healthy 96 years with out any disease. Julia Child cooked the equally unhealthy, sauce and butter heavy French cuisine and lived into her mid 90s as well. She coined the phrase: everything in moderation. Duh ["Paula Deen's Food Network shows," 2012, February 8].

The "life's too short" argument echoed through comments in support of Deen and her recipes. However, some tweeters addressed Deen's disclosure by going further and referring to type 2 diabetes as the result of a "good, delicious meal." For instance, Nish said, "Just put Paula Deen's pumpkin crunch cake in the oven. Pretty excited about getting diabetes later" (2012, November 22). Similarly, Sunu wrote, "Making Paula Deen's Sweet Potato Bake for the fam's Thanksgiving lunch on Friday. With any luck, we'll all have diabetes by Saturday" (2012, November 20). Of course, we recognize the quite strong potential for such tweets to be attempts at humor as well as bids to emphasize freedom to choose such dietary options. However, again, such tweets not only mistreated the severity of type 2 diabetes, but they constructed type 2 diabetes as an illness that does not need to be taken seriously but, rather, celebrated as a life lived well. At the very least, such tweets minimized the risk from consuming such foods as individuals scoffed at the possibility of developing type 2 diabetes by merely indulging. For instance, Rich scoffed, "I've had more sugar in the past 3 days than Paula Deen has had in her entire life. What now, diabetes? What now?" (2012, December 26).

Some tweeters acknowledged potential health concerns while baking Deen's recipes such as her baked macaroni. Jasef shared, "Using a Paula Deen recipe for baked macaroni. This better be worth the diabetes, y'all" (2012, December 24). This tweet speaks to the acknowledgment that this food may not be the wisest health choice but implied that it may be worth the risk of negatively influencing one's health. These tweets not only used humor as a mechanism to excuse unhealthy behavior, but such discourse also mirrors a Western individualistic culture. Celebrating diabetes, or the potential to obtain diabetes, suggests that some tweeters plan to disregard health safety as they choose to eat what they want. Such tweets reflected embedded American/Western cultural ideologies to overly consume and to not let perceived risks or someone else to influence their decision-making practices. As in *Fast Food Nation* (Schlosser, 2012), these tweets speak to the *Man vs. Food* culture of the United States. At the same time, the tweets implicitly (although, perhaps not seriously) treated type 2 diabetes as a good time and victorious achievement in which one has put food "in its place."

<h2 style="text-align:center">INSPIRATION</h2>

Our analysis of tweets also revealed a collection of individuals who praised Deen for helping them with their own struggles regarding type 2 diabetes. For example, Teresa wrote, "@Paula_Deen I want to say you are a great inspiration to all of us who has type 2 diabetes. Just wish I had the support as you did" (2013, April 4). Teresa noted that Paula inspired her, and others, with type 2 diabetes and bemoaned a lack of social support for her own struggle with type 2 diabetes. Paula's inspiration offered such support to the public, mirroring findings about the potential for celebrities to inspire (see also Beck et al., 2014; Niederdeppe, 2008). For instance, Genny wrote, "@Paula_Deen Yes you are inspiration to all of us ... I have type 2 diabetes ... gonna try some of your recipes, thank you Paula" (2013, April 4). Genny noted that Paula's inspiration encouraged her to try some of her diabetic recipes to help her manage her own struggle with type 2 diabetes. Additionally, Paula's own openness about her struggles and 30+–pound weight loss encouraged others. Genny tweeted, "@Paula_Deen I'm new to all the diabetes stuff, but I have learned. Have lost 54 pounds and still going :-)" (2013, April 4).

Other individuals acknowledged Paula Deen as part of broader educational conversations about type 2 diabetes, even if they did so by humorously invoking her as a punch line. Morgan reported that "'Paula Deen has reversed her diabetes.' The things we talk about in anthropology class #haha" (2012, November 6). Jim also tweeted, "[t]oday is health class we talked about diabetes, so for how to avoid them I said don't watch Paula Deen's cooking show" (2013, January 30). Liz shared, "Accidentally wrote in my food paper that Paula Deen has developed 'type 32' diabetes. She uses that much butter" (2013, March 6).

Conclusion

Nearly a year after her admission that she has type 2 diabetes, in June of 2013, the Food Network elected to part ways with Paula Deen, purportedly because she made racial slurs, but at least two reporters also noted a decline in ratings as a potential reason for the split (Arnowitz, 2013, June 27; Testa, 2013, June 26). According to Testa, "All this racial brouhaha just provided a convenient out so they could replace Deen with a younger, more ratings-friendly star without any backlash" (para. 12). Arnowitz concurred, sharing that "[a] source with knowledge of the Food Network's ratings said the Southern cook's show was not even among the network's most-watched daytime series" (para. 4). However, both Arnowitz and Testa pointed to shifts in viewer preferences regarding format (competitions versus traditional how-to shows) as opposed to a declining interest in Deen's style of cooking.

The choice to cut Deen has not shown clear results for the Food Network. Indeed, in 2014, St. Clair argued that "the Food Network is at a crossroads. Its ratings in 2013 were already sagging when it decided to dump Paula Deen, further sending its numbers downward" (May 28, para. 3). Meanwhile, Paula has rebounded with plans for "the new Paula Deen Network, a subscription Web site that will feature cooking shows, recipes and tools" (Stelter, 2014, June 11, para. 1). Stelter quoted an official with Deen's company as asserting that, with this new online forum, Deen "would gain 'a greater level of direct access to her millions of fans' and 'full creative control of the shows, recipes and content'" (para. 10). Clearly, Paula Deen continues to participate in public conversations about diet, nutrition, and, by extension, type 2 diabetes.

As we reflect back on Deen's emergent health narrative, we wonder about the extent to which Paula Deen bears some responsibility for the behavior of her viewers. In a case such as this one—where a celebrity essentially engages in and promotes something related to health that could eventually cause harm—at what point should a celebrity disclose a personal impact? When do their stories become our stories to the extent that we must know their private information? Individuals take risks in eating high-fat foods. Such risk takers may impose burdens on society as a whole, especially if public tax dollars support their health costs (Guttmann, 1997; McLeroy, Gottlieb, & Burdine, 1987; Veatch, 1980).

Deen's diagnosis and disclosure prompt another question as well: Did this culture make Paula, and if so, why is the public, as demonstrated in tweets, upset with her delivering the type of U.S.–Southern food they craved, desired, and couldn't consume enough? Especially given our societal emphasis on food and nutritional issues, Deen's narrative holds implications for outlets like the Food Network in terms of ethical responsibility. To what extent do shows and chefs need to divulge nutritional information or offer cautions about potential health implications over cultural and personal preferences?

Although Deen claimed that she never intended for someone to eat like she cooked every day, her cooking shows constructed an "excited to get diabetes" (or "life's too short") mentality as demonstrated throughout various tweets. Such response spoke to the opposite of Guttman's (1997, 2000) depriving dilemma. Instead of deprivation, the ideology of mass consumption is perceived to be encouraged. In fact, this ideology resulted in numerous fans and followers who claim to be excited for sweet taste-bud sensations which they would soon eat, just ate, or were currently baking. This chapter, therefore, extends Guttman's (1997, 2000) health communication ethical considerations to include an "indulging dilemma."

The indulging dilemma is on the opposite end of a dialectical expression of Guttman's (1997, 2000) depriving dilemma. Rather than asking what risks are associated with asking individuals to deprive themselves of certain behaviors and practices, the indulging dilemma raises the question: To what extent might encouraging overconsumption and/or indulging practices encourage unhealthy behaviors and/or practices which may contribute to individual/group health concerns? Individuals with greater resources and access to certain foods and/or products may be at greater risk to "indulge." At the same time, "indulging" may be inexpensive. Indulging in overly processed, enriched foods may actually be cheaper than indulging in organic, locally grown fresh fruit. In spite of attempts to combat overindulgence, such as the documentary *Super Size Me* (which chronicles Morgan Spurlock's 30-day journey of eating nothing but McDonald's), our fast-food culture flocks to shows such as *Man vs. Food*, which depicts man in a heroic light when he conquers indulgent food challenges. The danger of the indulging dilemma is not that it, necessarily, poses a great risk of being ostracized, but it contributes to overconsumption and reinforces the cultural significance of women and men conquering all, even their bodies. Indulging may pose personal and societal health risks. Therefore, such should not be celebrated. Further research should consider ways in which the indulging dilemma constructs an ideal image for participants who willingly participate in its propagation.

CHAPTER SIX

Celebrity Body Image Narratives and the Media
A Framework for Personal Health Disclosure?

"I knew I wasn't anorexic, but maybe my body is somehow not right…. When you're going through a period where you're really getting a lot of criticism, you go, maybe all this is right!"—Keira Knightley as cited on FoxNews.com regarding her cover on *Allure Magazine* ("Knightley talks," 2012, November 13, para 5).

Keira Knightley's celebrity status continued to grow after she appeared in *Star Wars: Episode I—The Phantom Menace*, considered by F. Smith (2014) as her first "high profile" role (para. 1). Since then, Knightley has starred in films such as *Bend It Like Beckham, King Arthur, Atonement, Pride and Prejudice, Love Actually*, and, probably her most well-known role as Elizabeth Swan, in *Pirates of the Caribbean: The Curse of the Black Pearl* (IMDB, 2014e). With each role, fans have become more and more interested in Knightley's life. For example, she purportedly worried about managing publicity of her private wedding ceremony when she married James Righton ("Knightley talks," 2012, November 13).

Intersections between private life and celebrity status also emerge in Knightley's highly publicized (and contested) narrative pertaining to body image. As we detail throughout this chapter, Knightley has been criticized for being too thin and even accused of having the eating disorder, anorexia. Dominant celebrity health narratives in the media often involve body weight, shape, and size, and we question such a prevalent mediated discourse that emphasizes such issues over other attributes and even good health. The 2011 selection for Sundance Film Festival, *Miss Representation*, tackles the socially constructed perspective of women and power in the media, arguing that "[i]n a society where media is the most persuasive force shaping cultural norms, the collective message that our young women and men overwhelmingly receive is that a woman's value and power lie in her youth, beauty, and sexuality, and not in her capacity as a leader" ("Synopsis," 2014, para. 4).

Notably, attention to female body features in the media is not new (see related work by Austin, 2012; E. Burke, 2006; Horner & Keane, 2000; Press, 2011; Reed & Saukko, 2010; Ross, 2012; Saukko, 2006; Weitz, 2003) nor limited to the United States (see, e.g., Austin, 2012; Ibroscheva, 2013; Luo, 2012). At least one of our co-authors recalls the craze for Farrah Fawcett pinup posters in the 1970s and 1980s, and, of course, the annual infamous *Sports Illustrated* swimsuit issue endures in popularity, now marking its 50th anniversary of spotlighting women (and even Barbie) in often skimpy swimsuits (Boren, 2014, February 18; "Magazines Shape Culture," 2012, Winter). However, our current hypermedia society facilitates a culture of public critique about private matters, such as body weight and structure (especially with the ease of tweeting on Twitter and posting on Facebook), that we believe warrants exploration in this volume.

This chapter extends earlier work by Beck et al. (2014) in terms of the "implications of blurring boundaries when celebrities choose to interweave their private health narratives with public discourses about health, healing, and well-being" (p. 244). We argue that Knightley's challenge in positioning "her" personal body and health intensified as fans/observers asserted a "right" to speculate/judge/label public images as problematic or "too thin." Notably, Knightley has not overtly said that she supports women and body issues, and she has not created a campaign or anything on that public level. Instead, we are intrigued by her struggle in refuting criticism and reclaiming "her" narrative regarding "her" body image and overall health. Knightley's situation prompted us to wonder about how much control celebrities do (or can) have over their respective narratives when they are criticized for their weight by the media and how social media help to form a positive method/framework for noncelebrities' conversations about health and body image. First, we share a brief review of body-image issues related to dissatisfaction, eating disorders, and media. Next, we consider the intersection between the aforementioned ideas and the case study of Keira Knightley's narrative and media reports and responses to criticism about her weight. Finally, we conclude by highlighting implications for public and private conversations regarding body-image issues, especially with regard to other celebrity narratives related to body image and weight loss.

Body Image in the Media

Ideas related to body image, body image dissatisfaction, and body disturbance have been expansively studied (see, e.g., Austin, 2012; Bergstrom &

Neighbors, 2006; E. Burke, 2006; Cohen, 2006; Grabe, Ward & Hyde, 2008; Groesz, Levine, & Murnen, 2002; Herrman & Tenzek, 2011, November; Holmstrom, 2004; Horner & Keane, 2000; Lopez-Guimera, Levine, Sanchez-Carracedo, & Fauquet, 2010; Press, 2011; Reed & Saukko, 2010; Ross, 2012; Saukko, 2006; Weitz, 2003). In this chapter, we follow Bergstrom and Neighbors' integrative review on body image disturbance and social norms approach, which used Grogan's (1999) simplistic definition of body image as "a person's perceptions, thoughts and feelings about his or her body" and body image disturbance as "a person's negative thoughts and feelings about his or her body" (p. 976).

The media has been associated with issues surrounding body image, especially regarding media use and perceptions of self. How we feel about and understand ourselves leads to positive or negative self-esteem and differing levels of body image dissatisfaction. Kubic and Chory (2007) found that more exposure to television self-makeover programs led to higher perfectionism and body image dissatisfaction and lower self-esteem. This study further supports a trend in research examining body image dissatisfaction where the more exposure women have to television programs leads to lower body satisfaction (Eggermont, Beullens, & Van den Bulck, 2005). However, scholars hesitate to claim only media as an influence on women's dissatisfaction with their bodies. Accordingly, body image involves many facets, such as eating pathology, body dissatisfaction, and body size estimation and self-esteem (Bergstrom & Neighbors, 2006; Holmstrom, 2004). When scholars combine media exposure with peer influence, lower body satisfaction tends to be the outcome (Clark & Tiggemann, 2006). Similarly, Van Vonderen and Kinnally (2012) argued that media has an indirect relationship on body dissatisfaction and recommended further consideration of peer influence and social/environmental factors on self-esteem. One explanation for why women experience such low body image satisfaction after watching television programs and commercials, as well as after reading magazines, stems from the social and cultural pressures surrounding individuals to conform to what is considered the thin ideal (Billhartz, 2002, March 5).

THIN IDEAL

The inclusion of media into our perceptions and enactment of self and body image have created a vehicle for conversations about the thin ideal. A review of literature examining the drive for thinness noted that "[t]he thinness ideal has been repeatedly transmitted through popular culture, especially through media" (Cohen, 2006, p. 61). Therefore, common ways of studying the thin ideal involve different media including television, advertisements, magazines, and commercials and even sports. Results of a meta-analysis further supported the argument by stating, "Exposure to media images depicting the thin-ideal body is related to body image concerns for women" (Grabe et al., 2008, p. 460). It is oftentimes difficult to disentangle the sole cause of body image dissatisfaction, as results of Botta's (1999) work found; media, directly and indirectly, influence adolescent girls' body disturbance through processing and promoting a thin ideal, respectively. Further support for the contention that media exposure to the thin ideal negatively influences women's body dissatisfaction included results that found "[e]xposure to fat-character television, thin-ideal magazines, and sports magazines predicted eating-disorder symptomatology for females, especially older females" (Harrison, 2000, p. 119).

Not all scholarship supports this line of reasoning. One study, in particular, supported the counter argument that women who look at thin ideal media actually experienced higher body satisfaction (Knobloch-Westerwick & Crane, 2012). Knobloch-Westerwick and Crane claimed that, for the young American women in the study, after exposure to thin ideal—content messages, behaviors such as diet and exercise changed, leading to higher body satisfaction. However, they acknowledged that the "full-page ads and articles" (p. 96) used in their study differed from other investigations, accounting for some variance. Additionally, long-term effects should be taken into consideration as some women's behaviors may have changed at the time of the study, but the long-lasting effects may be unknown. However, health should be juxtaposed with body-image preferences (see related works by Austin, 2012; E. Burke, 2006; Saukko, 2006; Spitzack, 1993). The quest to become thin may be taken too far when eating disorders become part of an individual's health narrative. Cohen (2006) argued that this quest for thinness and striving toward a thin ideal pertains specifically in women with eating disorders.

EATING DISORDERS

According to the National Association of Anorexia Nervosa and Associated Disorders (ANAD) website, 24 million people in the United States suffer from an eating disorder; however, only one in ten receive treatment, and almost 50 percent are depressed ("Eating Disorder Statistics," 2014). According to the National Eating Disorders Association's (NEDA) website, both men and women experience a variety of eating disorders with serious consequences ("General Information," n.d.). Common eating disorders include anorexia nervosa, bulimia nervosa, and binge-eating disorders. The enactment of manipulating food intake and possible purging pose serious health implications. Anorexia nervosa changes the body in many ways as, overall, it weakens, including decreasing heart rate. Blood pressure becomes lower; muscles decrease in strength; bone density lessens, and possible dehydration and death can occur, if individuals do not seek treatment. Therefore, health issues constitute a serious concern for those living with an eating disorder.

With the social pressures for celebrities to achieve and maintain that thin ideal and image of acceptable beauty, quality of life and notions of health seem to be lost in the quest for thinness (see Saukko, 2006). According to a Healthline article online, the pressure to be thin can prompt celebrities to alter eating patterns and, for celebrities such as Paula Abdul, Victoria Beckham, Karen Carpenter, Princess Di, and Jane Fonda ("Famous Faces," 2011, July 6), the development of eating disorders (see also E. Burke, 2006; Saukko, 2006). Additional stars who have revealed struggles with eating disorders include Katie Couric, Lady Gaga, and Demi Lovato (Stone, 2013, March 2). Angelina Jolie also reportedly struggled with eating disorders earlier in her life (Freydkin, 2005, June 8). A telling example of the interconnectedness among celebrity body image, technology, and health is evident in pro ana and pro mia websites.

Pro Ana and Mia Websites

Pro ana and mia websites offer a community for people dealing with body issues. Scholars have researched these websites in a variety of ways, including messages and expressions of uncertainty for online participants (Herrman & Tenzek, 2014, April), language use (Wolf, Theis, & Kordy, 2013), and imagetexts (Jensen, 2005). Arguments against pro ana websites claim that this online space promotes eating disorders and unhealthy behaviors. Others assert that the websites actually function as a space for those struggling with or recovering from eating disorders to support one another and help others in the same position stay healthy and continue the process of recovery. Balter-Reitz and Keller (2005) contended that pro ana websites constitute a positive online community, offering support for those struggling with eating disorders, and provide insight to site content:

> The sites feature discussion boards and chat rooms, where viewers can exchange information and diary entries; picture galleries that exhibit stick thin models or individuals in late stages of anorexia as beauty ideals; and exchanges on such topics as: how to hide uneaten food; how to use laxatives or other products to promote weight loss; how to deny hunger; and how to cope with social isolation [p. 79].

On these websites, online participants disclose private information into a public setting for potentially millions to see and respond. Part of the disclosure process involves visual images. Within the media, images are incredibly powerful, and visual representations open the door for an additional layer of context to be added to narratives.

Jensen (2005) examined the pro ana lifestyle and contrasted it with professional medical opinion that eating disorders comprise serious health concern and psychological illness that require treatment. Conversely, part of the pro ana community believes that ana and mia are lifestyle choices. Jensen argued that, rhetorically, the images present within the pro ana community hold argumentative power in combination with text to support pro ana as a lifestyle. For example, with "thinspiration," striving for the thin ideal, online participants work toward becoming thin through posting, sharing, and critiquing pictures of thin celebrities or themselves as inspiration to keep losing weight and become thinner (Cohen, 2006; Collins, 2004, November–December; Heffernan, 2008, May 25; Herrman & Tenzek, 2014, April; Norris, Boydell, Pinhas, & Katzman, 2006). According to one blogspot website ("Thinspiration pictures," n.d.), which claims a separate identity from pro ana websites, the title reads "Thinspiration pictures, Thinspiration photos of real girls, models and celebrities." Participants post photos of thinspiration in a manner that shows weight loss through before and after body images. Keira Knightley's picture oftentimes appears in sections of pro ana online communities, suggesting she is thinspiration and a fellow ana community member. Based on the visual argument of Knightley's extremely thin body, image presence, and association with thinspiration, media controversy flourished over accusations of anorexia ("Keira Knightley Disappointed," 2012, November 13; Jessen, 2007, May 2; Johnson, 2012, November 13; Luafik, 2012, April 5; Serpe, 2012, November 13). The next section details boundaries of disclosure as a lens through which to examine Knightley's narrative of body-image struggles and the fight for control over her personal health information.

Communication Privacy Management

As we have discussed thus far in this book, at the heart of privacy disclosure is control over personal information and the decision surrounding revealing and concealing private information (Petronio, 1991, 2000, 2004, 2007). This type of decision in disclosure has been in the health context examining HIV status (Tenzek, Herrman, May, Feiner, & Allen, 2013; Yep, 2000) and public versus private narratives (see Beck, 2005; Harter et al., 2005).

Communication Privacy Management theory offers a framework to aid in the decision-making process of disclosure (Petronio, 2007) and emphasizes concepts such as boundary formation, co-construction of boundaries, and rule-breaking.

For Knightley's case, the concept of "turbulence" warrants attention, given that it "reflects situations where there are intentional rule violations, privacy dilemmas, and when the boundary lines are fuzzy" (Petronio, 2004, p. 204). Knightley's attempt to enact control over disclosure of personal issues (such as body-image issues, eating disorders, and self-esteem) did not begin with her decision to disclose, but, instead, it was socially and culturally constructed through audience participation in conversations about celebrity health using technology to diffuse information. Therefore, Knightley was forced into a defensive role in terms of body image and health related information.

Keira's Story: The Quest for Control

Based on the results of our thematic analysis, we discovered the overarching theme of struggles for control between the media and Knightley regarding the "truth" about her health, with various co-stakeholders challenging the legitimacy of Knightley's claims about her body (see related arguments by Fisher, 1984, 1985a, 1987a). The following paragraphs explain a narrative quest to integrate her personal narrative of being healthy (i.e., not having an eating disorder) with the media's accusations, as she attempts to regain control.

THE ACCUSATIONS

In news stories related to the actress and eating disorders, Knightley has constantly defended herself against accusations against rumored anorexia. As early as 2006, Knightley has been accused of having eating disorders (L. Roberts, 2008, June 16). An article in *The Daily Mail* entitled "It's itsy bitsy teeny weeny Keira Knightley" includes a photo of Knightley on the beach wearing a swimsuit that revealed her thin frame (Simpson, 2007, January 8). Simpson began with "[s]he wasn't exactly curvy to start with, but Keira Knightley seems to be shrinking daily" (para. 1) and continued to highlight accusations that she had anorexia. Knightley countered: "I've got a lot of experience with anorexia—my grandmother and great-grandmother suffered from it, and I had a lot of friends at school who suffered from it, so I know it's not something to be taken lightly and I don't. But I don't have it, I am very sure of that" (para. 13). However, the controversy didn't stop there.

Rumors, tabloids, gossip, and chatter continued, referring to Knightley as "too thin." Sophie Mazurek's mother, Rosalind Ponomarenko-Jones, essentially blamed Knightley, a public figure who was too skinny and should not be a role model for young girls, for her anorexic daughter's death. The mother argued that "[i]f you can see someone's ribs then they have a problem. When they are in the public eye it is not just unhealthy for them, it is an extraordinarily bad message to give out to youngsters who want to be glamorous too and follow their example" (Simpson, 2007, January 8, para. 7–8).

More controversy surrounding Knightley surfaced three days later (January 11, 2007) as *The Daily Mail* reportedly ran a story that posted a picture of Knightley in a swimsuit with a caption blaming her for Sophie Mazurek's death. Foxnews published an Associated Press article with the claim, "[i]f pictures like this one of Keira carried a health warning, my darling daughter might have lived" ("Keira Knightley wins anorexia libel claim," 2007, May 25, para. 4). We were unable to find the actual article from *The Daily Mail* on January 11, 2007, but other sources indicate that the article prompted Knightley to sue the newspaper (Brook, 2007, January 22; Jury, 2007, January 23).

As Perry asserted in a January (2007, January 23) issue of *People* magazine, "Actress Keira Knightley is suing a British tabloid, saying that it implied she lied about having an eating disorder" (para. 1). A statement made by the actress' legal firm claimed that:

> Ms Knightley will argue that the Mail's article suggests that she has dishonestly sought to mislead the public about whether she has anorexia or similar eating disorder, and will show that she does not have anorexia; and further will challenge the suggestion that she is responsible and to blame for the tragic death of the teenage girl by setting a bad example [Brook, 2007, January 22, para. 5].

Ultimately, Foxnews ("Keira Knightley wins anorexia libel claim," 2007, May 25) reported that "Kate Wilson, representing the publisher of the Daily Mail, Associated Newspapers, told a court Thursday the newspaper accepted that Knightley was not responsible for a death, and that Knightley 'does not have an eating disorder, and has not misled the public'" (para. 3).

Narratives surrounding the accusations embody Knightley frustrated at the media's public statements on her health and stronghold on her private information. While news reports claim that Knightley was not at court, she did end up winning the case (Dowell, 2007, May 24; "Keira Knightley wins damages over weight slur," 2007, May 24), and she intended "to donate the settlement to Beat, an eating disorder and mental illness charity" ("Keira

Knightley wins anorexia libel claim," 2007, May 25, para. 6). While the case closed on this legal battle, the accusations did not end there. Jessen wrote in *People Magazine* (2007, May 2) that "Knightley has long denied eating-disorder rumors, and Knightley told *People Magazine* in January: 'Whatever people say about my weight they are all wrong'" (para. 6).

SHARING CONTROL: FRIENDS AND FAMILY SUPPORT

While the conversations between media and Knightley ebbed and flowed in an accusation and response pattern, Knightley continued to act in films; her body remained in the spotlight, and concerns about her diet and health ensued. She claims that she has worked with doctors to help maintain a healthy diet, but she also acknowledged that the rigorous filming during *Pirates of the Caribbean* absolutely led to weight loss. Yet, she steadfastly denies any eating disorder, and friends and family support her stance.

As Petronio's (2007) Communication Privacy Management theory indicates, private information can be shared, and who knows the information can be negotiated. While Knightley maintains control over her body and information regarding her health, Knightley's friends and family have stepped in to offer support in this public dialogue as co-narrators. For example, a good friend of Knightley's, Sienna Miller, was quoted as saying "She is a really good friend of mine, she is a wonderful girl. Eats like a pig for everyone out there who calls her anorexic" (L. Roberts, 2008, June 16, para. 19).

Knightley's mother released statements too, defending her daughter against the accusations. She spoke out to assure fans that her daughter does not have an eating disorder but is just naturally "thin" (L. Roberts, 2008, June 16, para. 5). She explained that her daughter has a skinny frame, similar to Knightley's father; therefore, her daughter's thin body isn't the result of an eating disorder, but, rather, family genetics. Scholarly work in the area of privacy and confidentiality of genetics raises concerns and challenges in a variety of contexts such as legal, social, and even ethical implications of sharing genetic information (see Rothstein, 1999). In the case of celebrity health, references to genetics pose an interesting foci for consideration as the private information within a family context may become public and challenged by the audience. Of course, mentioning a family member's body structure isn't exactly confidential, but, in this case, doing so works to entangle that person in the ongoing public construction of the emergent narrative about Knightley's body image.

In this case, Knightley's mother came to her daughter's defense, contending, "It's a playground situation that we're looking at with the Press—it's a form of bullying—but what can we do?" (L. Roberts, 2008, June 16, para. 9).

Her claim that starting rumors and making accusations about her daughter's personal health and lifestyle function as forms of bullying work to reclaim the narrative, suggesting that the press should not assert power over such information or "bully" her daughter into questioning her body or threatening litigation, but, as she asked in the L. Roberts' article, what can be done?

Beyond Anorexia: The Struggle
for Control Continues

Knightley explained in interviews with *People Magazine* that she appreciates the seriousness of anorexia and that she has known many people who have had it (Jessen, 2007, May 2; Perry, 2007, January 23; Pisa & Silverman, 2006, July 4). Because of those relationships, she affirms that she knows that she doesn't suffer from the eating disorder. While Knightley has spent a lot of time defending her naturally thin physique to those who label her as anorexic, the struggle for control over her body-image narrative has taken a toll. Knightley admitted that, at some point, she began to wonder, is something really wrong? Accepting and making sense of other people's criticism certainly marked a power struggle for control over one's own story (for related work, see Petronio, 2002, 2004).

Knightley's quotation at the beginning of this chapter reveals that charges of not having the "right" body, being too skinny, ultimately prompted her to question what she knew about herself: "I knew I wasn't anorexic, but maybe my body is somehow not right…. When you're going through a period where you're really getting a lot of criticism, you go, maybe all this is right!" ("Knightley talks," 2012, November 13, para. 5). Throughout her journey, Knightley has purportedly sought help to put on weight from doctors, but, according to Knightley, the plans have failed, due to her naturally thin frame. Knightley shared, "I went to the doctor to be checked out and asked him what I could do to put on weight. He told me that, for someone of my body type to get to a size 12, I would have to eat a lot of s*** food, stop exercising and drink loads. Basically, my body type is naturally thin. There is nothing I can do about it" (L. Roberts, 2008, June 16, para. 15).

Featuring Knightley in a bathing suit caused great consternation and turmoil as it was the crux of controversy in 2007 that led to legal involvement over body image and personal information. In a more recent report, Knightly noted that she hates going to the gym. As Knightley shared, "The very thought of a diet makes me want chips and ice cream, and I just hate going to the gym…. The most exercise I get is turning on the TV" (Chang, 2014, February 3, para. 4). Through such comments, Knightley interjects "evidence" into the public conversation that she is not anorexic or health-obsessed because she does not like to work out or avoid high calorie foods, striving to make her narrative as a "healthy" (not anorexic) person more credible and convincing to onlookers (for related arguments on narrative rationality, see Fisher, 1984, 1985a, 1987a).

Petronio (2007) argued that an individual has power and control over their personal information and can make decisions about disclosure. Knightley has sought to manage boundaries and rules regarding her body as a public figure. In the first excerpt from an *Allure* magazine interview, which was posted in many different media outlets (e.g. Chang, 2012, November 15; Gorgan, 2012, November 14; Z. Johnson, 2012, November 13; "Keira Knightley Disappointed," 2012, November 13; "Knightley talks," 2012, November 13), Knightley discussed three normatively private areas of information: breasts, which are part of her body; anorexia, dealing with her private body image and physique, and marriage, an intimately private discussion between her and her fiancé. Yet, all three appear in press for the public to consume, critique, and debate. A sentence in one particular media story began with "the normally private Keira Knightley" ("Knightley talks," 2012, November 13, para. 1) and demonstrates the presence of a blurred boundary in which Knightley may normally have control over her private life and information, but she routinely grants entirely private body and health matters as interview content for an audience of potentially millions of readers. Knightley has been on magazine covers (*Allure, Marie Claire*) and movie posters, which implicitly underscore visual aspects of body image and health.

VISUAL ASPECTS OF EATING DISORDERS

In a *Shape* magazine article by Michele Luafik on April 5, 2012, titled "Celebrity Weight Loss: Did These Stars Get Too Thin," Knightley was 19 of 21 celebrities that the media questioned their body image. Magazine covers of Knightley are often physically revealing, affirming public perception of her body as available for general conversation and scrutiny. Being visible to the public is part of being a celebrity, whether paparazzi photos or planned celebrity photo shoots; individuals cannot always control what parts appear (and in what form) and what stays private and invisible.

In one interview, Knightley explained the power artists have to airbrush her body, and she expressed disappointment at the digital manipulation in her *King Arthur* movie poster. Z. Johnson (2012, November 13) quoted Knightley as saying, "They always pencil in my boobs. I was only angry when they were really droopy" (para. 4). In the same interview, Knightley clarified that she has certain rules for what is acceptable to show on camera and what should remain private. Even though Knightley has attempted to affirm what constitutes acceptable in terms of the visibility of particular body parts in front of the camera, with or without clothes, her body has become a public conversation. Further, social media has opened the door to the continuation of controversy surrounding privacy, health, and body image. In the next section, we explore examples of social networking sites (such as Twitter) and comments sections of news reports as a popular space where the power of conversation about the body image and health of Keira Knightley is left to the digital participants.

POWER OF THE PEOPLE

Especially with social media, fans and onlookers have become empowered to contribute to public narratives, even ones that involve personal health information of (and speculation about) celebrities. With each interview, Knightley implicitly expands her privacy boundaries as well as invites additional commentary—both positive and supportive as well as negative and evaluative.

In response to the magazine articles (*People*, *Allure*, etc.), threads of "Keira Knightley Disappointed By Weight Accusations And 'Droopy' Boobs," "Keira Knightley Goes Topless and Talks Body Image in Allure: … http://bit. ly/X2memc," and "Keira Knightley Body Secret and Weight Loss Tips http:// bit.ly/15wAdoi" have been tweeted and retweeted multiple times by many people. These online venues create the space for people to share in Knightley's narrative through comparison, support and criticism.

As we note in several other chapters as well, through Twitter, individuals routinely compare themselves to celebrities, and they certainly have done so with regard to Knightley and their own respective size. For example, a tweet from December 27, 2012, claimed, "Ugh, Keira Knightley stop being so cute with your British accent and that whole no fat on your body thing you've got going on, #itsnotfair." Another person likened herself to Knightley, tweeting "Keira Knightley is so thin and attractive. Why can't I be more like her." Others considered Knightley in relation to other celebrities. In October 2012, one person posted, "Haha … I just realised Keira Knightley is also a 'KK'. She and Kim could be the two ends of the Female Body spectrum." Another commented, "If only Georgina Dorsett had the body of Georgia Salpa and the voice of Keira Knightley #PerfectFemale" (March 2012). A popular tweet that was retweeted numerous times also highlights the quest for a perfect female body: "Is Kim Kardashian Really The 'Ultimate Woman'?: Body parts of Megan Fox, Angelina Jolie, Keira Knightley and roy … http://dld.bz/aDxch" (January 2012).

Fans expressed support through tweets about her career, her beauty, and even that thin ideal. One fan noted, "I think it's much better to go with the flow and embrace your body, whatever shape it is, and just be happy.—Keira Knightley" (August 2012). One male Twitter user supported Knightley's body and referenced her physical attractiveness: "I stopped watching Triple D from my DVR and Bend it Like Beckham was on. All I have to say is Keira Knightley's body = #damn" (December 2011). From a Caraway Clinic, a support clinic for individuals with eating disorders in the United Kingdom, another person tweeted, "Keira Knightley slams #anorexia talk and says the rumors make her insecure http://ow.ly/fqLW3" (November 2012). The lines between support and critique may have been permeated at times, as evident in the following tweet: "i adore keira knightley and everything about her but she has gotten too thin."

Twitter users also employed technology and social media to critique Knightley's body. Some posts described her as "too thin." Additional commentaries involved her body, face, teeth, eyebrows and even acting career. Critiques included: "Keira and her million teeth. She's still one of my favourite actresses" (February 2012); "Keira Knightley's body is too anorexic to be appreciated. I always want to cover her up and give her meat to eat" (April 2012), and "Reckon if my teeth were crooked, I had a 12-year-old boys body and an overbite I could be the next face of Chanel. Keira Knightley #lemmebeu" (September 2012). One tweet, in particular, suggested that the individual wanted to change her body type to be more like Knightley, but then upon reflection, realized that she would never obtain a similar body type because she enjoys eating too much: "new years resolution = get a body like keira knightley. begins right after this bacon and cheese sandwich #nom #whoamifooling" (December 2011).

As these tweets illustrate, Knightley has sought to articulate a narrative of health and control of her own body while reporters and social media users have advanced their own sense-making of Knightley's health and body image, in relation to their own experiences and concerns. Discussions of Knightley have led to comparisons between her body image, the images of other celebrities, and assumptions about what constitutes an "ideal" frame. In the next section, we consider implications of such a battle for control and blurred lines between private and public health information.

Implications

A-list actress Keira Knightley's health narrative has revolved around media accusations, with competing explanations for her thin body other than "simply skinny." The media's involvement even escalated to comparing a picture of Knightley's body and blaming her for the death of an anorexic teenager. Knightley has worked to shape her own personal health narrative, amid public speculation and, sometimes, scorn about her body image, thin ideal, and rumored eating disorders. Her response to the dialectic pull between personal and public control has been one of defensiveness. Knightley even tried Twitter, but her use of the social media did not last ("Why Keira Knightley lasted 12 hours on Twitter," 2013, December 30), ironically, given her preference for privacy. We argue that Knightley's act of disengaging in the use of social media comprises a strategy for regaining privacy control, yet removing her voice from Twittersphere could not silence the rumblings, scrutiny, and uncertainty about her health that has plagued her public persona.

Fisher's (1984, 1985a, 1985b) work on narrative provides a possible theoretical explanation for public skepticism pertaining to Knightley's preferred interpretation of her body size. The press, fans, and public onlookers have actively challenged the plausibility of Knightley's "it's just my body type" argument, relying on her appearance as "evidence" and implicitly disputing the credibility (and "narrative rationality") of the narrative that she has struggled to affirm (see Fisher, 1984, 1987a). Individuals who look to Knightley as thinspiration bring a different lived reality to their evaluation of the emergent narrative. For them, Knightley's claim that she does not have an eating disorder, in spite of her quite thin frame, might well run counter to their assumptions about weight loss, dieting, exercise, and maybe even pro ana behaviours to obtain a certain body image (such as Knightley's).

Of course, we cannot label any of these vistas as "Truth," nor do we want to proclaim one vantage point to be more "real" than another. Regardless of the legitimacy (or lack thereof) in terms of claims and counterclaims, this case exemplifies the complications that celebrities encounter when they put themselves in the public eye, by virtue of their celebrity status. Especially when others decide to debate reasons for changes in physical appearance, available behaviors, etc., celebrities inherently confront obstacles in controlling their own narratives, particularly when those others contest the "accuracy" of celebrity explanations or even interpretation about what types of body image might look "healthy" or "sexy" (or "too thin" or "too plump") or action seem reasonable. As Fisher (1984, 1985a, 1985b, 1987) argued, accounts or behaviors that might seem quite acceptable or appropriate to some may well not "ring true" to others, and, to borrow from the classic tale of Goldilocks, "just right" truly does depend on each individual's perspective.

Jennifer Lawrence, of the *Hunger Games* movies, has overtly addressed the traditional Hollywood emphasis on body image. Lawrence noted that "[w]e have control over this image, we have control over this role model. Why would we make her something unobtainable and thin?" (Tyley, 2013, November 22, para. 2). In so doing, Lawrence employed the pronoun *we*. In this era of social media, perhaps more than ever before, "we" comprise diverse stakeholders with varied perspectives, interests, and agendas, fostering a complicated cultural, societal, and gendered landscape in which celebrities must perform their public and private lives. Referencing pressure to lose weight, "Lawrence says it's 'dumb' to go hungry to make other people happy" (Trout, 2014, March 5, para. 21). Yet, as we have illustrated through responses to Knightley, those "other people" inherently flavor a celebrity's personal (and health) narrative as they co-author it through the near constant barrage of comments, critiques, and sometimes wisecracks in the press and on social media.

Conclusion

Keira Knightley has struggled for ownership over her private health information amid public scrutiny of her body image. Many more celebrities have also publicly been criticized for weight issues, such as Oprah, Kirsty Alley, Melissa McCarthy, and Kate Hudson. According to Brook (2007, January 22, para. 6), "Kate Hudson accepted an apology and damages from the UK edition of the *National Enquirer* after it implied in a story that the actor had an eating disorder and was 'looking like skin and bones.'"

The narrative of body image in the media will likely continue, fueled by increasingly invasive and pervasive traditional and social media. With more and more individuals joining public conversations about weight, "the" narrative of "ideal" body image has become fragmented, with tensions between praise for fitting a thin ideal and being beautiful, criticism and speculation about possible eating disorders, and resistance to thin as an "ideal" standard for all.

Individual celebrities stand in the crossfire of frenzied discussions and debates about their respective bodies and even health. Even though Knightley spoke out against those accusations about anorexia, Twitter feeds and news stories continue to highlight her tiny frame and thin body. As we noted, by virtue of her presence in the public eye, Knightley no longer owns her narrative; others can (and do) analyze and scrutinize her photos and add their own twists to her story (for related argument, see Petronio, 2007).

Moreover, as those individual narratives unfold, they reflexively reify, perpetuate, and, perhaps, contest a priori perceptions of the public about body image "ideals," healthy eating, self-esteem, eating disorders, and agency for making changes or opting to stay the same. In so doing, they hold the potential to impact not only celebrities but also others who participate in co-constructing these emergent treatments of body image, as well as still others who observe and reflect slightly beyond the fray.

CHAPTER SEVEN

Celebrity Death Narratives in the Media

College Student Perceptions on Conversations and Disclosure

"you were simply GREAT!! … simply a legend … love you…"—(Facebook post, January 1, 2013, on Heath Ledger's profile).

"Heath has touched so many people on so many different levels during his short life, but few had the pleasure of truly knowing him,"—(Ledger's father as cited by Feyerick, Chun, Susana, and Pontz, January 2008, January 22, para. 14).

Tweet: "John Mayer: I think we'll mourn his loss as well as the loss of ourselves as children listening to Thriller *on the record player. Dazed in the studio. A major strand of our cultural DNA has left us. RIP MJ"*—("Celebs react to Michael Jackson's death," 2009, June 26).

"we should all walk the steps that michael jackson did we should all share the love and heal the world, and make this world a better place" —(Facebook post, October 6, 2013, on Michael Jackson's profile).

Tweet: "Queen Latifah @IAMQUEENLATIFAH Oh Dear Lord! Hurting so Bad!!! MY Sister Whitney!!!!!!! Newark please Pray!!! World Please Pray…. Wyclef Jean 'The voice of an Angel, the Heart of a Lamb, the spirit of a Lioness, the presence of a Goddess, love you R.I.P Whitney Houston'"—("Mariah Carey on Twitter," 2012, February 11).

Russell Brand ✔@rustyrockets "Love and prayers for Philip Seymour Hoffman's family. Addiction kills, I hope all who need it have access to abstinence based recovery…."
Anna Kendrick ✔@AnnaKendrick47 "Philip Seymour Hoffman. Unbearably, shockingly, deeply sad. Words fail to describe his life and our loss"—(Lin, 2014, February 3).

These four celebrities made their mark on their profession and had loving, supportive fans when news of passing away too soon began to fill newsfeeds. Unfortunately, not only did celebrity status link these people together, but narratives related to drug addiction, overdose, and death also connected them. These narratives have become increasingly prevalent in news stories, headlines, and Twitter feeds. For example, Mickey Rooney died at the age of 93 in April 2014. His professional career flourished, but reports indicate his personal life was not as accomplished (Duke & Leopold, 2014, April 7). As with the passing of Philip Seymour Hoffman, whose official autopsy report indicated drug related overdose (Sanchez, 2014, February 28), fans often express a sense of sadness at death coming too soon and lives ending too quickly. However, celebrity struggles with drugs and alcohol are not a new health-related topic. One website, Drugs.com, listed celebrities who have died of drug-related overdose, starting with Sigmund Freud in 1939, as he passed away from prescription drug overdose. The list also includes widely known actors and musicians such as Hank Williams, Sr. (1953), Marilyn Monroe (1962), Judy Garland (1969), Elvis Presley, (1977), Truman Capote (1984), Kurt Cobain (1994), and within the last decade, Heath Ledger (2008), Michael Jackson (2009), Whitney Houston (2012), and Cory Monteith (2013) (Drugs.com, 2014).

With each new story that breaks about a celebrity death related to drug overdose, fans question how such a tragic event could happen. While death is often considered to be a private event, celebrity status challenges the lines between private and public life. As we consider the passing of a celebrity because of drug overdose, we wonder about the value of these narratives in the media shared as news stories in terms of sparking productive conversations about healthy behaviors. Celebrity narratives are not just shared by other celebrities, but noncelebrities as well, as details become part of public discourse. By reflecting on these celebrity death narratives and new media through the lens of Communication Privacy Management theory (Petronio, 2007), we ask how social media continue or constrain interpersonal conversational topics about difficult conversations, especially in terms of perceptions of death in the media under such circumstances and the health-related implications of drug and alcohol misuse.

In this chapter, we explore the taboo nature of engaging in difficult discussions, such as death and dying along with drug and alcohol addiction. Next, we highlight how social media functions as a communicative vehicle to share difficult information. This chapter is unique because we include responses from college-aged students about their perceptions related to celebrity death, social media, and interpersonal conversation. Integrating four celebrity narratives of death due to drug-related use and abuse with college students' responses affords us an intriguing perspective on the intersection of celebrity death through drug overdose and social media and audience reactions.

Difficult Conversations

DEATH

Conversations surrounding death and dying are often taboo in nature and difficult to discuss (Keeley & Koenig Kellas, 2005). Cultural attitudes regarding death have changed and shifted throughout history (O'Gorman, 1998). Death is a natural part of being alive and used to take place in the home, a very private family event. As time passed, medical advances progressed, and people began to visit the hospital more to be cured from illness, and the once private, natural event has become more public and mechanized, which complicates how we make sense of death and dying (Kaldhusdal & Bernhagen, 2011; Navasky & O'Conner, 2010, November 23). Current trends indicate that hospice is an option, that, for family members where the loved one wants to die in their own home surrounded by family and friends, should continue to grow and be embraced (Twycross, 2007). While people often indicate that they would like to die in their own homes, they do not always get to do so (Kaldhusdal & Bernhagen, 2011), and the struggle for social control lies within competing perspectives at end-of-life, juxtaposing death with dignity and life at all costs (Du Pre, 2014; Hart, Sainsbury, & Short, 1998). We may be faced with death in our personal lives, but scholarship has also examined death in the media.

Niemiec and Schulenberg (2011) began with the argument that "[t]he portrayal of death is one of the most common themes in movies and is often unrealistic, promoting misconceptions to the public" (p. 387) and proceed to describe different ways that film depicts death. They conclude with the argument that films have great educational value because "movies are one means of positively influencing death attitudes, with the potential to increase death acceptance and lessen death anxiety" (p. 403). Hilden and Honkasalo (2006) studied end-of-life conversations in the media (newspapers and television). They found that the consumerism approach to health care was evident in doctor-patient interactions and the media's role in spreading information and advocating for patients. For the celebrities mentioned in this chapter, substance abuse led to untimely death. Avoiding conversations about preparing for or discussing the end-of-life process is irrelevant because drug-related overdose has resulted in death. The power and control of the individual to have these conversations, which may open the door to death with dignity, has closed, and the celebrities' voices are lost. However, drugs and addiction also constitute difficult conversations to engage in with a loved one.

DRUG USE

According to the National Institute on Drug Abuse (2014), results of the 2012 National Survey on Drug Use and Health (NSDUH) indicated that illicit drug use is on the rise. The report indicated that marijuana was the cause for the higher percentage, and other illicit drugs have remained the same or even decreased (e.g., psychotherapeutic drugs, cocaine, heroin etc.). Alarmingly, prescription drug abuse is more common in teenage drug use than illegal substances (Foundation for a Drug Free World, 2014). Of great concern about drug use, according to the Centers for Disease Control, is that instances of drug overdose have continued to rise over the past 20 years ("Prescription Drug Overdose," 2014), and, disturbingly, according to another report, "[m]ost people use drugs for the first time when they are teenagers (para. 6).... Drug use is highest among people in their late teens and twenties (para. 8).... There continues to be a large 'treatment gap' in this country" (para. 17) (National Institute on Drug Abuse, 2014).

A study conducted with the 2010 data from the National Survey on Drug Use and Health found that, among college students, alcohol and prescription-drug use for nonmedical purposes were related to mental health in terms of illness and provision of care (Lo, Monge, Howell, & Cheng, 2013). The study also sought to understand the gender dynamic in college-aged students' drug and alcohol misuse and found the relationship between alcohol abuse and mental health was stronger for women than men. Results of a study focusing on college-aged students concluded that "college students with low self-control are at an increased risk for binge drinking, marijuana use, and prescription drug misuse" (J. A. Ford & Blumenstein, 2013, p. 65). These results also added support to the argument about a connection between "individual characteristics (self-control) and social environment (opportunity and peers)" (p. 65). Related to our conversation of celebrity death narratives, social media, and interpersonal conversation, we were intrigued to connect celebrity narratives of death due to drug use and noncelebrity conversations.

In 2009, over a stretch of several days in June, 23–28, four celebrities passed away ("4 Celebrities Die in One Week," 2009, June 28). With varying levels of status and stardom, Billy Mays, Ed McMahon, Farrah Fawcett, and Michael Jackson passed away that June. Fawcett passed away just hours before Michael Jackson, and the media seemed to bounce from one narrative to the next, the coverage "somewhat overshadowing the in memoriam specials news stations had already planned for Farah Fawcett" (Ekberg, 2009, June 25, para. 1; see also Goodman, 2009, June 26). During the *NBC News with Brian Williams*, a report began with Michael Jackson coverage, and, as Williams even explained, "We were preparing a remembrance of Farrah Fawcett … and now this confirmation tonight that he [Jackson] has died" (June 25). Even though celebrities pass away for a myriad of reasons, with some related to health and the aging process (Fawcett—anal cancer, McMahon—86 years old), others are unexpected (e.g., Paul Walker in a car crash); the level of perceived control over the process varies greatly, with some passings related to risky behaviors (such as drug overdose) rather than "unavoidable" illness or aging. Notably, Brian Williams indicated an expectation that he would soon be doing a tribute to Farrah Fawcett, who had been in declining health due to her public battle with anal cancer. Yet, he expressed shock and surprise about Jackson, who had been rehearsing for another world tour.

When combining the difficult conversations of drug use and death, issues of control over a celebrity's narrative shifts as news stories begin to break, and media coverage features information about the celebrity and their lives and their deaths. A CNN report (Respers France, 2013, July 4) shared 32 celebrity photos with narratives of those individuals' respective struggles with substance abuse. Stories of drugs and alcohol abuse, rehab and continued struggles appear in an open online space. A repetitive thread in the narratives is that the stars were often unhappy during what appeared to be very successful moments in their career. As audience members, we obtain access to those narratives through news stories and interactions on social media.

Social Media Use

Not surprisingly, social media trends have changed that the way people communicate. According to a report by the Pew Internet Research Project (Duggan & Smith, 2013, December 30), around 73 percent of adults use some form of social media online. While Facebook remains still the dominant form of social media, adult users participate in a variety of different forms of social media in addition to Facebook. Twitter, a microblogging method of communicating, boasts 255 million users that are actively engaged in this form of social media (Twitter.com, 2014). As stated on Twitter's official website

(2014a), the mission of Twitter is "[t]o give everyone the power to create and share ideas and information instantly, without barriers" (para. 1). When we apply the mission of Twitter and knowledge about other social networking sites, the possibilities for sharing information become seemingly endless.

As we have mentioned throughout this book, the functionality of social networking sites complicates boundaries between personal and public health information. Chou, Hunt, Beckjord, Moser, and Hesse (2009) claimed that changing trends in social media use and age groups require consideration for health communication. Sadly, celebrity death narratives related to drug misuse, abuse, and overdose provide a sad but rich context for exploring blurred lines between public image and private lives.

Celebrity Narratives: Part 1

Heath Ledger (1979–2008) (IMDB, 2014d). Ledger was a well-known Australian-born Hollywood actor whose more notable roles included *A Knight's Tale, The Patriot, Monster's Ball,* and Oscar nominated performances in *Brokeback Mountain* and *The Dark Knight.* The young talented actor seemed to live in a world of endless possibilities and a bright future, which came to an end on January 22, 2008.

Michael Jackson (1958–2009) (IMDB, 2014g). Michael Jackson started his career with the family group, Jackson 5, then began his solo career with his most famous album, "Thriller," and was directly in the public's eye. However, as the decades ensued, Jackson began altering his behavior and appearance; through lawsuits and even more plastic surgeries, he became more private. An *NBC News Nightly Report with Brian Williams* referred to Jackson as a "shooting star" leading a "very troubled" and "private life" (*NBC News,* 2009, June 25).

Whitney Houston (1963–2012) (IMDB, 2014j). Celebrity singer Whitney Houston achieved multiple award-winning albums, Grammys and accolades for her role in the film *The Bodyguard.* Houston's struggle with drugs seemed to be part of her narrative intermixed with struggle and success in the music industry. "She was twice admitted to rehab and declared herself drug-free in 2010 but returned to rehab in May 2011" (IMDB, 2014j, para. 7).

Philip Seymour Hoffman (1967–2014) (IMDB, 2014h). Hoffman was an actor on the big screen and stage and directed theater as well. He was in a variety of films and plays leading to what IMDB calls his breakout role in *Boogie Nights* (1997) and continued his success leading to his Oscar-winning performance in *Capote* (2005). Hoffman was no stranger to drug use and addiction as he shared with *60 Minutes* in a 2011 interview that he used drugs, and, at the age of 22, fear prompted him to sober up (Prokupecz, Karimi, Turner, & Sanchez, 2014, February 5). According to *TMZ*, unfortunately, after 23 years, in 2013, Hoffman started using again and entered detox, as he admitted, "It started slowly with prescription pills, and recently escalated to snorting heroin" ("Philip Seymour Hoffman entered detox," 2013, May 31, para. 2).

PRIVATE YET PUBLIC LIVES

Petronio's work on the control and flow of private information provides a framework for self-disclosure (2002). Communication Privacy Management has been used in a variety of contexts, including the parental decision to disclose HIV status to children (Tenzek et al., 2013), college students' disclosures of revealing behaviors (Venetis et al., 2012), and college students and their decision to reveal or conceal nondrinking status (Romo, 2012). A study employed CPM and self-disclosure to understand behaviors on Twitter, and results indicated that "[p]rivate information regarding daily lives and entertainment was disclosed easily and located at the outermost layer of the disclosure onion. In contrast, health-related private information was concealed and located within the innermost layer of the disclosure onion" (Jin, 2013, p. 813). The dynamics of information shared through Twitter fit nicely with our investigation into celebrity death narratives and social media use.

According to Petronio (2007), five principles can be applied to communication that promote knowledge and comprehension of disclosure processes. First, private information is controlled by the individual or owner of that information. Second, the owner has the power to disclose or withhold that private information from others. Third, the theory suggests the owner has control of the creation of rules and boundaries for sharing information. The next principle suggests that, after one has made the decision to share information, an opportunity exists to reconstruct and negotiate rules and expectations for co-ownership of the original private information. Finally, in terms of control and flow of the once private (now shared information), if the co-constructed and negotiated boundaries are violated, boundary turbulence may result (p. 219). Jin (2013) connected CPM to Twitter and articulated that users have control over information flow and boundaries.

We can apply this framework of disclosure of private information to celebrity death narratives in two ways. First, death from drug-related misuse comprises a very private matter, but it becomes public when news stories alert a larger audience who, in turn, spread it to others through social media.

Second, we wonder how the flow of formerly private information gets reshaped and negotiated through conversation with others at an interpersonal level (see related work by Petronio, 2007).

In the next section, we weave the four celebrity narratives together with research participant voices (indicated by the use of pseudonyms—such as Taylor, Pat, and Sam—for clarity, consistency, and gender neutrality). The celebrity deaths implicitly involved private information shared with the public, which then became part of an online conversation. Similarities among the celebrity death narratives included initial responses to the death and verification from the coroner with an "official" report of death. The celebrities were found at home in either their bedroom or bathroom, arguably very private places in the home. Once the stories became public, multiple threads of information emerged about how the celebrity died, different news sources and family perspectives, police perspectives, health perspectives, and the public's response using social media.

As we detail, college-age students attempt to make sense of celebrity death narratives through the use of social media by enacting a dialectical tension straining between positive and negative perceptions of social media. Further, we explore how celebrity death narratives, social media, and interpersonal conversations about prescription drug use intersect through boundary extensions in interpersonal conversation.

Celebrity Narratives Part 2: Death

INTEGRATING NARRATIVES: CELEBRITY DEATH AND COLLEGE STUDENTS' PERCEPTIONS

The quotation below illustrates the media's involvement in sharing the news that a celebrity has died. Notions of privacy boundaries surface, and appropriate levels of involvement in the celebrity death narratives emerge. One of our research participants, Taylor, commented,

> I believe that media coverage surrounding the death of a celebrity is actually the only time the media has respect. There are many instances where the media respects the family's need for privacy. However, there are some instances where they do cross the line by interviewing any and everyone who knew or had contact with that celebrity to make a story. I believe that a celebrity's death certificate and autopsy results should not available to the public unless it allowed by their family members.

News reports started flying (from sources such as CNN, *Time*, and *New*

York Times) that actor Heath Ledger had been found unresponsive in his Manhattan apartment bedroom, and the cause of death was reported as possible overdose but was not confirmed right away (Chan, 2008, January 28; Feyerick et al., 2008, January 22; Luscombe, 2008, January 22). In February 2008, reports from the New York City Medical Examiner's office indicated that "Heath Ledger died from an accidental overdose of prescription medications including painkillers, anti-anxiety drugs and sleeping pills" ("Ledger's death caused by," 2008, February 6, para. 1). Ledger's death narrative and Taylor's insight illustrate that oftentimes private celebrity information is shared with the public before any sense of "Truth" or the "real story" has been confirmed. In the next section, we pursue the contradiction between rule formation and turbulence as respondents try to make sense of celebrity death.

How Do College Students Make Sense of Celebrity Death through Social Media Use?

Another research participant, Sam, asserted that "[i]t's important in that it [social media] brings about discussions of mental health awareness, but … it also invites a lot of unfair criticism." Sam references the tension between benefits and negative aspects of social media use and celebrity death and demonstrates a push and pull between how the participant makes sense of death in the media. On one end of the spectrum, college students' responses suggest that celebrity death narratives do have a place in the public eye, and, on the other side of the spectrum, participants believed that social media has no place discussing or sharing celebrity information.

Tensions in Sense-making

The tension between opposing views seemed to be illustrated in the dynamic between openly sharing information and having people involved in the conversation in the media and celebrity death narratives remaining closed off from outside audience members. For example, Pat shared insight to the constructive aspect of social media helping make sense of information to a point until it becomes impersonal. Pat noted, "While I do believe that it may be constructive for others to learn about the causes of deaths in different people, I also believe that in the case of a celebrity death, media coverage becomes impersonal and sometimes insensitive about others' private lives." Taylor highlighted the battle between audience engagement, voice, and participation in an online discussion and acknowledged that those voices may bring criticism against the celebrity and/or family in a public forum:

I think that it's good to know for those who are fans of those celebrities, but it also invites unfair criticism and judgment by complete strangers, especially on the Internet, essentially it gives everyone a voice to their opinion on the subject. I also think it's unfair that the media doesn't typically respect the privacy of the family.

The next example advances the positive nature of social media in terms of power to increase the rate of sharing information. Audience members know almost in real time when celebrity events happen, but, with that speed, come negative words and possible false information. Sam explained, "News travels fast since almost everyone uses some form of social media. Within hours a celebrity's death will be posted on twitter. However, there will always be people who spread rumors, harsh words, and comments via social media about the deceased celebrity."

In the next section, we strive to disentangle the dialectical strain by separating responses into negative and positive.

Negative Responses

Given the advent of social media, celebrity death narratives emerge quickly and quite publically, and the time to process and understand may become compromised. Celebrity Whitney Houston had been a long-time drug addict, working through rehab and becoming sober. Unfortunately, the narrative did not have a happy ending. Houston was found drowned under water in a hotel bathtub in Beverly Hills, Los Angeles. Reports claimed her death was caused by drowning, but reports also confirmed that she had heart disease, and cocaine was found in her system (Murphy, 2012, March 22).

According to an ABC video report led by Bill Weir (n.d.), Houston's case included threads of known addiction, stints in rehab, and living a drug-use lifestyle before drug abuse claimed the life of this celebrity singer. On the website *Mashable,* Murphy Kelly (2012, February 12) wrote that Twitter reported Houston's death 27 minutes before any news station or website had the information. Although such private information should flow within the family first, that confidentiality disappears when the news story hits social media. Pat explained,

I don't think there is any [value]. The celebrity has passed (will never see written hashtags or posts) and I highly doubt kind words from #1 fans will comfort the grieving family! I'm pretty sure the last thing parents, siblings, and friends of the celebrity would want to do is read pages and pages of comments about what complete strangers think and assume!

Sam concurred: "I think mourning should be a more private event. Let the families miss their loved ones in peace, you didn't know that person."

Sam continued by sharing that "[social media] makes it harder for the loved ones to cope in such a public light, no privacy." Emotionally arguing that we should keep death private and away from social media speculation, Pat asserted that "[i]t's useless and stupid because the people on the sites are generally uneducated on the subject and spread false information." Sam seemed angered/irritated at the open-endedness that social media allows in terms of audience participation if users are uneducated and pass false information forward. Notably, in each of these exemplar celebrity narratives, authorities did not release the actual cause of death right away, but rumors, stories, and speculation about how the celebrity passed away spread rapidly.

Participants also responded negatively to the media's framing of celebrities that have died from drug overdose as victims, and the narrative of undesirable outcomes of drug-related behavior seems to get lost. For example, Taylor commented that "[t]hey over publicize the situation and sort of make it seem okay to everyone even though it's horrible they did drugs or alcohol to begin with." Sam asserted, "I think sometimes the media over glorifies death of celebrities. We forget the reason why they've passed is because of drug overdose, etc., and I think a lot of times the media coverage over romanticizes it." Sam further tried to make sense of Whitney Houston's passing away from drugs by talking with friends and family, recalling that "[w]hen Whitney Houston died, my friends and family discussed how long she had been addicted to drugs and other things and why she never stopped." For Houston, her private life as an addict was exposed in the spotlight as she struggled to overcome drug use. At the time of her death, sharing information through social media may have blurred the lines of reality and truth, but she was still proclaimed as being an amazing influential singer. Along the same lines, not all sense-making efforts about celebrity death narratives and social media were negative. We offer positive responses toward social media's value in sharing celebrity death narratives in the following section.

Positive Responses

Positive social responses from our participants included ideas related to the continuous flow of and rate at which information can be distributed. For example, Taylor mentioned that "[s]ocial networking sites are frequently checked and updated, making news travel pretty rapidly." Our participants acknowledged that transmitting information through social media allows for topics to gain popularity in different ways. Pat pointed to "[t]rending topics on Twitter; News articles shared on Facebook; pictures of the celebrity on Instagram." As Pat noted, social media "spreads the word more quickly."

Whispers of Jackson's death began online and were shortly thereafter confirmed by *LA Times*, Associated Press, *NBC News* and continued to spread from there (Coyle, n.d.). Reports claimed Jackson experienced a heart attack and died shortly after ("Michael Jackson," 2011, November 9; "Michael Jackson Dies," 2009, June 25). While Jackson passed away on June 25, the Los Angeles coroner's office report indicated that he died of two drugs, propofol and lorazepam, nearly two months later on August 28 (Duke, 2009, September 4; "Michael Jackson," 2011, November 9). While controversy ensued over what actually took place and who was to blame, Jackson was laid to rest in Glendale, California.

Our college-student participant narratives about positive aspects of social media that helped make sense of celebrity death build on the ability to spread information quickly and involve opening the door to conversations that connect people in a way that may not have been possible otherwise. For example, Sam expressed that "[p]eople discuss them to get attention and more followers/likes; as well as start conversations and make friends." Additionally, Pat explained that social media "[m]akes the death more known and the causes of the death more public knowledge." In doing so, the flow of information could challenge preconceived notions about celebrity health and drug use.

According to a CNN report, Hoffman was found dead, with a syringe in his arm, in his apartment bathroom and "died of acute mixed drug intoxication, including heroin, cocaine, benzodiazepines and amphetamine" (Sanchez, 2014, February 28). Surrounding Hoffman were syringes that had been used and empty bags that most likely had contained heroin. Taylor's response sheds light on how social media can be used to make sense of celebrity death by drug overdose and also learn more about difficult topics. Taylor explained that a narrative such as Hoffman's "[b]rings drugs out in the open and puts a face to drug addicts. It shows that it's not always the stereotypical people you would expect to do drugs."

Finally, college students made sense of celebrity death through social media in a positive way by considering the implications that the narrative had for drug-use outcomes and presenting a way for people to get help if they needed it. For example, as Sam shared, celebrity death narratives in the media "[s]how what drugs do to the body, make me want to stay away." Pat offered a similar sentiment, noting that it "[c]ould show the followers that the use of drugs is dangerous and has serious consequences." Taylor speculated, "Maybe helps some teens out seeing how some celebrities got help and are going through the same problem they are and can help them get through it."

These quotations illustrate threads of negative responses in the way that college students reflect on celebrity death and the role of social media in sharing the narrative. At the other end of the dichotomy, our participants acknowledged some positive aspects, noting that such public narratives might spark conversations with others about the topic and even raise important health information that may not have been discussed previously, including death in general. The following quotation by Sam succinctly embodies the tension between positive and negative information. Sam claimed that the media over exaggerates coverage, but recognized its power to raise awareness and provide helpful information for someone who may be experiencing a health-related issue, that coverage "[s]ometimes is ridiculously overdone, but sometimes it can be helpful when it's a tragic mental health or drug related death because it can create awareness and sometimes makes it easier for the average person to begin coping with a problem appropriately."

Upon reflection, narrative sense-making of celebrity death illustrates Petronio's (2007) process of information flow through disclosure in the social media outlets and online participants. The next section further extends the boundaries of celebrity information through social media to interpersonal contexts to better understand how audience members, such as college students, use celebrity death to spark conversation and engage with others.

Connecting Celebrity Death Narratives, Social Media and Interpersonal Conversations

While the prior section highlighted celebrity death narratives, we now detail the ways in which celebrity deaths sparked conversation for our participants with others in their own personal lives. Therefore, this section focuses solely on participants' narratives about celebrity death as they engage in interpersonal conversations. Some respondents indicated that simply having conversations about a celebrity death from drug overdose did not influence their perceptions of drug use. Responses of this nature include "not really," "it hasn't," and "no influence, still the same thoughts." Conversely, other respondents indicated that conversations about celebrity drug misuse did influence their perceptions about drug and alcohol use. The rationale behind these responses also varied. Reactions included acknowledgments that the conversations did not influence their perceptions because they already felt strongly about the issue, did not drink or do drugs, or the narratives reinforced their ideas about the topic. For some respondents, the conversations were connected because of personal experience using drugs or learning to know their limits regarding drug or alcohol consumption.

Boundary Extensions
in Interpersonal Conversation

Our participants noted that they tended to interact with family, classmates, and friends about celebrity death narratives, in addition to following more public conversations on social media. By bringing the topic of particular celebrity deaths into private conversations, individuals not only expand boundaries of those specific narratives to include family, friends, and classmates. They prioritize such narratives as something of relevance and potential usefulness to their own lives.

Family

Our participants noted that celebrity narratives of drug overdose prompted them to set new boundaries or reinforce personal boundaries of drug and alcohol use because of family history. Sally wrote,

> These conversations about celebrity death influenced my perceptions of drug and alcohol use in that I will never ever use drugs because I know that they can really ruin my life and also I have family members that use to be drug addicts and I know for a fact I will never go down that road ever. Now alcohol, I do drink, but I do not always drink everyday all day because I need to still stay focused on school and also I know that it is not good for your health if you drink alcohol every day.

Jane recalled discussing the death of Amy Winehouse with her stepmother:

> I was talking about the cause of Amy Winehouse death with my step-mother. And she said that this is why celebrities should not be anybody's idol, she said make an idol of yourself, family or even a friend. People that you really know should be the ones you look up to not the people on television who look phenomenal all the time and have talent because you don't know their actual daily lifestyles.

Participants expressed boundaries in terms of not idolizing celebrities because, as audience members, we cannot access the "Truth"; we can only glimpse segments and therefore, must rely on others with more information as they identify more reliable role models and idols.

Classroom

Because we visited with college students between the ages of 18 and 24 years, some of the responses referred to discussions related to drug overdose that took place in the classroom. Bob shared that "[u]sually these conversations come up in class discussions. Usually things are discussed as to why people pay more attention to these deaths than other deaths." As Bob noted, a celebrity death triggered a classroom conversation as well as critical reflections regarding why a celebrity death would be different from anyone else's passing.

Joe explained, "We talked about it in one of my high school classes with my teacher. They were really saddened by it because that is someone's role model." The same thread of celebrities as role models was a part of the above quotation, and, while Jane's conversation with her stepmother promoted setting up boundaries for role models, Joe's rule formation situated the celebrity as a role model and therefore, upon hearing about passing away, caused great sadness, almost as with the loss of a "friend" (see Meyrowitz, 1985, for background work on parasocial interaction as well as other related arguments throughout this book).

Friends

Claire confided her perspective on conversations with friends about drugs as a relatable narrative because of the effect of drug use on their hometown. Claire shared, "If you hear in the news about a celebrity dying from a drug overdose, it definitely gets me and my peers talking. Many of us come from towns that are really hard hit from drugs, especially heroin. It's just another reminder of our friends at home." Max indicated that conversations within the online community and peer group allow for pause and reflection that death due to substance abuse does not discriminate, celebrity or not:

> When Corey Monteith died it brought up many discussions in my peer group. When you think of the type of person who would overdose on drugs, the image of Corey Monteith does not come to mind. He was handsome, young, and talented in many ways. It was almost impossible to not know about Cory's [sic] death because of how much it was trending through social media. Fans reached out to him and his significant other Lea Michele by tweeting at them with support. It is amazing how much support you can get from people you don't even know. When celebrities pass away from drug or alcohol usage, my friends and I always say how you never think it will happen to you, but you just never know.

Discussion

Within the framework of Petronio's (2007) work, celebrities have their own personal health information, but, when details (such as an untimely death) leak into social media conversations, the floodgates crash open to further interpersonal communication exchanges, speculation, and debate.

Although we acknowledge the problems inherent to violated privacy boundaries, we recognize great potential power for positive health-related messages to be exchanged online, especially when lessons can be taught about life-altering (or life-ending) consequences of drug and alcohol abuse. In this discussion, we note implications for celebrity death narratives and use of social media, public versus private boundaries, celebrity status, and responsibility.

Public versus Private Boundaries

According to Jin (2013), social media, especially Twitter, embody dialectical tensions between concealing and revealing information. Boundaries change and become renegotiated throughout the communicative interaction. Celebrities certainly tread the line between public and private information as their true impressions, personalities, and identities are often masked or distorted by media outlets, and, as this chapter sadly reveals, turbulence and misinformation continue amid rumors of drug use and reports of a celebrity death. What information should appropriately be shared about the autopsy in relation to the drug overdose? How is the perception of the star influenced when negative information is shared?

Our participants' responses highlight a boundary struggle between lived experience and expression and the way we remember death and dying. Additionally, we, the receivers of private information about celebrity death, often only get pieces of information, not an entire narrative at one time, but piece by piece. The function of social media in this case seems to open the door for critique and judgment of the celebrity narrative without verification of information. Because of the fragmented nature of social and mainstream media (and, indeed, contemporary public/private discourse in this postmodern era, see Gergen, 1991), impression management, public face, celebrity identity, and public image might well conflict with realities of a problematic private life involving drug or alcohol abuse, ultimately leading to death. As we detailed in this chapter, subsequent efforts to reconcile public images and discourse during our private interactions can be challenging, confusing, affirming, or enlightening, depending on available information, personal perspectives, and interpersonal dynamics.

Revealing and Concealing Drug Use

Respondents indicated that celebrity death from drug overdose can come as a surprise. Because the private information of celebrity drug habits does not always emerge as a media story until death, the privacy boundaries are permeated, not by the individual, but the media. In death, the celebrity loses his or her ability to make decisions related to sharing information, and ownership shifts. Interestingly, some respondents claimed that the family of the celebrity who passed away should be left alone and able to grieve privately away from the public eye. For example, each of the celebrities that we have discussed thus far in this chapter left behind children—Ledger: daughter "Matilda Rose" (Feyerick et al., 2008, January 22, para. 29); Jackson: children "Prince Michael I, Paris, and Prince Michael II" ("Michael Jackson dead at 50," n.d., para. 11); Houston: daughter "Bobbi Kristina" ("Singer Whitney Houston dies at 48," 2012, February 11, para. 28): and Hoffman: children "Cooper Alexander Hoffman," "Tallulah Hoffman," and "Willa Hoffman" (IMDB, 2014i, para. 36, 37, 38). Boundaries and sharing of private information reach many levels, opening the door for caring and criticism that becomes part of the children's narratives. Yet, electronic "grapevines" (such as Facebook and Twitter) crash through privacy boundaries and inherently expand those walls to encompass fans and others "with an inquiring mind" who seek and scroll for information by merely clicking a mouse.

A second aspect of the revelation of drug use seemed to present as almost a fear appeal. Multiple respondents claimed that, because of the celebrity death from drug overdose, they were scared to try drugs. The narratives reinforced the negative consequences of doing drugs, and participants viewed the potential of social media to be positive if educational messages were shared. Finally, the introduction of drug use into a celebrity health (or death) narrative challenged the perception that celebrities "differ" from others. Messages from social media about celebrity death narratives functioned as an equalizer—drug use behavior has consequences, and it does not matter who you are, even purported "role models."

Responsibility

The topic of "responsibility" surfaced at many levels throughout our conversations with participants. We asked questions related to celebrities as responsible for serving as role models, responsibility of social media use, and responsibility in our inter(personal) relationships. Etherington's (2006) work demonstrates that life stories constitute one way in which we can understand drug misuse and how identities change during the course of experience. Etherington expressed the power of life narratives as a means to make sense of lived experiences where "an individual's subjective experiences can show how social environments and the wider social/cultural resources help people make sense and meaning of their lives" (p. 233). In this chapter, each celebrity crafted (intentionally and inadvertently) their own unique narrative, complete with accomplishments, flaws, and untimely death, and "outsiders" attempted to make sense of their passing as they became "insiders" and "coauthors" of the emergent death narratives.

When people have private information, Petronio (2007) argued that they are able to decide when and with whom to share any information. However, the very nature of being a "celebrity" works to remove privacy boundaries from the individual's control, especially when they no longer live to give instructions, offer explanations, or guard secrets. Social media further complicates disclosure due to the ability to share information quickly and with an infinite number of people who have access to it. Amid these negative consequences for celebrities and their grieving families, we argue that social media holds much positive potential to pass on celebrity death narratives, opening a space for sense-making, grieving, and, perhaps, even reflections on the positive contributions of the celebrities (Sanderson & Cheong, 2010). While the chapter has discussed CPM and traditional interpersonal disclosure, participating in online conversation can be distinguished by emotional bandwidth. High et al. (2014, p. 80) argued that "manipulation of technological affordances on Facebook enables people to control the transmission or disclosure of information about their affective states, a capacity henceforth referred to as 'emotional bandwidth.'" Connecting emotional bandwidth and celebrity death narratives provides a new avenue for future scholarship. Ultimately, online conversations could be extended to interpersonal relationships between peers and families, offering possibilities for new boundaries, rules, and information sharing about important topics.

College students' insight and perceptions to celebrity death narratives and drug misuse open the door to important conversations and an understanding of how social media can work to promote positive messages and interpersonal discussion, while simultaneously hindering a sense of narrative truth for the celebrity. If people interact about these types of taboo topics using social media, then health campaign scholarship and promotion could benefit from future examinations of the potential use and benefits of social media to encourage healthy behavior of society.

Chapter Eight

No "I" in Team

Impression and Boundary Management
in Illness/Injury Narratives
Involving Sports Celebrities

Peyton Manning lives in Denver now. Indeed, Schwab (2014, March 3) reported that Manning earned $20 million when he played quarterback for the Denver Broncos, the team that he led to a Super Bowl in the 2013 season, in 2014.

However, Manning's presence remains strong in Indianapolis. Quarterback for the Indianapolis Colts from 1998 to 2011, Manning set records and won recognition, including 13 Pro Bowl appearances and Super Bowl MVP (http://en.wikipedia.org/wiki/Peyton_Manning). Although Manning sadly parted ways with the Colts after a neck injury threatened his storied career, he did not break off ties with the community, and he remains beloved by many in the greater Indianapolis area (Haythorn, 2013, October 19).

Denver area reporter Russell Haythorn (2013, October 19) noted that "[t]he Peyton Manning Children's Hospital is now the cornerstone of Manning's charitable work in Indianapolis. And the young people being treated there not only idolize him, many know him" (para. 4). According to Haythorn, Manning's visits to young hospital patients began in 1999 and continue, in spite of his move from the area. Haythorn reported that "[i]t turns out Manning doesn't just talk the talk here. He didn't just donate big bucks to get his name on this hospital. As moms and hospital big wigs will tell you, he walks the walk. Up and down the halls that display his jerseys, popping in on patients all the time" (para. 12).

As Kassing (2013, p. 431) noted, "Sport and advocacy have a long shared history," and, certainly, Peyton Manning exemplifies a commitment in the National Football League to civic engagement, community service, and, quite simply, giving back a bit of what players have received by virtue of their status as professional athletes and spokespeople. The National Football League website affirms that "[f]ootball and community are the twin pillars of the NFL. Whether nationally at the league level, locally at the team level, or individually through the volunteerism and philanthropy of owners, players, coaches and club personnel, there exists a powerful NFL-wide commitment to giving back" ("NFL and the Community," 2014, June 3, para. 1).

A 2012 *Forbes* report revealed much potential for "giving back." As of 2012, players in the National Football League averaged 1.9 million dollars per year. Their colleagues in the National Hockey League earned, on average, 2.4 million dollars, contrasted with the average Major League Baseball salary of 3.2 million. Players in the National Basketball Association topped the list at average salaries of 5.15 million dollars (M. Burke, 2012, December 7). Coupled with visibility from nationally televised games (plus some hefty commercial deals), many professional athletes attract considerable public attention and attain financial benefits that allow them to enjoy lavish lifestyles. Amid such a lucrative and sensational backdrop, fans easily recognize favorite athletes by name and face—Peyton. Lebron. Beckham. Tiger. Sports buffs can easily recall "greats" such as Magic and MJ—players who stand out on the star quality merits of their talent, personality, and visibility (see related works by Boyle & Haynes, 2000; Harris, 2013; Sandvoss, Real, & Bernstein, 2012; Smart, 2005; Teitelbaum, 2005; Whannel, 2002). Indeed, according to Sandvoss et al., "In this age of global celebrity, few public personae enjoy greater popularity and recognition than professional athletes" (p. ix).

Although coaches admonish children from the very beginning of peewee soccer that "there's no 'I' in 'team,'" spotlights on individual athletes transform the "I" into a prominent dimension of college and professional team sports. Further, as this chapter will detail, consideration of "team," in relation to a specific group of sports professionals and in the context of broader communities, constitutes a major component in the accomplishment of illness or injury narratives for celebrity athletes.

This chapter will, first, explore challenges for sports figures in balancing personal health concerns in light of preferred professional persona and relationships. Second, we discuss the ways in which athlete disclosures about health issues transition individual narratives into ones with much broader implications, invoking fans and teammates as part of an extended "team" against the health-related foe. In so doing, we describe how the expanded narrative can serve as a base from which to rally that expanded team into advocacy and appeals for action and funding (both private and public).

Private Pain and Public Personas
in Professional Athletics

In his memoir, former professional football player Nate Jackson (2013) noted:

> We lift and run as we are told. No one asks us how we feel. It's assumed that we feel fine and that we are ready to push on, harder and faster. There simply isn't time to pay attention to the individual athlete's body. It's the industrial football complex. Here's the program. Go [p. 137].

Jackson's book chronicles pushing forward in spite of injuries, ignoring pain, pursuing the prize—playing another game in the National Football League. Jackson recalled,

> The next morning we leave for Kansas City. I'm in a lot of pain, possibly the most painful injury I've ever played with. Another 6 milligrams of Toradol into my ass the night before the game but it doesn't help.... Warm-ups are so painful that I'm considering the unthinkable: telling my coach I can't play. The Toradol, the adrenaline, and my access to the pain switch: none of them can override this invisible injury. But my pride won't let me pull the plug. I suit up and tell myself, once again, that I am a warrior, and this is my war. I stare at myself in the mirror and fight back the fear. It is dangerous to be on the NFL field if you're not healthy. Trained killers are coming for you. As I run on the field before each play, I ask myself: how are you going to get through this? And after each play, I ask myself: how are you going to get through the next one? Eventually the game is over" [p. 212].

Erving Goffman (1959, 1963, 1967) described the integral nature of impression management in public performance. In the "front stage," we strive to present ourselves as preferred types of individuals, implicitly affirming taken-for-granted assumptions about what characteristics should be enacted to "pull off" our preferred persona. According to Goffman (1967, p. 168), "Of the various types of object the individual must handle during his presence among others, one merits special attention: the other persons themselves. The impression he creates through his dealings with them and the traits they impute to him in consequence have a special bearing on his reputation." To "give in" to injury or hurt defies the "tough guy" image essential to enacting the role of NFL football player. As Goffman (1959, p. 48) noted, "A performer tends to conceal or underplay those activities, facts, and motives which are incompatible with an idealized version of himself and his products."

Jackson's (2013) narrative reveals the decisions that he made in order to present himself as a legitimate or "real" football player—tough, tenacious, fighter, "warrior." (For related research on identity construction in sports, see Beamon,

2012; Carless & Douglas, 2013a, 2013b; Cushion & Jones, 2014; Houck, 2006; Martin & Horn, 2013; Roderick, 2006; Sandvoss, 2012; Steinfeldt & Steinfeldt, 2012; Tasiemski & Brewer, 2011; Yoo, Smith, & Kim, 2013.) In their work, Carless and Douglas (2013a, 2013b) emphasized that involvement in athletics, growth as an "athlete," and, indeed, formulation of sports communities sculpt and, implicitly, reify emergent individual and collective narratives that reflexively and artfully communicate meanings and expectations. Micro-level choices by individual players, coaches, teams, leagues, and fans do important identity work, shaping the ongoing (overt and underlying) stories of what it means to be part of a particular sport and to perceive and present oneself as a "legitimate" member. (See related work by Billings, Butterworth, & Turman, 2012; Brookes, 2002; Bryant & Cummins, 2010; Carless & Douglas, 2013a, 2013b; Cinoğlu & Arikan, 2012; Earnheardt, Haridakis, & Hugenberg, 2012; Garfinkel, 1967; Goffman, 1959, 1963, 1967; Hundley & Billings, 2010; Roderick, 2006; Schirato, 2013; Steinfeldt & Steinfeldt, 2012; Young, 2008). For example, Schirato argued:

> The sight of male athletes staggering or collapsing while finishing a race effectively reinscribes and naturalizes the link between competitiveness, endurance, resilience and self-overcoming, and masculinity; in other words, a semiotics of distress, pain, suffering and discomfort is what is expected of, and commensurate with, the male athlete [p. 5].

Jackson's (2013) book underscores American football's tradition, indeed, culture, of not whining about the hits, not complaining of every physical misfortune, not quitting. Indeed, Jackson recounted one coach's admonishment that "[y]ou must choose the pain of discipline or the pain of regret" (p. 230) and observed declarations "on the training room wall, 'Durability is more important than Ability.' As if the injured guys don't feel bad enough already. Might as well say, 'If you're reading this, you're a pussy'" (p. 230). As a line from the Academy Award-winning song *Let It Go* emphasizes, "Conceal, don't feel, don't let them know.... Well, now they KNOW."

THE CASE OF TRAUMATIC HEAD INJURIES

As Jackson (2013) shared in his raw account of life in the NFL, only a "pussy," a wimp, a whiner, a quitter, a loser, gives in to pain or acknowledges injury. If not tough enough, get out. The next young and fit guy can step in, take the hit, and replace the weak, old, and injured. This context undergirds the challenge to improve safety in the NFL, especially with regard to invisible or chronic injuries such as concussions (Berezow, 2013, December 11; Fainaru-Wada & Fainaru, 2013; Goldberg, 2013; Kerr, Marshall, Harding Jr., & Guskiewicz, 2012; King, 2010, November 1; Van Natta, Jr., 2013, October 2).

This chapter cannot do justice to the truly riveting reporting in *League of Denial: The NFL, Concussions, and the Battle for Truth* (Fainaru-Wada & Fainaru, 2013). However, we touch on the saga surrounding concussions in the NFL as a means of illustrating the critical importance of impression management, illness narratives, and professional sports.

King (2010, November 1) described reactions by players in a locker room to an NFL training video about new rules on types of hits allowed during games:

> "It was like a bad B movie," says 49ers linebacker Takeo Spikes. "Guys were booing, throwing stuff at the screen. They were mad. You heard stuff like, 'Did this guy [Ray Anderson, NFL executive VP of Football Operations] ever play?'" (Anderson was a receiver and kick returner at Stanford.) ... Even the Players Association was angry about what seemed to be an attempt to make the game safer. "The skirts need to be taken off in the NFL offices," said union president Kevin Mawae on ESPN radio [p. 35].

According to Fainaru-Wada and Fainaru (2013), Dave Duerson, an 11-year veteran of the NFL, repeatedly defended the league and the game, even in Congressional testimony, before eventually committing suicide purportedly due to long-term effects from prior football-inflicted head trauma. Fainaru-Wada and Fainaru wrote, "If there was a point when Duerson became conflicted by his own worsening condition and his disdain, public and private, for the claims that football caused brain damage, he didn't show it. Nor did he hide his contempt for what he saw as the softening of the game" (p. 299). Fainaru-Wada and Fainaru recalled,

> Duerson had a radio show, *Double Time with Double D*, that ran on VoiceAmerica. On October 21, 2010, Duerson told his listeners, "I'm pissed today." He lamented the NFL's crackdown on dangerous head-to-head tackles. He read one of his own Facebook postings: "The Big Hit has been told to turn in his pads and jockstrap." He read several comments from readers ridiculing the league for trying to "sissify" the sport [p. 299].

Yet, as Solotaroff (2011, May) detailed, in spite of his fervent protests about "softening" the often brutal game, Duerson also increasingly struggled with memory, relational, and financial issues:

> Once a man so acute he aced his finals at Notre Dame with little study time, he found himself now having to dash down memos about what he was doing and when. Names, simple words, what he'd eaten for dinner—it was all washing out in one long wave. No one had to tell him what those symptoms implied or what lay in store if he stuck around. Once a savage hitter on the best defense the game has ever seen, Duerson filled the punch list for chronic traumatic encephalopathy (CTE), the neuron-killing condition so rampant these days among middle-aged veterans of the National Football League [para. 2].

According to Schwarz (2011, May 2), "Duerson shot himself Feb. 17 in the chest rather than the head," explaining that "[h]is final note to his family finished with a handwritten request: 'Please, see that my brain is given to the N.F.L.'s brain bank'" (para. 2). Duerson's demise mirrored the tragic end of other professional athletes who suffered CTE, yet Duerson's decision to wait until his death to publically acknowledge his mental (and related relational and financial) trials seemingly reflected his conundrum—counter his fervent claims about the pivotal role of big hits for players and the game ... or concede that, perhaps, the impact might just be more than players and American professional football could (or should) handle in the long run.

Fainaru-Wada and Fainaru (2013) asserted,

> There has never been anything like it in the history of sports: a public health crisis that has emerged from the playing field of our twenty-first-century pastime.... Football's health crisis featured not millions of anonymous victims but very public figures whose grotesque demises seemed almost impossible to reconcile with their personas [pp. 6–7].

Moreover, this situation stems from and works to underscore rhetorical (and, subsequently, physical) choices by league officials, players, and, to some extent, fans and sponsors to perpetuate the nature of American football. As Fainaru-Wada and Fainaru discovered, the league continues to minimize links between concussions and this condition, resisting efforts to "sissify" a sport that depends on stops, hits, and tough tackles. Players continue to ignore risks and even injuries, and fans cheer for their favorite teams and players to do whatever it takes to win.

However, the ugly, dark side lurks in the shadows as former players deal with consequences long after the crowds grow silent, the fame fades, the fat paychecks end. At that point, the potential stigma of speaking out pales in contrast to desperate pleas for help. Indeed, Fainaru-Wada and Fainaru (2013) shared that, as of the publication of their book,

> nearly 6,000 retired players and their families were suing the league and Riddell for negligence and fraud.... One week before the start of the 2013 season, the NFL settled the case—agreeing to pay the players $765 million, plus an expected $200 million in legal fees. The NFL did not admit wrongdoing, but the settlement hardly resolved the question at the core of [the league's concussion crisis: How dangerous is football to one's brain? [p. 7].

However, for our purposes, another riveting and important question emerges: how do individual players, with lives (and futures) beyond the field or court, juxtapose personal health concerns with identity issues intricately embedded in enacting professional roles and responsibilities?

Privacy Management

Once again, Sandra Petronio's (2000, 2002, 2004, 2013) work on Communication Privacy Management theory provides a useful theoretical lens for understanding the intricacies of navigating privacy boundaries. Petronio (2004, p. 202) argued,

> CPM theory presumes that people believe they own their private information. Individuals need to control that information because it has the potential to make them vulnerable. In addition, control is also important because people feel they have the right to determine what happens to their private information. Consequently, ownership and control are rudimentary to understanding the way people define and handle their private information [p. 202].

As Nate Jackson's (2013) narrative reveals, football players carefully protect internal flickers about physical ability to play and/or fears about getting hurt to preserve preferred perceptions by teammates or coaches. Further, as Fainaru-Wada and Fainaru (2013) found, in a "tough guy" sport like football, vocal resistance to labeling hard knocks to the head as dangerous, for the love of the game, can also work to silence concerns. Would a "real" football player/fan/owner want to "sissify" the sport by overtly acknowledging the legitimacy of claims about concussions, even if each has a reason to wonder? Moreover, as the following cases illustrate, a dispreferred, potentially stigmatizing, diagnosis can be challenging to reconcile with other aspects of an individual's identity, such as sports hero, champion, or competitor.

Arthur Ashe

In a world trying to make sense of HIV/AIDS, tennis player Arthur Ashe had reason to hesitate before disclosing that he had contracted AIDS due to a blood transfusion. In an August 28, 1992, interview on *CBS This Morning*, Ashe noted,

> Well, the reaction to me has been positive. I haven't had any untoward or negative reactions from anybody—families, friends, commercial affiliations, what have you. To me, it's been terrific. But I keep reading in the paper that ordinary people with AIDS or who are diagnosed as HIV positive are not treated that way. And even acts of violence committed against HIV-positive people have increased, according to some informed sources. So I am just being treated differently [para. 3].

Clearly, by virtue of his status as a celebrated athlete, Arthur Ashe wasn't "ordinary," and others did not categorize (nor respond to) his condition as typical. As Ashe acknowledged, his health narrative differed from others who could not claim a "special case" or an exemption from being lumped in as one of "those" AIDS patients. He managed to avoid treatment as "one of them," reject a potential "victim" label, and emerge as a hero. Capitalizing on goodwill and wishes from other athletes and fans, Ashe founded the Arthur Ashe Foundation for the Defeat of AIDS and enlisted fellow tennis players to participate in benefit matches as a means of raising money. Only a little over five months after the *CBS This Morning* interview and benefit tennis tournament, Ashe passed away on February 6, 1993, at the age of 49.

Ashe was no longer a professional tennis player when he announced the AIDS diagnosis. He could have opted to remain silent and allow rumors about his health to circulate without addressing them. When he came forward, he risked negative public reaction but in terms of his reputation and legacy, not the potential of impacting a current career. Conversely, two other individuals wrestled with disclosing a potentially stigmatizing (and potentially career-ending) condition while in the prime and spotlight of their respective jobs as professional athletes.

Greg Louganis

Greg Louganis, an Olympic diver and medalist, kept mum about his status as HIV-positive prior to competing in the 1988 Olympics. In an excerpt in *People* magazine from his book, *Breaking the Surface*, Louganis (1995, March 6, p. 66) wrote, "Before the '88 Olympics, I had debated telling Dr. Puffer [the team physician] about my HIV status. It was irresponsible for me not to, but I didn't want him to have the burden of keeping such a difficult secret." After Louganis cut his head on a preliminary dive, Dr. Puffer attended to his injury without wearing gloves. Louganis recounted, "I wanted to warn Dr. Puffer, but I was paralyzed. All I could do was cry" (p. 66). Later, Louganis subsequently took to the podium, received another gold medal, heard the crowd applaud, and wondered, "What would the people cheering for me think if they knew I was gay and HIV-positive? Would they still cheer?" (p. 74). Louganis didn't take the chance on disrupting his status with fans or his team, revealing his diagnosis six years after he retired from competition. (According to Louganis, Dr. Puffer subsequently tested negative for HIV.)

Magic Johnson

Conversely, Magic Johnson chose to retire from the National Basketball Association very soon after learning of his HIV-positive status. Notably, Johnson's fairly immediate decision to retire reflects his at least initial assessment that this diagnosis disqualified him as a legitimate player in the league, i.e., affirming the viewpoint that someone in this health situation should/could not compete due to the possible risk to others. No coach or owner told him that he had to step off of the court. He did so of his own accord, implicitly acknowledging a perceived incompatibility between this particular illness narrative and his then current trajectory of playing basketball as a professional athlete.

Johnson contested that perspective when he initiated a return to the NBA months later, after researching more about the nature of his condition and the ways in which it could be transmitted, but his peers balked. McCallum (2001, August 20, p. 77) noted that "[m]edical expert after medical expert insisted that the chances of his infecting another player though incidental contact were infinitesimal, but that did not allay the fears. A number of NBA players … voiced strong concerns over Magic's playing." As McCallum reported, Johnson soon quit again, noting in his statement that "[i]t has become obvious that the various controversies surrounding my return are taking away from both basketball as a sport and the larger issue of living with HIV for me and the many people involved" (p. 78). Through their negative responses, stakeholders in the league reified Johnson's immediate gut reaction—a person living with HIV does not "fit" within the context of competition in the NBA.

Yet, Johnson still sought to compete for his life, both physically and personally, amid the societal and medical uncertainties of the early 1990s. Johnson made his dual decisions to retire and disclose the reason for the retirement quickly but not without apprehension and subsequent consequence. In an interview on *Face to Face with Connie Chung*, Johnson admitted his first reaction of fear, sharing, "Well, I—I was scared, yes. You know, I'd be lying if I didn't say I was scared, but I didn't think about—really, dying and death. The main thing was my wife, telling her, first of all" (Chung, 1991, December 11, para. 4). Johnson's wife, Cookie, responded with hurt, shock, and apprehension about her own health and that of their then unborn child. (Cookie and their child subsequently tested negative). However, Cookie's concern shifted swiftly to potential public reaction regarding Johnson, given the stigma surrounding the disease (Samuels, 2011, May 23).

In her interview, Chung referred to rampant rumors about Johnson's sexuality, length of time that he had known about the disease, and, even, the status of his condition, and she noted,

> Martina Navratilova said if she had gotten AIDS, people would have said: Oh, she's gay. She had it coming to her…. Also if a woman—a heterosexual woman had gotten AIDS—they'd say—from sleeping with people—they would have said: Oh, she's a whore, she's a slut and the corporations would have dropped her like a lead balloon [Chung, 1991, December 11, para. 65–67].

Johnson acknowledged the treatment of others in society who had been wrestling with the physical and societal consequences of an HIV/AIDS diagnosis, noting, "I understand completely. And I really—you know, I feel for them, really, because they've been fighting this and saying this for a long time. And even I had not been listening, you see?"

Soon, Johnson had to hear and confront personally unprecedented challenges as others continued to dispute his account of how he contracted the disease—what are the odds that a heterosexual male could contract HIV through sex with a woman? Perhaps even more than the perceived incompatibility of this illness narrative with the role of professional basketball player, some could not accept the idea that healthy, heterosexual males put themselves at risk for HIV/AIDS through sex with women. (For related work on narrative rationality, see Fisher, 1984, 1985a, 1985b, 1987a.) McCallum (2001, August 20) detailed,

> At least one influential journalist, Dave Kindred of *The Sporting News*, demanded that Magic "tell the whole truth about how he acquired the AIDS virus." For weeks the newspapers were filled with stories about how one of Magic's close friends, who turned out to be Isiah Thomas, had spread rumors that Magic was bisexual. Magic lost nearly all his endorsement deals after announcing he was positive. "And that was just what the public knew about," says Lon Rosen, Magic's former agent and a close friend. "What he went through in private—the things people said to him, the letters he got—was horrible." He had to deal with something else as well: the looks of pity [p. 78].

USA Today columnist Ian O'Connor (2001, November 7, p. 13C) commented that "[w]e all counted him as a dead man walking.... Then a strange thing happened on the way to the funeral.... The disease that would suck the life out of Arthur Ashe, among the great noblemen of sport, could not steal the light in Magic's eye." Johnson prodded through the stigma and conflict regarding *how* he became infected to flourishing—personally, professionally, and socially. Now 23 years since his fateful announcement, Johnson continues to thrive as a businessman and sports analyst (see magicjohnson.com) and to maintain his good health, a credit to carefully crafted pharmaceutical cocktails that prevent his condition from progressing to AIDS (see Hadhazy, 2011, November 7). He has also used his experience to enlighten others.

Writing at the 10-year milestone, McCallum (2001, August 20, p. 82) noted that Johnson "and Cookie believe he was chosen to get the disease 'because God needed someone and He picked me.'" According to Adler et al. (1991, November 18, p. 61), "The gist of Johnson's initial message has been that if *I* got it, everyone must worry about the AIDS virus." Soon after his disclosure, Adler et al. pointed to the potential for Johnson to be a powerful force as an advocate for HIV/AIDS activism:

But if the nation was saddened, it was galvanized, too. "If you tried to come up with the perfect person to carry the message of AIDS awareness to the people it ought to reach," said New York AIDS activist Rodger McFarlane, "you couldn't do better than Magic Johnson." The National AIDS Hotline lit up with 40,000 phone calls on the day of Johnson's announcement, instead of the usual 3,800. At the Centers for Disease Control in Atlanta, AIDS-related calls, which usually average 200 per hour, jumped to 10,000 in a single hour on a Thursday night [p. 59].

Magic had just joined another team.

Educating and Empowering the "Team"

Petronio (2002) explained that disclosing personal information reflexively and concurrently expands intimacy boundaries. Just as Magic had honed his skills as a professional athlete and contributed to the Los Angeles Lakers as an all-star basketball player, his revelation to the world that he had contracted HIV transitioned him from "only" an athlete to an individual with connections to broader communities—certainly, various global efforts to enlighten people about safe sex and HIV/AIDS as well as the smaller collection of individuals who continue to be linked by the results of a blood test. Magic was not merely a former Los Angeles Laker, sharing the traditions, values, and goals of that organization (see related work on teams by Cotterill, 2012; Syer, 1986). Magic's public disclosure, and subsequent work to raise awareness about HIV/AIDS prevention, shifted his focus from playing basketball to empowering others to avoid his mistakes (see B. Brown & Baranowski, 1996; Hollander, 1993; Kalichman & Hunter, 1992; Leerhsen et al., 1991, November 18). The ever inspiring Magic embraced a new team.

As we detail in this section, athletes who struggle with health-related challenges weigh potential consequences of disclosure for their careers amid possible benefits (both personally and societally) of revealing details to the public. Those who choose to transform private health narratives into public ones perform important work on behalf of health-related "teams" and, often prompt fans to take action as well.

INSPIRING THE "TEAM"

Throughout this chapter, we have described the challenge for athletes in navigating privacy boundaries while competing in professional sports—how should one negotiate personal health-related struggles while enacting the role of "athlete" to teammates and fans? In some cases, illness or injury end careers, and, as we mentioned earlier with Jackson and Louganis, the risk of losing chances to compete (or attain/maintain lucrative endorsements) can silence athletes or end careers. Yet, especially in this heavily mediated era, privacy cannot always be preserved, and, even if they could stay quiet, some athletes choose to utilize their fame and health experience as a means of helping others in some way ... altering their life narrative to "play" for and perhaps inspire a new "team."

Dave Dravecky

For over a year, Dave Dravecky, then pitcher for the San Francisco Giants, fought to return to the pitcher's mound, combatting cancer in his pitching arm and rehabbing to return to form (Dravecky, 1990; Dravecky & Dravecky, 1992). In his introduction to Dravecky's book, *Comeback*, Pastor Chuck Swindoll wrote:

> The whole sports world watched in amazement as the all-star hurler returned to the mound, confident and sure as ever. Many called it a miracle as he was reunited with his team, the San Francisco Giants.... Dave Dravecky was suddenly a synonym for *comeback*.... His next game was in Montreal. Excitement was at an all-time high. Throwing with a strange tingling sensation in his arm, Dave pitched well enough through five innings to be ahead 3–0.... In the bottom of the sixth ... Dave took his set, stared at first base to restrain a runner, pivoted, and, kicking high, he pushed off the rubber and let it fly. He didn't realize that it would be the last pitch of his life. A dull, sickening crack could be heard across the unusually quiet stadium.... Little did he realize, as he writhed in pain upon the ground, that he had delivered "the pitch heard round the world" [Dravecky, 1990, p. 16].

Dravecky retired from baseball and beat the cancer, but with a high price—the eventual amputation of his arm. Dealing with the loss of his arm, career, and dream weren't easy, but, through faith and determination, Dravecky persevered, and he now serves as a motivational speaker and co-founder (with wife Jan) of the Dave Dravecky Foundation of Hope for others who have been affected by cancer (http://express.howstuffworks.com/extraordinary-dravecky.htm). In his book, *When You Can't Come Back: A Story of Courage and Grace*, Dravecky recalled a scene from classic baseball movie, *Field of Dreams*, and positively reframes his cancer journey:

> In another scene from Field of Dreams, the hero, Ray Kinsella, tracks down an old ballplayer named "Moonlight" Graham, whose career in the majors was so short it wasn't even a flash in the pan. Graham was an old man now. He had become a doctor and had dedicated his life to alleviating suffering in the small town where he lived. Kinsella couldn't get over how short Graham's baseball career had been.

"For five minutes you were *that* close," Kinsella marveled. "It would kill some men to get that close to their dream and not touch it; they'd consider it a tragedy."

Graham looked him in the eye and with a wistful smile said, "Son, if I'd only gotten to be a doctor for five minutes, now that would have been a tragedy."

When I look back over the past four years and see all I've learned from other people who have suffered, all I've experienced of their love and all God has shown me of his mercy, I think: if I'd have continued as a ballplayer and missed that, now *that* would have been a tragedy [Dravecky & Dravecky, 1992, pp. 194–195].

Scott Hamilton

Figure skater Scott Hamilton has also shared his cancer journey with others, raising awareness about testicular cancer and prompting expressions of concern and well-wishes. In the introduction to Hamilton's 1997 *People* magazine article, fellow skater Kristi Yamaguchi noted that "I'd be at an appearance, and the first thing people would ask me was, 'how's Scott?'... It was amazing to me how many people wanted to know how he was feeling and to see him back on the ice" (Hamilton, 1997, September 8, p. 99).

Fan letters to the editor of *People* in a subsequent issue illustrated warmth for the skater as well as pointed to Hamilton as an inspiration. Caryn wrote, "As an oncology nurse I find that so often patients hear of only the horror stories of those who have cancer. Scott's story showed that cancer has the potential to be beaten with chemo, courage, and determination. Scott is not only a sports hero, but a hero to all cancer survivors" ("Mail," 1997, September 29, p. 4). Jeff wrote an even more personal tribute:

After reading your article I did a self-examination. Being a very healthy 28-year-old male, I figured what could I lose? That night I found a lump, and I was diagnosed with testicular cancer after a few visits to my doctor.... I often think what would have happened if I had not caught it early. I credit your magazine for heightening my awareness. Though very rare, testicular cancer has a 90 percent cure rate. I have no doubt I will be in that 90 percent ["Mail," 1997, September 29, p. 4].

Both Dravecky and Hamilton's upbeat survival stories contribute to broader narratives about cancer, empowering others through information, awareness, and alternate vistas from which to approach this illness. These athletes' willingness to share their struggles and successes with others beyond their intimate circles enables their individual journeys to serve as sources of hope and inspiration for many that they will never meet in person. Their public health narratives can also spark activism and advocacy.

RALLYING THE TEAM

As we argued in an earlier work (Beck et al., 2014), celebrity health narratives can provide a powerful platform for public conversations about particular diseases and health-related conditions, encouraging individuals who also face similar situations and lending a rallying cry for awareness, prevention, and additional research. In so doing, those athletes captain different sorts of teams—collections of individuals striving for a cure … the chance to live (if not play) another day … competing on a new, unfamiliar playing field for precious medical and financial resources. For example, the Cleveland Clinic, where Hamilton received care for his cancer, heralds Hamilton's activism:

> Scott Hamilton then turned his experience with cancer into an opportunity to help others with cancer and is now a lifetime spokesperson for the Cleveland Clinic Taussig Cancer Institute and the founder of the Scott Hamilton CARES Initiative, the Cancer Alliance for Research, Education and Survivorship. Through CARES, Scott champions the 4th Angel Mentoring Program, promotes ChemoCare.com and helps raise money for breakthrough cancer research. It is Scott's vision to eradicate cancer within his lifetime, and his mission remains to help find strategies to improve the quality of life for individuals with cancer ["About Scott Hamilton," 2014, June 3, para. 5].

Hamilton certainly isn't alone in efforts to channel a personal health challenge into something of value for the public good. Upon learning that his daughter (as well as others in her hospital unit) needed a bone marrow transplant, baseball player Rod Carew, "taking advantage of his Hall of Fame stature … began calling reporters, inviting TV crews to her ward and appearing in marrow donor drives" (J. Howard, 1996, May 16, p. 76). According to J. Howard, "Since then, the National Marrow Donor Program has experienced a threefold increase in calls to its 1–800-MARROW2 hotline. Enrollment in the program has leaped by 277,635" (p. 76).

Professional football player Chris Spielman and his wife, Stefanie, established the Stefanie Spielman Breast Cancer Research Fund after her diagnosis with breast cancer (Crane, 2001, p. A1). Indeed, as a result of the couple's intense advocacy efforts, one reporter referred to her as "the woman whose name has become synonymous with breast cancer survival and efforts to find a cure" (Crane, 2001, p. A1). Saunders (2009, November 19) saluted Stefanie's commitment to activism from the very beginning of her illness:

> With his wife facing chemotherapy and a mastectomy, Chris wanted to skip his upcoming professional season with the Buffalo Bills but debated how to explain his absence to the public. Stefanie saw the situation as an opportunity to serve her community. "Tell them I have breast cancer," she recalled telling her husband. "It may make one guy go home and say: 'Honey, my favorite football

player's wife has breast cancer. You got to remember to make that mammogram appointment'" [para. 10–12].

Sadly, Mrs. Spielman passed away in 2009 (Saunders, 2009, November 19), but the foundation continues and exceeded $11 million in donations in 2013 (https://chrisspielman.com/charities/stefanie-spielman-fund-for-breast-cancer-research/).

Major league baseball pitcher and cancer survivor Eric Davis set up a foundation to raise money for colorectal research; golfer Arnold Palmer spoke about his battle with cancer; boxer Muhammad Ali created the Muhammad Ali Parkinson Center. In tribute to his son, former NFL quarterback Doug Flutie formed the Doug Flutie, Jr. Foundation for Autism. Former NFL Hall of Fame quarterback Jim Kelly testified before Congress and founded Hunter's Hope Foundation in honor of his infant son who suffered from Krabbe Disease. After his death from cancer, Chicago Bear legend Walter Payton's widow spoke before the House Government Reform Committee as part of hearings on Integrative Oncology and established the Walter Payton Cancer Fund. Arguably one of the most famous athletes-turned-advocate, Tour de France winner Lance Armstrong won his battle against testicular cancer and championed the Lance Armstrong Foundation (subsequently the Livestrong Foundation), offering resources for cancer patients and survivors.

These cases all reflect a common trajectory—celebrated athletes experience a health-related challenge off of the field, course, or court and then embrace their fame as an opportunity to engage in dialogue about their particular illness, injury, or condition. Notably, athletes are uniquely situated to reframe personal health narratives as public conversations about an illness for two reasons. First, sports fans tend to be intensely loyal and intimately knowledgeable about their favorite athletes and teams (see, for example, Earnheardt et al., 2012; Hugenberg, Haridakis, & Earnheardt, 2008; Hutchins & Rowe, 2012; Sanderson, 2011). Second, as the following cases exemplify, individuals who dedicate years to perfecting pitches or plays can attack illness or injury with the same tenacity, seemingly adopting a sports model (i.e., complete with competitive and team-oriented rhetoric) for tackling the problem orientation. For example, invoking language such as "we" can "beat" or overcome the common "opponent" of cancer, Alzheimer's, or other conditions that affect millions and await a champion in the public sphere.

Pat Summitt

In her 2013 memoir, Pat Summitt chronicled her life from farm girl to legendary coach and detailed her agonizing decision to retire. When one physician recommended that she "needed to quit, and get myself out of the public eye as quickly as possible, or I would 'embarrass' myself and ruin my legacy" (Summitt, 2013, p. 17), Summitt responded with characteristic courage and spunk.

As long-time co-author and friend Sally Jenkins (2012, June) wrote, "Summitt has accepted the word 'can't' in only one instance of her life: On April 18 she was forced by her diagnosis of early-onset Alzheimer's to step aside as the women's basketball coach at Tennessee after 38 years and eight national championships" (p. 8). Yet, Summitt now brings her trademark tenacity and drive to her new team. Henderson (2013, November 10–16) reported:

> When not cheering on her beloved team, she is sharing her inspiring story and using her fame to fight a new opponent: Alzheimer's disease. In 2011, she launched the Pat Summitt Foundation to promote public awareness, advocate for patients, and fund research into the progressive and debilitating brain disease for which there is no known cure. "It is in my nature to be forthcoming, to confront things head-on," Summitt says. "I do not want a pity party for me. I want to use my energy and determination to help win the fight against Alzheimer's. I want my foundation to be part of the national team finding a cure for this disease" [p. 3].

According to Henderson, "instead of going into hiding, Summitt immediately began using her renown to shine a light on the disease she shares with 5 million Americans" (p. 8), implicitly sending the message that individuals with Alzheimer's and their loved ones don't have to hide, and they don't need to quietly accept their fate.

Through her foundation, book, and public engagements, Summitt has rallied others (even non-basketball fans) to the cause and inspired them to join the team against Alzheimer's. Henderson (2013, November 10–16) shared the following comment from the executive director of the Pat Summitt Foundation, Patrick Wade:

> On a daily basis, we hear from people who are donating that have no connection to basketball whatsoever or to Tennessee, but they've heard of Pat Summitt and are fans of hers just because of who she is and what she's doing…. Her celebrity status is bringing awareness to Alzheimer's in a way nothing else could have done [p. 6].

Boomer Esiason

Upon learning that his young son had cystic fibrosis, Boomer Esiason's first impulse was to retire. According to G. Smith (1993, October 4, p. 24), "Everything would have to change now. All the film study, practice sessions, football games, appearances, commercials, interviews, reunions, laughs … it would have to end. All the time and energy it took to be Boomer would have to go to the little boy." However, Esiason soon came to a different realization.

> He drove past Riverfront Stadium on the way home from the hospital.... A sad song was playing on the radio. He kept looking at the stadium. It just didn't feel right, turning inward to fight this war, becoming smaller. He snapped off the sad song. "No," he decided. "I'm not going to quit. They won't listen to me if I quit or have a bad year. I'm going to have a great year. I'm going to go on a crusade. They'll listen to me if I have a great year. They'll *have* to listen. They'll *have* to" [G. Smith, 1993, October 4, p. 24].

One fan responded to the *Sports Illustrated* article with a letter to the editor, voicing the public support that Boomer hoped to attain:

> After reading your story about Boomer and Gunnar Esiason, I've decided to root for the Jets. If their success will give Boomer a better forum for raising funds for cystic fibrosis, I can't think of a better reason to become a fan. As a father of two, I'd like to express my gratitude for their good health by helping Boomer beat this thing. Would you please print the address of the Cystic Fibrosis Foundation? ["Letters," 1993, October 11, p. 8].

Building on his work on the football field and subsequent media attention, Boomer founded the Boomer Esiason Foundation to raise money for research and even testified before Congress, appealing for federal funds. Like Pat Summitt, Boomer continues to use his famous face as a means of attracting attention to a cause that might otherwise not garner public interest or understanding. As Beck et al. (2014, p. 251) noted, "As celebrities march up Capitol Hill, they symbolically lead the charge for others who confront the same health circumstance but lack the social, cultural, and/or political clout to warrant an invitation into the hallowed halls of Congress."

Just over 20 years after Boomer began the most important drive of his career, we're delighted to share that, as we finalize this book, "[f]or Gunnar Esiason, the clock is still running—and for Boomer Esiason's kid, that means he is winning the game of life" (Herzog, 2013, June 18, para. 1). No, Gunnar has not been cured of this (thus far) incurable disease. Yet, his younger sister remarked, "When I wake up and I'm not feeling well or if I just don't want to start my day, I think about him and I know he's feeling 10 times worse than I am and he's always upbeat and doing all the things everyone else is doing or should be doing'" (Herzog, 2013, June 18, para. 10). A recent college graduate considering law school in the future, according to Herzog, Gunnar has "discussed with Boomer taking an expanded role in the foundation. 'I'll continue my poster boy role. I've accepted that.... Who better to do it than me? I can see that being a career for me, living as the poster boy and making sure the disease is eventually cured'" (para. 8).

As Boomer Esiason was grasping his son's diagnosis and beginning his fight against cystic fibrosis, some 20 years ago, another relatively young and famous sports professional, with children of his own, heard the life-altering words, "Coach.... I'm 90-percent sure this is cancer" (Vitale, 1994, April, p. 81), and former North Carolina State University basketball coach Jim Valvano responded by recruiting an all-star team against the deadly disease ("Our Story: 'Don't give up ... don't ever give up,'" 2013).

Jim Valvano

Notably, the three featured cases in this section—Pat Summitt, Boomer Esiason, and Jim Valvano—epitomize narratives that explicitly embrace a competitive sports orientation. Especially in the latter case, Valvano employed language directly borrowed from sports discourse. He referred to "beating" an opponent (the illness), "recruiting" others to "join a team," referring to eventual "victory," and even acknowledging the implicit competition between various advocacy groups for precious, limited research dollars.

To begin, Valvano actively joined the team of individuals struggling with cancer, continuing to appear in public and exposing the ravages of this illness. He did not "sugarcoat" or mask the toll that cancer (and related treatments) took on his formerly strong, athletic body. One of his daughters, Jamie Valvano Howard, (2013, May 16) wrote:

> He spent the final ten months of his life giving the world personal insights into the life of a cancer patient in the hope that he could bring some attention to the disease that affects millions. He was not afraid to let others witness his weakening body or the tears that he shed when he spoke of his certain death during interviews and public appearances [para. 9].

As sports writer Gary Smith (1993, January 11, p. 14) observed, "He lived in a land where people vanished when they became terminally ill," yet Valvano refused to quietly slip away. Smith quoted Valvano as commenting, "I want to help every cancer patient I can now. For some reason, people look to me for hope. I'm feeling half dead, and they're coming up to me in the hospital for *hope*. I don't know if I can handle that, but it's the only conceivable good that can come out of this" (p. 20).

Yet, much more good could (and did) come from Valvano's very public health narrative. Valvano expressed outrage about what he considered to be complacence about funding for cancer research, especially when compared to celebrity attention to other more popular causes:

> *Half a million people* die of cancer every year in America, one out of every four of us will get it, and there's no moral outrage; we *accept* it. I'm all for AIDS fund-

ing and research, but how can the government give 10 times as much per AIDS patient as per cancer patient? Barbra Streisand isn't singing for cancer, Elizabeth Taylor isn't holding a celebrity bash for cancer [Smith, 1993, January 11, p. 20].

According to Kreis (2013, May 16), "Friends like Mike Krzyzewski comment, 'Jimmy formed the V Foundation during the last couple months of his life.... One night he said, "I want to try to fund cancer research. I want you to be on my team!" He recruited me during that time. His wisdom and his ability to think beyond his life was incredible'" (para. 2). Only a few months before he would succumb to his illness, on March 4, 1993, a very fragile Valvano received the first ever Arthur Ashe Courage and Humanitarian Award at the ESPY Awards ceremony. His friend, Dick Vitale, recalled later that "[t]he cancer had advanced, and Jim thought he might not make the ceremony.... He looked weak, his skin a pale olive color ... [yet] Jimmy drew from some final reserve of energy, deep in his heart, as if his life wouldn't be complete without sending out his message one last time" (1994, April, p. 82). Giving one of the most memorable and powerful speeches in sports history, Valvano stood at the podium, expressed gratitude for the award, and then implored others to join him in the fight against cancer:

> Now I look at where I am now and I know what I want to do. What I would like to be able to do is spend whatever time I have left and to give, and maybe, some hope to others. Arthur Ashe Foundation is a wonderful thing, and AIDS, the amount of money pouring in for AIDS is not enough, but is significant. But if I told you it's ten times the amount that goes in for cancer research. I also tell you that five hundred thousand people will die this year of cancer. I also tell you that one in every four will be afflicted with this disease, and yet somehow, we seem to have put it in a little bit of the background. I want to bring it back on the front table. We need your help. I need your help. We need money for research. It may not save my life. It may save my children's lives. It may save someone you love. And ESPN has been so kind to support me in this endeavor and allow me to announce tonight, that with ESPN's support, which means what? Their money and their dollars and they're helping me—we are starting the Jimmy V Foundation for Cancer Research. And its motto is "Don't give up, don't ever give up." That's what I'm going to try to do every minute that I have left. I will thank God for the day and the moment I have. If you see me, smile and give me a hug. That's important to me too. But try if you can to support, whether it's AIDS or the cancer foundation, so that someone else might survive, might prosper and might actually be cured of this dreaded disease [1993, March 4, para. 8].

Vitale (1994, April, p. 82) noted that [i]n the months that followed, Jimmy's speech rallied support for cancer research and inspired thousands of cancer victims, who heard the message that Jimmy Valvano had spent a career telling his players: *Don't give up. Don't ever give up."* Nineteen years later, his daughter, Jamie Valvano Howard (2012, November 27) commented on the V Foundation website,

> As a daughter and cancer survivor I will carry the memories of that night with me forever, but I continue to be astounded by the individuals from all over the country that have been changed by his words. Just a few months ago I was reminded again of the impact of the ESPY speech. The middle school where I teach has the "Don't Give up.... Don't Ever Give Up" quote painted on the gymnasium wall. When I shared with my students that I was Jimmy V's daughter, one girl became teary. She revealed that every year her entire family watches the ESPY speech to celebrate her Dad remaining cancer free [para. 4].

To this day, Valvano's speech (and that classic line) echo through cancer and sports communities, and his foundation has thrived. Colleagues in the college basketball and broadcasting communities did, indeed, join his team, hosting special events (such as golf tournaments) and donating money for three-point shots during an annual cancer awareness week near the beginning of each college basketball season. In spite of the fact that Coach Valvano passed away over 20 years ago, his team against cancer continues to rally and fight on his behalf. The V Foundation website proclaims Valvano's legacy and success in building a team that endures and prospers two decades later:

> Although Jim lost his battle with cancer less than two months after delivering the ESPY speech, his dream of a cure lives on through research grants.... The V Foundation has awarded more than $100 million to more than 100 facilities nationwide and proudly awards 100 percent of direct donations and net event proceeds to cancer research ["Our story: 'Don't give up ... don't ever give up,'" 2013, para. 4].

Discussion

Tough. Tenacious. Resilient. Strong. Fit. Success in collegiate or professional athletics mandates careful and artful attention to sculpting and training bodies that can compete and excel. As the stories of athletes in this chapter illustrate, illness narratives introduce jarring disruptions to lives in progress, and diagnoses (and subsequent struggles with treatment, rehab, and/or other challenges) can be especially difficult to reconcile with attributes of strength, endurance, and drive, all intricately interwoven with athlete identity.

Certainly, the unexpected twist of a broken arm, diagnosis of a chronic condition, or battle with a life-threatening illness shifts attention, momentarily or permanently, from assumed, mundane, often taken-for-granted abilities and moments to prioritizing medical issues (and negotiating health-related obstacles)—for nonathletes and athletes alike. However, enacting what would otherwise entail a private health narrative in a very public arena poses threats to an athlete's preferred (and painstakingly cultivated) identity amid the potential stigma (not to mention loss of income, endorsements, and fame) that could come from not being able to perform as expected (or at all).

To what extent has a deeply rooted culture of playing through pain impacted discourse about traumatic head injuries, for example? What messages do athletes send as they navigate physical concerns (visible and not), face preferences, and social responsibility to admirers (including young people) and others who wrestle with similar challenges? Our conversation in this chapter about identity management in light of illness/injury narratives for sports professionals underscores the complexity of co-negotiating physical, emotional, financial, and social concerns during private yet quite public health sagas.

Although difficult, the interruption of an individual's journey as an athlete or sports professional with an illness or injury also affords unique opportunities for advocacy. Societal and mediated attention to professional athletes positions them on a prominent stage for raising awareness about the importance of early detection and treatment options and provides them with a loud megaphone for "recruiting" a "team" or encouraging donations to a cause. Although we acknowledge the good that has come from public-service efforts by teams and individuals, we herald the efforts of athletes who become vital parts of new "teams," by virtue of a common affliction. As we have documented throughout this book, personal stories, especially from celebrated athletes, become persuasive and powerful contributions to public dialogues about health.

CHAPTER NINE

Blurring "Real" Life
and "Reel" Life

Integration of Daytime Drama Actor Illnesses into Soap Opera Storylines and Health Promotion

Jeanne Cooper portrayed Katherine Chancellor on the daytime drama *The Young and the Restless* for more than 40 years—from the show's premiere on March 26, 1973, until her death on May 8, 2013, at the age of 84. Over four decades, audiences watched Cooper's riveting performances as Katherine lost her husband to a much younger woman, struggled with alcohol, and then thrived as a businesswoman, friend, and mother, not, of course, without much more sudsy plot turmoil along the way.

In 1984, viewers also witnessed an unprecedented event on television—Cooper's real-life face-lift. In her autobiography, *Not Young, Still Restless,* Cooper (2012, p. 102) explained, "More and more often, I found myself looking in the mirror and wondering where 'I' had gone. Rather than seeing fifty-five year old Jeanne Cooper, I kept staring at someone who was wearing every hurt, every moment of stress, every disappointment ... and I hated it."

After deciding on the procedure, Cooper discussed the implications of the decision for her character with *The Young and the Restless* cocreator, Bill Bell. Rather than attempt to ignore the actress' actual face-lift, they forged ahead with the plan not simply to acknowledge it but to integrate the face-lift journey into Katherine's storyline as well. Cooper (2012, p. 103) explained,

> Bill Bell was ecstatic and readily agreed to my demand that it be shot documentary style—no special effects, no "prettying it up" for the cameras. "If we're going to do this, let's do it right, let's do it for 'real,' and let's do it honest," I said. "Let's have Katherine show people who are afraid of plastic surgery exactly what it's like and what a difference it can make."

Cooper (2012, p. 103) acknowledged that "[a]s had happened more times than I can count over all these years, Katherine and I had hit simultaneous low periods in our lives. She was feeling as 'used up' as I was." Cooper recalled one particularly pivotal scene in crystalizing Katherine's motivation to get a face-lift:

> Katherine slowly began disassembling herself, removing her glittering gown ... her makeup ... her false eyelashes ... at that moment in time, as far as she was concerned, the whole carefully constructed disguise she wore to trick people into thinking she was still an attractive, vibrant woman.... As she looked in the mirror, her façade crumbled, exposing the flawed, fading, empty shell she felt she'd become [p. 104].

Episodes of *The Young and the Restless* featured the actual surgery, becoming, as Cooper (2012, p. 107) asserted in her book, "television's very first reality show." In so doing, the on-screen face-lift not only bolstered ratings and addressed Cooper's (and Katherine's) new appearance. It also sent a message of inspiration and reassurance to viewers about the possibilities of plastic surgery. Cooper noted,

> I got literally thousands of letters from people all over the United States and Europe telling me that watching Katherine Chancellor's face-lift defused their fears of plastic surgery—a big accomplishment in the 1980s when it wasn't nearly as common as it is today. It was even more gratifying that, as I'd hoped, the vast majority of mail came from men and women who'd been considering plastic surgery not for the sake of vanity but to correct some birth defect or trauma-induced disfigurement that had created a barrier between themselves and their God-given right to enjoy full, confident lives [p. 106].

Jeanne Cooper could have been just one more actress to quietly enhance her appearance through a face-lift. However, by allowing her experience to be interwoven with her character's saga on the show, Cooper brought plastic surgery out of the shadows and into the spotlight. Notably, as we detail in this chapter, the nature of the soap opera genre affords performers and writers a very prominent and personal platform for educating viewers who continue to "tune in tomorrow."

For over 70 years, daytime dramas have entered homes daily via radio, television, and, now, the Internet, and actors, such as Jeanne Cooper, routinely continue their roles for decades (Ford, De Kosnik, & Harrington, 2011a, 2011b; Hinsey, 2011). Thus, instead of an episode of a prime-time show or television movie about a face-lift, *The Young and the Restless* embedded this storyline in a continuing drama, about a character who had been on the air for over a decade and who remained on the show for nearly 30 more years. Moreover, fans did not simply care about the character; they loved Jeanne, as a person.

Soap fans connect strongly with long-term soap opera actors, especially as they read about them, interact with them (during personal appearances, exchanging letters, and now through social media), and, quite frankly, age with them as both fans, characters, and actors embark on their respective (yet intertwining) life journeys (see Beck, 2012).

This chapter highlights the unique opportunity for soap opera actors to employ not only their celebrity status but also their roles on daytime dramas to bring attention to and understanding of a health condition, especially when that issue affects them personally. In this chapter, we describe the willingness of some performers to blur boundaries between "real life" and "reel life" and integrate actual health situations into storylines on the show, enabling soap operas to wrestle with issues such as bipolar disorder, cancer, ALS, diabetes, substance abuse, weight issues, and, yes, even a face-lift, with added realism and humanity (see also related work by Beck, 2012). After providing background on intersecting life narratives between long-term soap opera actors and their characters, we offer exemplars of celebrity health narratives that blur public-private boundaries on daytime dramas and, in so doing, richly contribute to health education and promotion. The chapter concludes by highlighting implications of these deeply personal storylines for edutainment, health promotion, and health advocacy.

Intersecting Narratives: The Unique Case of the Soap Opera Genre

As Ford et al. (2011a, 2011b) detailed, the soap opera genre constitutes a unique form of entertainment, literally spanning decades and touching the lives of millions of viewers across generations. Ford et al. asserted that "[t]he longevity of soaps, as well as certain characteristics of soaps' narrative structures, has given rise to forms of committed viewing that few other television genres can rival" (2011a, p. 5). In this section, we argue that years of long-term storytelling uniquely situate soap operas for telling stories that matter to fans and for enabling those stories to resonate with fans because they care about the actors as well as the characters.

STORIES THAT MATTER

Scholars have documented the exceptional investment of soap opera fans to "their" stories (see, e.g., Brunsdon, 2000; Harrington & Bielby, 1995; Hayward, 1997; Hobson, 2003; Matelski, 1999; Morton, 1997; Spence, 2005;

Williams, 1992; Wittebols, 2004). Others have investigated the captivating, enduring narratives that inspire viewers to "tune in tomorrow," year after year, decade after decade (see, e.g., Matelski, 1988; Mumford, 1995; Scodari, 2004).

Over those decades, soap opera writers have entertained viewers with tales of "love in the afternoon" as well as educated audiences. As Hinsey (2011, p. 162) noted, "Interracial romance, homosexuality, divorce, alcoholism, mental illness, unwanted pregnancy, abortion, impotence, addiction, incest, Down Syndrome, suicide, anorexia, HIV/AIDS, rape, adultery … you name it. Daytime has dealt with it. NO other form of entertainment has so effectively addressed social issues."

On *General Hospital*, viewers mourned little BJ after her school bus collided with a car driven by a drunk driver, witnessed the bittersweet moment when BJ's heart saved her young cousin, Maxie's, life, and learned valuable lessons about drunk driving and organ donation in the process. *As The World Turns'* Mac (and, more recently, *Days of Our Lives'* Caroline) developed Alzheimer's disease, and viewers observed as Mac, his wife, Nancy, and their family and friends struggled with the diagnosis, devastating symptoms, and his eventual death. *Bold and the Beautiful, Young and the Restless, All My Children*, and *General Hospital* have all poignantly woven HIV/AIDS story-lines on their respective canvases.

For example, Mumford (1997) described *General Hospital's* HIV/AIDS storyline in which Robin Scorpio, a teen-ager whom audiences literally watched grow up before their eyes, became HIV-positive after unprotected sex. Mumford explained that "[t]he choice to make Robin, a regular character for more than a decade, HIV-positive personalized the issue for viewers who had grown attached to her through the years as well as serving the didactic purpose of stressing the risks of unprotected sex" (p. 107).

General Hospital's Monica and *Guiding Light's* Lillian both fought breast cancer, impacting the fictional communities of Port Charles and Springfield, respectively, as well as actual fans of these cherished core characters. In her book, *Changing Shoes*, Tina Sloane recalled the overwhelming response to her character, Lillian's, breast cancer storyline on *Guiding Light*:

> This was the first time that breast cancer had been dealt with on daytime television, and the story went on for about a year and helped millions of women by raising awareness.… After each show, I would appear in a public service announcement and urge women to check for breast cancer, and the response was phenomenal. Phone calls and letters poured in, and I received multiple awards, including one from the American Cancer Society for raising awareness and inspiring the largest turnout for mammograms in their history. Women who had survived breast cancer told me that in crying for Lillian they were finally able to cry for themselves [2010, p. 79].

In their related research, other authors have commented on the powerful use of soap operas, especially beyond the United States, to enlighten viewers about health issues and to motivate them for social change (see, e.g., de Block, 2012; Gesser-Edelsburg & Endevelt, 2011; Kennedy, Beck, & Freimuth, 2008; Kennedy, O'Leary, Beck, Pollard, & Simpson, 2004; Klein, 2011, 2012; Mohammed, 2001; Moyer-Gusé, Chung, & Jain, 2011; Nariman, 1993; Redmon, 2013, July–August; Singhal, Cody, Rogers, & Sabido, 2004; Singhal & Rogers, 1999, 2003; Vaughan, Rogers, Singhal, & Swalehe, 2000; Vu & Lee, 2013; Wang & Singhal, 1992). Notably, U.S. soap operas do not typically fit the criteria for "entertainment-education" in that storyline decisions prioritize entertainment and do not usually privilege expanding "audience knowledge about an educational issue, create favorable attitudes, and change overt behavior" (Singhal & Rogers, 1999, p. xii; for additional work on entertainment-education, see also Gesser-Edelsburg & Endevelt, 2011; Klein, 2011, 2012; Petchauer, 2012).

However, in a rare exception, in consultation with the Hollywood, Health, and Society program based at the University of Southern California, *Bold and the Beautiful* (a soap opera that is produced in the United States but broadcast throughout the world) deliberately crafted a storyline featuring Kristen, a member of the core Forrester family. Her fiancé, Tony, revealed that he tested HIV-positive. Although the family wrestled with the unhappy news, Kristen decided to marry Tony anyway (and they eventually adopted an AIDS orphan from Africa). The show also produced and aired PSA announcements after select episodes and encouraged viewers to call hotlines for more information (see Kennedy et al., 2008; Kennedy et al., 2004; O'Leary et al., 2007), and viewers lit up the phone lines.

The *Bold and the Beautiful* HIV/AIDS storyline underscores the rich potential of soap operas to provide information in a powerful and intimate manner. Whether strategically planned for educational or persuasive purposes or not, soap opera storylines hold great potential for impacting viewers. As Sloan (2010) noted, fans care about the characters (and the actors who portray them), and, when something happens to their on-screen "families," they respond.

Connecting with Characters and Actors

The sheer longevity of soap operas contributes to another distinctive feature of the genre—the long-term portrayal of a character by a single actor for decades. As Eileen Fulton wrote in her autobiography (1995, p. 230), she spent "over three decades of living in Oakdale [as] Lisa Miller Hughes Eldridge Shea Coleman (almost Hadley) McColl Mitchell." Fulton celebrated her 40th anniversary on *As the World Turns* just prior to the show's cancellation in 2010. When cast on *All My Children*, Susan Lucci (2011, p. 65) noted that she "knew, without a doubt, that Erica Kane was 'the part of a lifetime.'" Yet, as Lucci shared in her memoirs, "I had no idea that this expression would end up being so literal in my case," with her work on the ABC soap opera spanning four decades, 21 Emmy nominations, and one Emmy award for best actress.

The winner of four Emmy awards for best actress, Kim Zimmer developed the iconic role of Reva Shane on *Guiding Light* in 1985, and, even though she was "only" on the show for 26 years, Zimmer heralded the interconnections between the lives of the fans, characters, and actors. Zimmer introduced her 2011 book, *I'm Just Sayin'! Three Deaths, Seven Husbands, and a Clone! My Life as a Daytime Diva*, with the following passage:

> I thought many times about writing a firsthand account of life as a "daytime diva," but as with many things, procrastination set in and my schedule was substantially full and eventually the desire faded. However, all that changed on the morning it was announced that *Guiding Light*, the oldest show in broadcast history, was being cancelled after a seventy-two-year run....
>
> I wanted to have something that I could share with the lifelong and devoted followers of *Guiding Light*. You are the generations of viewers who got to share our stories with us. There were times when I was honored to meet as many as four, or occasionally even more, generations of viewers at an event, all of whom were so proud to tell me about passing this show down from generation to generation within their family! I was a fan of the show too, and as you will read, just as hurt and confused by its cancellation as everyone else [p. ix].
>
> So it's with great pride and appreciation that I present this book to all of you who stuck with us through thick and thin, eight presidents, five major wars, innumerable marriages, divorces, births, deaths, and so much more! Please enjoy this fanciful and thoughtful journey through the parallel lives of Kim Zimmer and Reva Shayne [p. xii].

Bill Hayes and Susan Seaforth Hayes met on the NBC soap opera *Days of Our Lives* in 1970, and they married in real life in 1974. Hayes and Seaforth Hayes (2005, p. 87) also pointed to parallel life journeys between their real and reel lives, disclosing in their joint memoir that "[t]he viewers wanted a happy ending [for their characters]. 'We know they're married in real life, so why not on the show?' the producers' mail kept whining.... Ultimately the producers caved in and made the most of the obvious." Although not the focus of a current storyline on *Days*, they continue to make occasional appearances on the show, some 40 years later, with frequent absences explained by the couple's love for travel. As Mary Stuart, who portrayed Jo for years on the daytime drama *Search for Tomorrow* acknowledged in her autobiography, *Both of Me*, "What was happening in each life off the show became inevitably a part of the daily episode in some way" (1980, p. 130).

Beck (2012) posed a theoretical argument for the passion of soap opera fans, contending that part of the commitment to soap operas by long-time viewers involves the interwoven nature of life narratives by fans, characters, and actors. Although others have examined the usefulness of soap opera storylines to communicate health information as characters experience health challenges, in the rest of this chapter, we affirm that soap opera actors who allow their actual health situations to become part of their characters' storylines also embrace an opportunity to underscore the relevance and consequentiality of those conditions for viewers who are fans of the show, the character, and, indeed, the actor.

Exemplars of Blurred Boundaries in Daytime Drama for Health Education and Promotion

Only two days after Jeanne Cooper passed away at age 84, *The Young and the Restless* announced that she would be the focus of yet another unprecedented event. Usually, daytime dramas do not "break the fourth wall" by acknowledging and addressing an actor's death during an actual episode of a show. (Soap operas do routinely dedicate an episode to a fallen cast or crew member with a note at the beginning or end of a given episode.) Although *The Young and the Restless* planned to address the character's death at a later date, show officials decided that they needed to allow time for fans and colleagues to mourn Jeanne first. Thus, they devoted an entire episode on May 28, 2013, to a tribute of Jeanne Cooper's life by inviting fellow cast members to tell real-life stories about (and in remembrance of) the cherished matriarch of the 40-year-old soap opera. An official at CBS noted that "[t]he cast will honor their longtime friend, family member and coworker in the greatest way possible, as we celebrate her life and vibrant spirit and share it with the audience who loved her as much as we did" (Gennis, 2013, May 10, para. 3).

Although daytime dramas had never before paused "reel-life" stories to create space for a "real-life" memorial service, writers and producers routinely face the challenge of somehow addressing actual situations involving actors as they become evident to the audience. For example, fans know that *Bold and the Beautiful's* Darlene Conley passed away from cancer in 2007, but her character, "Sally Spectra," lives on by traveling the world off-screen. However, the blurring of "real-life" and "reel-life" becomes even more consequential when actors remain with the show while confronting a physical challenge and, as Cooper did with her face-lift, suggest that their characters embark on that same life trajectory. In so doing, as the following sections elaborate, that blurring results in a dual focus on the issue as both the actor and the character face implications and complications, both on- and off-screen.

RAISING AWARENESS ABOUT COSMETIC ALTERNATIVES

When *Guiding Light* transitioned from radio to television, the actors wondered how audiences would react to seeing them, not just hearing them. In the special 70th anniversary episode that aired on January 25, 2007 (http://www.imdb.com/title/tt0950929/), cast members reenacted reactions to news that they would be airing live television broadcasts as well as performing the same episode, also live that same day, on the radio in the usual time slot, with more than one questioning if actors would look as audience members had envisioned them. Indeed, when listeners heard radio broadcasts, they could only imagine the images to go with character voices. With *Guiding Light*'s move to television on June 30, 1952 (http://en.wikipedia.org/wiki/Guiding_Light), immediately, actor (and character) appearance became important production considerations.

Caitlyn Van Zandt

In 2006, *Guiding Light* introduced "Ashlee," a smart, loyal teen who happened to be overweight. However, in 2008, after two years of portraying one of the few heavier characters on daytime drama, Caitlin Van Zandt told producers that she had decided to undergo lap band surgery. Believing that she could positively influence viewers, Van Zandt asked if her real-life choice could be woven into her character's storyline.

In a *TV Guide* interview with the actress, interviewer Michael Logan noted, "Lap-Band surgery isn't controversial. It's minimally invasive, unlike gastric by-pass, and considered safe—yet your choice to have it stirred up controversy" (Guiding Light star weighs in on weight-loss story," 2008, May 28, para. 1). In that same article, Van Zandt responded:

> Celebrities talk about everything from their drug rehab stints to the people they've slept with, yet I've gotten flack on the Internet for doing the Lap-Band as if I'm somehow being a bad role model. A lot of the fans relate to me because I'm real-looking—which I think is wonderful—but they also had this predisposed notion that I was proud of the way I looked. Truth is, I've been self-conscious about my weight since I was a kid. I haven't worn a bathing suit since I was 6—we even used that as a line on the show [para. 2].

Other than the bathing suit line (and a bit of self-doubt during a breakup), fan surprise could be attributed to the character's apparent acceptance of her weight. Indeed, according to Tan (2008, May 26), Ashlee was created to be "a full-figured character" (para. 3). Yet, after receiving approval from the show, Van Zandt underwent the surgical procedure that dramatically altered her own, as well as Ashlee's, appearance, prompting a strong reaction from some fans. According to Tan, "While she remains sensitive to her fan's concerns, Van Zandt—who has dropped 41 lbs and is down to a size 14—says she has no regrets. 'I chose to take control of my life and raise awareness that you can be healthy'" (para. 4). Indeed, the actress uploaded a video diary on YouTube of her weight-loss journey and also became a spokesperson for "The Moment is Now," an obesity health education campaign ("Guiding Light star talks about her weight loss surgery," 2008, September 30, para. 1). Even viewers who did not necessarily like or agree with the changes for "Ashlee" on *Guiding Light* could learn about positive ways that the procedure impacted Van Zandt because of her willingness to share her experiences beyond the scripted storyline on the show.

Alison Sweeney

Like Van Zandt, Alison Sweeney ("Sami," *Days of Our Lives*) struggled with her weight both on and off camera. As Sweeney wrote in her 2004 book, *All the Days of My Life (So Far)*, the show brought her on with a bulimia storyline already in mind, not aware that the actress had been "absolutely obsessed with and fixated on my weight" (p. 81). Sweeney wrote,

> At the time, newspapers and magazines were filled with articles about Tracy Gold ... who had gone public in 1992 about her personal struggle with self-induced starvation (anorexia nervosa) beginning at age twelve. So at *Days* ... everyone was more sensitive than usual about the dieting obsessions and the devastating eating disorders that can occur with young actresses. They wanted to make sure that in playing a bulimic, I didn't become so immersed in my character that I lapsed into an eating disorder in real life [p. 82].

Sami's battle with bulimia resonated with fans, and, in her book, as Sweeney (2004) expressed gratitude for being "involved in episodes like these that have confronted very important issues in the lives of our viewers, and really touched people's lives" (p. 84). Sweeney praised the producers for always accepting her body shape, even though she was a few pounds over her ideal weight. Yet, her size continued to be an issue for some in the press as well as "mean-spirited fans" (p. 164), casting directors, and even herself.

Yet, as Sweeney (2004), also now the host of NBC's *The Biggest Loser*, revealed, "Once I changed my primary goal from being superthin to being superhealthy—and once I stopped bashing myself and hating myself because of what the scale said—I lost a lot of weight" (p. 189), "and I was deluged with hundreds of letters and e-mails, with fans asking how I had slimmed down" (p. 192). Sweeney noted that "they've been motivated by my own success. Many have cheered me on. Or they've thanked me for publicly acknowledging that the battle to lose weight isn't an easy one" (p. 194).

Interestingly, Sweeney lost a good bit of her weight during the time that her alter ego was on death row for a crime that she didn't commit. Wearing loose fitting prison uniforms, "Sami's" weight loss wasn't apparent until after she was exonerated (as chemicals dripped into her body in the death chamber—long story) and released. Viewers could attribute the character's dramatic weight loss to the stress of prison and her impending sentence, and the actress has openly discussed her weight issues with fans during events, magazine interviews, and her book as well as through letters, e-mail, and now social media. With the decision to host *Biggest Loser*, Sweeney continues to provide valuable information and inspiration to others about successful strategies for healthy eating and exercising.

RAISING AWARENESS ABOUT ILLNESSES

In addition to acknowledging and addressing physical changes of cast members, such as weight loss, soap operas have also provided a platform for education and inspiration by linking "reel" and "real" health issues. As we share in this section, storylines become even more riveting (and powerful) when actors' actual health situations get woven on to the canvas as part of their respective characters' emergent narratives as well.

Linsey Godfrey

When Linsey Godfrey was hired on *Bold and the Beautiful* for the role of "Caroline," she figured that makeup artists would likely have to cover up the tattoo on the back of her neck. Indeed, according to Beagan (2012, July 1), "When she was hired, she was told her character did not have any tattoos" (para. 23). A childhood survivor of Hodgkin's lymphoma in real life, Godfrey had obtained the tattoo, a survivor ribbon, along with her mother and sisters, "in celebration of her recovery" (Beagan, 2012, July 1, para. 23).

The production staff did not know about Godfrey's history with cancer prior to coincidentally casting her as the namesake of an original character who had passed away from leukemia. Beagan (2012, July 1, para. 23) noted that "[w]hen producers saw the tattoo and learned Linsey's story, they rewrote the story line and incorporated the tattoo into an episode that aired in April." On the show, the character purportedly obtained the tattoo in honor of her late aunt for whom she was named, "Caroline Spencer."

Currently a celebrity ambassador for the Leukemia and Lymphoma Society (LLS), Godfrey has garnered attention from her role on *Bold and the Beautiful* into advocating for a cause very near and dear to her heart. In a mini-documentary with boyfriend Robert Adamson ("Noah," *Young and the Restless*) posted on YouTube (http://www.youtube.comwatch?v-P1AoNuL1We), Godrey and her mother emotionally described their experience with cancer and passionately encouraged others to support LLS and its fundraiser, "Light the Night 2013."

In addition to urging viewers to "join my team" for the event (see also http://pages.lightthenight.org/los/UCLA13/ohmygodfrey) , in the mini documentary, Godfrey referred to an online auction for a tour of the *Bold and the Beautiful* set and lunch in the CBS commissary as part of her personal efforts to raise money for the organization that she credits with sponsoring research that saved her life. One fan responded to the mini-documentary by commenting in the YouTube discussion section, "I got teary-eyed watching this video! Your story really touched my heart ... I really love your role as Caroline Spencer on B&B! You are truly an inspiration!"

Through her work on *Bold and the Beautiful*, Godfrey has a huge platform for bringing dual attention to LLS (as she portrays a character with a family history of cancer and shares her own story as a real-life cancer survivor). On December 10, 2013, CBS proclaimed that "[a]ccording to the most recent statistics and Guinness World Records, THE BOLD AND THE BEAUTIFUL is the world's most popular daytime TV soap opera. Since its first episode in 1987, THE BOLD AND THE BEAUTIFUL ... has established a daily viewership of 35 million globally" ("This just in," 2014, February 3).

Charita Bauer

Notably, on the show, Godfrey's "Caroline" has not suffered from cancer, but actual illness journeys have been written into character storylines to parallel an actor's diagnosis, with powerful messages for viewers. Over 50 years ago, in 1962, Charita Bauer portrayed matriarch Bert Bauer (last name coincidental) on *Guiding Light*. The show incorporated the actress' actual battle with uterine cancer into her character's storyline. Both character and actress survived. Years later, her obituary in the *New York Times* claimed that "Bert Bauer's struggle with uterine cancer helped provide information to many women.... She was credited with raising uterine cancer awareness among many women who watched the show. Many went on to get Pap tests, the standard screening test for the disease" (Craig, 2012, April, para. 3). As Bauer's entry in Wikipedia emphasized, "The storyline helped millions of women realize the importance of regular checkups and pap smear screenings. Bauer received a record amount of mail from fans" ("Charita Bauer," 2013, March 19, para. 6).

Two decades later, Bauer suffered a blood clot that resulted in the amputation of her right leg. Once again, *Guiding Light* allowed the beloved matriarch's journey to mirror the actress' actual health challenge, enabling "real" and "reel" events to educate and empower viewers. As Craig (2012, April) stressed, "Many TV stars do their share of public service announcements. Twice in her career, Charita Bauer turned her personal tragedies—cancer and a leg amputation—into public service announcements" (para. 1).

Colleen Zenk Pinter

Viewers certainly noticed and expressed concern when "Barbara" on *As the World Turns* started talking in an unusual way. According to Kroll (2007, October 28), "Online, fans wondered if the actress had suffered a stroke. Others thought that Pinter may have had some sort of dental work. Still, fans feared the worst and flooded soapcentral.com with messages asking what was going on" (para. 1). In an interview for *Woman's Day*, Colleen Zenk Pinter explained,

> The cameras were rolling and I was trying to say my lines, but I knew that I sounded like I'd had a stroke. For the last 30 years I've been playing Barbara Ryan, a feisty woman who's never at a loss for words, on *As the World Turns*. But now I couldn't get the words out clearly. Viewers started writing to the show and flooding fan websites, wondering why I sounded so awful. I knew I owed them an explanation, but I just wasn't ready. I was still digesting the bad news [n.d., para. 1].

After taking some time to process her diagnosis of Stage II oral cancer, Zenk Pinter announced her illness to fans and asked producers to craft a cancer storyline for "Barbara" as a springboard for enlightening viewers. A representative for the Oral Cancer Foundation praised this rich opportunity for exposing viewers to this disease and educating them about symptoms and treatments:

> Told with technical accuracy, the oral cancer issue will receive public attention for what will likely be many weeks of exposure on a daily TV show, as her character moves from diagnosis and the associated emotional issues, to treatments, and recovery. For a disease that has very low public awareness, this prolonged exposure of it in a mainstream daily TV series performs a valuable function in increasing public knowledge about a very dangerous and deadly disease ["Actress Colleen Zenk Pinter partners…," 2007, November 30, para. 5].

Moreover, Zenk Pinter joined forces with the Oral Cancer Foundation by giving interviews and appearing in public service announcements, urging others to seek screening. She emphasized that "[t]he irony is that my cancer could have been found and treated so easily long before it progressed.... I beg everyone who's reading this, please, go to your dentist and ask for an oral cancer exam. It takes less than five minutes, and it could save your life" (Zenk Pinter, n.d., para. 21).

Michael Zaslow

Like Zenk Pinter, Michael Zaslow also started to display symptoms on screen before revealing a real-life diagnosis. For decades, Zaslow played the part of "Roger Thorpe" on *Guiding Light*. Roger Thorpe was a strong, powerful, invincible, dastardly but charming villain, portrayed masterfully by engaging and compelling Zaslow. In his autobiography, cowritten with wife Susan Hufford, Zaslow recounted his realization that something might be amiss:

> "I'm not that man anymore." In September 1996, the moment I first noticed something was wrong with my voice was captured on videotape forever.... "I'm not that man anymore. Mananymore. Nanymore." My tongue would not negotiate that simple phrase. My voice sounded unfamiliar. Not me anymore. I tried the phrase on Maureen Garrett, the actress who played Holly, and a friend of longstanding. She said she couldn't hear any difference in my speech and neither did anyone else. It was only that one line [Zaslow & Hufford, 2005, p. 5].

Unfortunately, it wasn't just that line. Zaslow sought help from a speech therapist; another doctor ruled out a stroke. As Zaslow and Hufford (2005, p. 32) personally experienced, "ALS is a diagnosis by default, by process of elimination, of other less horrific neurological diseases. Many people with ALS (known as PALS) go from doctor to doctor for months, sometimes years, before a diagnosis is confirmed." Thus, as the symptoms continued, they searched for answers and for help.

Still without a clear idea about the cause of his problems, Zaslow faced the conundrum of needing to work to support his wife and young daughters, yet his symptoms could no longer be ignored or overlooked on screen. Zaslow shared,

> The night before what turned out to be my last show, I got up around 2 a.m. and wrote the producer a note. I reminded him that I had several times beseeched him to write my speech impairment into Roger's story. I reminded him about Charita Bauer, the talented and loved Guiding Light star who had cancer, which had necessitated the amputation of one of her legs. The writers successfully incorporated her disability into the storyline and the fans were grateful. I argued that the daytime genre was famous for including actors' health problems into their characterizations and storylines [Zaslow & Hufford, 2005, p. 34].

In this case, though, the producers refused and indicated plans to replace the actor instead, even asking him to "say nothing to the press.... For your own good" (Zaslow & Hufford, 2005, p. 35). For a time, he did stay mum, yet, after battling depression and desperately seeking financial retribution on his own, Zaslow decided to break his silence.

Under pressure from negative press (e.g., Lang, 1997, September 1; Lipton & Wang, 1998, June 1; "Michael Zaslow speaks out about his fight," 1998, January 20), fan outrage over treatment of the beloved and ailing actor, and an Americans with Disabilities–based lawsuit pending, Proctor and Gamble (owners of *Guiding Light*) eventually settled for an undisclosed amount. After the actor's condition deteriorated (and more and more tests and treatments proved inconclusive or ineffective), doctors ultimately determined that Zaslow suffered from ALS, amyotrophic lateral sclerosis or Lou Gehrig's disease, and Zaslow turned his attention toward raising awareness of the disease and seeking a cure. He found an ally in another soap opera.

During a previous time away from *Guiding Light*, Zaslow portrayed a character named David Renaldi on *One Life to Live*, and producers hired Zaslow to reprise his role. Zaslow recalled his conversation with an ALS expert about the chance to shine a spotlight on this disease:

> I explained how I was going to be a man living with ALS. Rather, David, the character I play, will be a man living with ALS instead of dying from the condition. We can show the public what it's like to lose your speech, to not be able to trust your own legs, but that the mind still isn't affected. We can prove that people with disabilities aren't their disabilities, but are still their former selves. I'm still me, Michael Zaslow. David Renaldi is still David, even though he can no longer play the piano or conduct. We can let the audience see how David struggles to communicate. We can raise awareness and money for research! [Zaslow & Hufford, 2005, p. 127].

At a press conference which heralded the return of Michael Zaslow to *One Life to Live* (as well as his character, David Renaldi), Zaslow praised the network and the show for the decision to proceed with this storyline, using a voice simulator, the Link, to utter the following statement:

> Thank you, Pat [ABC President Pat Fili-Knushel]. You and the people at ABC and *One Life to Live* have demonstrated that working for a giant corporation doesn't necessitate relinquishing one's humanity. ABC is exhibiting tremendous social responsibility in writing David Renaldi's return with ALS, something that has never been done before. I, and the 300,000 PALS living with ALS in the United States alone, thank you. You are giving us, and indeed, the entire neurological community, an opportunity to vanquish this disease and save our collective lives [Zaslow & Hufford, 2005, p. 156].

Fans praised Zaslow's return to daytime on OLTL and bashed CBS for its insensitive handling of Zaslow's condition, as the following sample of fan comments affirm:

> The staff of OLTL is to be commended for having the courage to bring Michael Zaslow back as David. The vignette on last Friday's 20/20 was so moving; I was in tears. I remember Michael as the powerful Roger Thorpe on GL; and now he is just as powerful as David on OLTL, only more so. I know that I speak for thousands of Roger/David fans when I say, you go Michael…
>
> I am so glad Michael is on OLTL again. I loved him as Roger Thorpe on GL as well as David Renaldi. Thank you OLTL for giving Michael the chance to show his great acting skills again. Guiding Light should be ashamed of themselves. They are truly cowards in every sense of the word. The scene with Dorian seeing David for the first time was so emotional and moving it brought tears to my eyes. Michael my heart is with you … you are truly an inspiration to all…
>
> Thank you so much for giving Michael Zaslow a chance to shine on "One Life to Live." I am thrilled that he is back on OLTL & I am now an OLTL fan. As a disabled person and a 17-year "Guiding Light" viewer, Mr. Zaslow's brutal dismissal from GL in April 1997 was devastating to his many fans and supporters. I saw the "20/20" profile and I was thrilled to see him on TV again. It was heartwrenching to see the hurt in his eyes and on his face when asked about the GL situation, but Mr. Zaslow is a true professional and a class act. I adore him and wish him & his family the best. Thank you, Mr. Zaslow, for hanging in there & being you. You are an inspiration to me … ["Applause, Applause," 1999, April 12].

Along with riveting performances on *One Life to Live*, Zaslow founded ZazAngels, an organization with the goal of a cure by 2000 ("Emmy-winner Zaslow dies," 1998, December 29; Lipton & Wang, 1998, June 1). Once silenced by CBS and *Guiding Light*, Zaslow reached out to fans for support and also testified before Congress, appealing for federal funding, even though, as the months passed, his ability to speak without the assistance of technology dwindled. Hufford described the scene as they arrived on Capitol Hill for the first ALS Advocacy Day in support of House Bill 2009, just after Zaslow returned to OLTL.

> Michael was amazing and, may I add, in his element. The ALS patients were greeting him, those who could shaking his hand, others emitting the same primitive sounds that now came from my husband. We had already appeared on several network television interviews, and his first show would be airing soon. Already, the public service announcements were playing on ABC, showing Michael as a man living with ALS. Never before had this disease been made visible to so many people. Just as I had turned away from some of the patients on ventilators, so the world had turned its back on this ugly disease. When we entered the room that day, Michael's presence electrified the ALS community. Faces lit up. PALS who could still speak called out their encouragement and gratitude. Everyone was smiling. Even those with the vacant expressionless masks that characterize PALS in the later stages of ALS conveyed a sense of joy.

They had a spokesperson. Feelings of hope were palpable, and love was all around [Zaslow & Hufford, 2005, pp. 157–158].

Guiding Light producers refused to address Zaslow's condition through "Roger's" storyline, implying that "Roger" was too strong to suffer such a fate (Lang, 1997, September 1). Ironically, through his advocacy and work on *One Life to Live*, Zaslow affirmed an extraordinary strength of spirit, will, and zest for life that proved inspirational and educational to viewers and others who heard of his journey (Lipton & Wang, 1998, December 21). Dedicated fans never accepted any other actor as "Roger" on *Guiding Light*, and writers quickly wrote the character off the canvas. Instead of seizing a chance to craft an empowering story, *Guiding Light* writers and producers allowed a once strong and central character to fizzle and fade quietly to the sidelines. Conversely, *One Life to Live* benefitted greatly (as did the public attention to ALS) by enabling viewers to understand ALS through the dual experiences of "David," the character, and Michael Zaslow, beloved Emmy award-winning actor.

Discussion

As this chapter reveals, daytime dramas (or "soap operas") hold much potential for impacting the lives of those who participate in the genre in front of the camera or the television set, especially in terms of health-care issues. Although critics bemoan the genre's melodrama and occasionally outrageous storylines, the heart of soap operas remains relationships, especially those between intensely loyal fans (who "tune in tomorrow," day after day, year after year) and committed actors who often quite literally grow old in their roles as beloved characters. Those relationships provide rich foundations for teachable moments as well as demonstrations of (and appeals for) support.

In 1985, Meyrowitz described parasocial interactions that occur when viewers believe that they have relationships with characters or actors on television, but, in actuality, viewers don't truly "know" the characters or actors in spite of any perceived bond. Nearly 30 years later, we argue that such connections have become much more complex than to be merely labeled "real" or "parasocial." To be sure, fictional characters hold no basis in reality, no matter how invested a fan might be in his or her "stories," and caring deeply about a character clearly fits within the realm of "parasocial."

Yet, as the exemplars in this chapter indicate, soap operas absolutely constitute a genre in which fans/viewers and actors routinely rip down the classic "fourth wall" of the theater, reaching out to each other through traditional forms of communication (exchanging letters) and, increasingly, interacting on discussion boards and through social media. Embracing contemporary technology and playing with the postmodern blurring of boundaries between "real" and "reel," individuals associated with daytime drama (especially actors and fans), perhaps more than any other genre on television, engage each other in varied ways and often grow to care about each other in ways that extend far beyond merely "parasocial."

Coupled with the intertwining life narratives of characters, actors, and viewers (see Beck, 2012), the interactive, dialogic nature of soap opera fandom fosters opportunities for sharing health and illness narratives in ways that could not be accomplished in other genres. As this chapter illustrates, when actual actor health situations have been written into scripts, shows and actors have received tremendous responses, in terms of ratings as well as expressions of support and concern. Fans care about fictional characters as well as feel for the actors in times of personal struggle. Moreover, in the context of these "real" and "reel" relationships, viewers gain valuable information about early warning signs, symptoms, diagnoses, treatments, and potential outcomes of diseases that can truly impact anyone at any time—even popular performers.

As we have mentioned, soap operas have been heralded as potential partners for educating and enlightening audiences about health issues through education-entertainment. This chapter suggests that multilayered health narratives on soap operas, when art imitates actuality for an actor, can inform and inspire viewers as well as permit the performer to take the particular illness or condition onto an even larger stage than the show. Notably, not all actors should feel compelled to blur private and public boundaries in this manner. However, those who are willing to reveal such intimate details with co-workers and viewers by disclosing a health situation and weaving it on to the show's tapestry, quite literally, hold the rich potential of saving and impacting lives through their "reel" and "real" health narratives.

CHAPTER TEN

A Tangled Web
of Health Troubles

Giuliana Rancic's Fight
for a Family Goes Public

The Italian-born television host (*E! News*, *Fashion Police*) and fashion designer Giuliana Rancic has battled two major health issues—infertility and breast cancer. For many years, Giuliana and her husband, Bill, struggled to get pregnant. After two rounds of in vitro fertilization (IVF), Giuliana's doctor recommended that she obtain a mammogram before starting a third round. The test revealed that she had breast cancer. Giuliana decided to undergo a double mastectomy and weeks of radiation therapy. With the help of a surrogate, Giuliana and Bill eventually welcomed a son, and, through their television show, they allow others to know about their life—each struggle and triumph. This chapter details Giuliana and Bill's quest to use their reality television show and speaking engagements as a platform for sharing their story of hope and positive attitudes about these health issues and educating others about early detection and the importance of routine mammograms.

Background

You know I've had some really tough times especially in the past few years; things that a lot of other women have been through, whether it's trying to have a baby and having struggles or being diagnosed with breast cancer, and I've realized that sometimes out the darkest of darks, the most beautiful light emerges. And in my case, I really had some dark moments, especially with the breast cancer. But then, you know, months later hearing we were finally having a baby [Giuliana gasps], was like the lightest of lights. So my favorite quote in the world and I live by this is "Everything will be okay in the end—if it's not okay, it's not the end." And it's very, very true [Giuliana Rancic as cited in an HSN (2012) interview (https://www.youtube.com/watch?v=nim2KAgf8sQ)].

The quote above from Giuliana Rancic suggests that, from the outside looking in, although she battled tough health problems, everything worked out. In a sense, Giuliana's quotation provides hope to other women who experience similar health problems (e.g., breast cancer, infertility, miscarriages, etc.). She has become a modern-day spokesperson for women's health issues, especially considering her job as an anchor on *E! News*. For the last 12 years, Giuliana has been a staple for the popular network, E!, or Entertainment. She is one of E!'s most popular network anchors, the star of *E!News*, as well as a co-host for the popular show, *Fashion Police*. On *E! News*, Giuliana worked alongside co-host Ryan Seacrest (from 2006 to 2012) and, more currently, Terrence Jenkins; this dynamic duo reports the latest celebrity gossip and news. *Fashion Police* is a show that shares and spills the hottest celebrity fashion trends of the week, as well as the celebrities that fell a bit short in terms of their look. In addition to her anchor and co-host duties, Giuliana, along with her husband, Bill Rancic, co-produce their hit reality television show, *Giuliana & Bill* (https://twitter.com/GiulianaRancic). Giuliana's most recent on-screen work extends to her newest show, *Beyond Candid with Giuliana*, where she sits down with a celebrity and conducts a raw, "gritty" interview with them about their life, career, and journey into stardom (Marquina, 2014).

When not in the limelight, Giuliana spends some of her free time working with the national nonprofit organization Bright Pink. Bright Pink focuses on risk reduction and early detection of breast and ovarian cancer in young women and also provides support for high-risk individuals (BrightPink.org, 2014). Giuliana creatively established her own charity, "Fab-U-Wish," where, together, Giuliana and Bright Pink grant wishes to women who are undergoing breast cancer treatment (Sizemore, Rott, Rancic, & Rancic, 2014b). She encourages women like herself to share their respective breast cancer stories. She explained its importance in season six, episode five, "Baby on the Loose," of *Giuliana & Bill*:

> Half the battle [referencing breast cancer] is the courage to share your story, because you have every right to keep it personal and private for the rest of your life.... You just never know when your story could change a life or even save a life, you know? [Sizemore, Rott, Rancic, & Rancic, 2013a].

Giuliana encourages women who are either survivors or pre-vivors (women who are currently in remission) of breast cancer to share their journey through cancer with other women. She follows her own advice as she uses her celebrity status and her hit reality television show, *Giuliana & Bill*, to convey information, hope, and support.

This chapter explores the journey that Giuliana Rancic took to have a baby. One woman's desire to start a family led to the discovery of multiple serious health conditions. Giuliana and her husband, Bill Rancic, employ social media, their reality television show, and public-speaking engagements as tools to connect with audiences and share their story in hopes of saving other women's lives. As with the rest of this volume, Petronio's (1991) Communication Privacy Management (CPM) theory and computer-mediated communication (CMC; see High et al., 2014) provide a valuable lens through which to understand the Rancic health narrative.

Communication Privacy Management (CPM)

Petronio's (1991) theory of Communication Privacy Management offers a helpful framework in understanding personal disclosure, or one's willingness, or unwillingness, to expose personal information to others, especially celebrity health disclosures to the mainstream audience. According to Petronio, this theory also facilitates identifying the parameters within which couples in a relationship regulate revealing and reacting to private information. As we have discussed throughout this volume, boundary management of private information enables individuals to preserve preferred levels of privacy and helps protect the self when disclosing to the other (Petronio, Reeder, Hecht, & Ros-Mendoza, 1996). These boundaries illustrate the way "tensions between telling and withholding private information are regulated to cope with potential vulnerabilities" (Petronio et al., 1996, p. 183).

Within Communication Privacy Management theory, two types of rules for disclosure emerge, regarding access and protection of disclosure (Petronio et al., 1996). Rules for access constitute the logistics of disclosure; these rules allow the individual to choose what information s/he discloses, to whom, when, and where. Access rules depend on the characteristics of the relationship, such as the individual's attraction for, liking of, or trust in, the other. With protection rules, the individual might not want others to know their private information, and in turn, guard against access and disclosure; lack of trust or a problematic situation can drive protection rules. Relative to intimacy issues, like trouble conceiving between two individuals, "protecting privacy may be one way to exercise control over the circumstance" (Petronio et al., 1996, p. 184). While some people may choose to keep personal health information between few people, other people may decide to share their experiences more publically. Either way, CPM serves as a powerful theoretical tool for understanding the relationship and communication strategies among individuals (Petronio 1991, 2002).

The blurring of public and private information is most certainly relevant when discussing celebrity limelight and intimate health topics such as infertility (Infertility, as defined by Jose-Miller, Boyden, and Frey [2007] is "one year of frequent, unprotected intercourse during which pregnancy has not occurred" [p. 849].) and cancer (Beck et al., 2014). The health-related struggles and openness from Giuliana Rancic—revealing her battle with infertility, which led to the diagnosis of breast cancer—exemplifies a celebrity who actively chooses to share private information with the public eye. In this chapter, we discuss Giuliana Rancic's struggles with infertility, her breast cancer diagnosis, and her efforts to encourage and inspire other women to get early detection of breast cancer. We use CPM to examine the ways in which Giuliana and her husband, Bill, face two difficult health issues—fertility problems and breast cancer—very much in the public eye (for related work, see Altman & Taylor, 1973; Bute & Vik, 2010; Petronio 1991, 2002).

Giuliana's Tangled Health Struggles—An Overview

As Giuliana's resume suggests, she started her career by reporting gossip and celebrity information, rather than revealing her own. In 2009, the tables turned when Giuliana and her husband Bill, a real estate developer and the season-one winner of Donald Trump's *The Apprentice*, signed on to star in their own reality television show on Style Network, *Giuliana & Bill. Giuliana & Bill* (still airing and on its 6th season) began as the couple struggled with infertility and attempted to conceive via in vitro fertilization (Curry, 2011, October 17; IMDB, 2014c). After three seasons focusing on this power couple's struggles to conceive (including two IVF treatments, one resulting in a miscarriage after carrying the fetus for eight weeks), the third season finale ends with Giuliana attempting IVF for the third time (Curry, 2011, October 17). As their fans anxiously awaited the news that her third time was the charm, some reached out to her, inquiring about a potential pregnancy. In an interview with Ann Curry, on the October 17, 2011, edition of the *Today* show titled "From E! to Reality TV—Real-life Struggle for Giuliana Rancic," Giuliana said,

> A lot of people have been asking, you know, we saw in the season finale [referencing season 3 finale] of your show that you went and got IVF, so what happened. Are you pregnant? But sadly, we've had to put that off because of the news [forthcoming information] [para. 16].

The seemingly private information about fertility that the couple willingly revealed to the public became even more personal during the *Today* show. Curry explained how Giuliana's fans expected her to announce a pregnancy, but, unfortunately, she had different news to report. Giuliana continued in a somber tone, confiding, "I do have other news. Through my attempt to get pregnant for the third time through IVF, we sadly found out that I have early stages of breast cancer, so, and it's been a shock because I recently found this out" (Curry, 2011, October 17, para. 16).

One short month after finding out that Giuliana had the early stage of breast cancer, she underwent a routine lumpectomy to remove the cancer cells in both breasts. When the lumpectomy failed to remove all cancerous cells, Giuliana and Bill had to decide if Giuliana would try to eradicate this deadly disease via a double mastectomy or via radiation and chemotherapy. Together, they engaged in this conversation on their show (season 5, episode 2—*Booby Trap*, aired April 10, 2012), and made a list of pros and cons for these two invasive options. Since the radiation and chemotherapy had the possibility of sterilizing her, they scheduled a double mastectomy with reconstruction for December 2012.

The cameras and America joined them in the hospital on the episode, "Surgery Day" (season 5, episode 4, aired April 24, 2012). The episode featured Giuliana moments before surgery and during her time in recovery. She granted a close-up view of her fluid drains under her surgical gown, holding nothing back from the camera. Giuliana truly strives to be an open book, unselfish in terms of exposing her experiences (good, bad, and the dirty). Her story unfolds even further when the couple receives news from the doctor that they should consider alternative options for conception because her body needs time to heal while she is on invasive medication (season 5, episode 5— "Baby Dreams"). The couple discussed alternatives on the episode and, ultimately, decided to go with a gestational carrier using Bill's sperm and Giuliana's eggs that they had opted to freeze years earlier.

In the wake of her courageous battle with cancer and infertility, Giuliana and Bill discovered that their private surrogate, publically known as Delphine, was carrying their baby. Giuliana gushed to Ann Curry on the April 23, 2012, episode of *Today* about the moment when she realized she was finally going to have a baby. Smiling, she said that "it was pretty much one of the best moments of my life, if not the best moment of my life. It was just another world, on another level" (Randee, 2012, para. 2).

As their story ensued, Giuliana and Bill welcomed their son, Edward Duke Rancic (referred to by Mom and Dad as "Duke"), into the world on August 29, 2012. Again, the cameras were in the private delivery room as

Delphine gave Giuliana and Bill the one gift that they could not give them-selves, a child. This emotional episode likely left many viewers crying happy tears of joy. Delphine and her family continue to be very much a part of the Rancic family's life, and they often appear in episodes of *Giuliana & Bill*. As we finish this book, Giuliana still takes medication to treat her breast cancer, and she will not be able to try to get pregnant for a few more years. With their dream of expanding their family out of their hands, Giuliana and Bill asked Delphine if she would be willing and able to carry their second child. In the season seven opener of *Giuliana & Bill*, titled "Home Alone," Delphine agreed to try another round of embryo implantation and attempt to carry a second child for Giuliana. So, as we go to press with this book, Giuliana and Bill's journey with cancer and fertility issues remain on center stage.

In response to Giuliana and Bill's public struggles to start and grow their family, messages poured in from their fan base (through Facebook, Twitter, the Home Shopping Network [HSN], *Giuliana & Bill*, etc.). Many of them expressed their words of encouragement and support while others used her stage as one to share their journey through similar experiences with Giuliana. For this chapter, we analyzed interactions between fans and Giuliana and Bill. First, we specify how Giuliana serves as a voice for women and the ways in which she encourages early detection of breast cancer and provides others with hope to move forward. Second, we consider how and why Giuliana (and sometimes Bill) share their story with others. Third, we reflect on this issue of co-ownership of private information as Bill and her fans function as co-owners of Giuliana's health story and the implications of Bill's role as a coau-thor to increase the reach of their messages and share "their" story with all different groups of people.

Public Service Announcement

Messages that promote healthy behaviors function as helpful calls to action by encouraging and promoting positive breast health and breast cancer aware-ness among women (Bender et al., 2011). Developing messages that will suc-cessfully hook the audience into its message comprises a challenge for health communication practitioners and scholars. O'Keefe and Jensen (2008, 2009) performed a meta-analytic review on the potential for loss-framed versus gain-framed messages related to disease detection behavior to produce message processing in those who listen to the message. A gain-framed appeal stresses the desirable significances associated with obedience with the directed view-point, such as early detection of breast cancer from mammography screening (O'Keefe & Jensen, 2009). A loss-framed message highlights the undesirable consequences associated with nonconformity with the directed viewpoint (O'Keefe & Jensen, 2008), such as messaging surrounding risk of not detecting breast cancer in its early stages when avoiding regular mammograms (O'Keefe & Jensen, 2009). These scholars found that gain-framed messages produced a slightly larger significance in message engagement being persuasive when compared to loss-framed messages, especially when considering messages around breast cancer detection (O'Keefe & Jensen, 2008, 2009).

Celebrity messages surrounding health-related issues are ever so apparent on social media sites like Facebook and Twitter. Thackeray et al. (2013) analyzed celebrity, health organization, and individual members' tweets on Twitter surrounding breast cancer awareness messages (BCAM) during breast cancer awareness month. They found that celebrities who tweeted about breast cancer had far more impressions on followers than organizations and other individual users since they typically have more followers. Celebrities were also more likely to mention BCAM in their tweets during this month over organizations and individuals, thus further increasing their reach of these powerful messages to followers on social media. Using high-profile celebrity spokespersons to spread the message about BCAM, especially if they have a connection to the disease (e.g., Giuliana Rancic) and have many followers on social media sites (e.g., Giuliana Rancic has ~3.3 million followers on Twitter), aids in engaging followers in a conversation about breast cancer and, in turn, may persuade them to seek preventive action (Thackeray et al., 2013).

With the cameras rolling during intimate life moments in Giuliana's life, she sought to raise awareness about women's health issues that were also affecting her. In a candid interview with *E! News* about her fertility problems, directly following a public reveal of her recent miscarriage, she said, "One in four women go through what I went through…. I'm just happy to be a voice for you" (EOL, 2010, September 30, para. 4). She allowed the camera to record in her private recovery room after her double mastectomy, in hopes that her experiences would help remove some of the stigma surrounding such intense surgery.

In the section that follows, we highlight how Giuliana's messages surrounding women's health topics help encourage women to be vigilant about their health. We detail how Giuliana Rancic's personal-yet-public health narrative serves as a voice for women, sends a positive message to others about early detection, and fosters hope.

A Voice for Women

In terms of managing private and public boundaries, Giuliana explained in a *Glamour* interview,

We've [referencing her and Bill] been given this incredible platform, and we think it was for a reason. I truly believe that. When I got my job at E!, I was the thirty-ninth person who auditioned. I wasn't the prettiest, I wasn't the smartest, I wasn't the most talented. And I always wondered why I got the job. Now I think God knew I wouldn't be a selfish little cow with this platform, and I'd actually try to do something good with it [Dunn, 2012, para. 26].

Clearly, Giuliana envisions her role in the public eye as entailing personal disclosures, especially if they could work to advance a "greater good." Similarly, two years prior to the quotation mentioned above, Giuliana revealed on E! News that she had a miscarriage. By revealing her own difficulties, Giuliana brought this challenging, otherwise private matter into public discourse. Giuliana's fans and followers applaud and appreciate her candor. The following posts appeared in an online blog area connected to the Glamour article. In response to the Today show interview about her double mastectomy, one fan, Jody, asserted, "Guilianna, you are living the purpose that God created for you—inspiring and encouraging others. God Bless you, Bill and your family in 2012. May all your dreams come true!" (2011, December 30). Norma also weighed into the conversation:

No matter what kind of cancer a person has it is a challenge. Your journey has been hard, but sharing it with others is a very courageous thing to do. I wish you a speedy recovery. I hope that your journey forward to have a child is successful and that you and Bill have many years of happiness, joy and peace from here on [2011, December 30].

Harpreet (2011, December 30) noted that "[m]any men and women suffer from some form of cancer. I applaud her for bringing breast cancer to the forefront of peoples' minds." Likewise, Chris (2011, December 30) commented, "I wish the best to Giuliana and I believe that anything that raises the awareness concerning breast cancer is a plus. I am in favor of highlighting the lives of the millions of women, like my mother..." As Lisa (2011, December 30) stated, "Thanks for getting your story out there as we little people don't have a way to do this." These posts attest to the gratitude of people who either have experience with or are concerned about breast cancer for Giuliana's willingness to be a voice for this deadly disease.

Message to Others—Early Detection

The simple fact that Giuliana's breast cancer was found in the earliest stage meant that she had a 98 percent survival rate (Curry, 2011, October 17). In her public address about her recent diagnosis of breast cancer, Giuliana expressed the importance of early detection in women who are not even at risk of breast cancer. During the October 17, 2011, Today show interview, Giuliana told her story to Curry, sharing how she and Bill decided to try their third round of IVF from one of the leading IVF clinics in the United States, located in Denver, Colorado. Their new doctor recommended that Giuliana get a mammogram. Giuliana recalled that she was defiant when it came to getting a mammogram, especially since she was only 36 years old, and in no way due for her first mammogram. She admitted, "I mean, I wasn't prepared to get a mammogram until I was 40 years old, like I've been told. And so I never in my wildest dreams expected anything would be wrong. And so I did go kicking and screaming to get a mammogram, to be honest" (Curry, 2011, October 17, para. 22).

Giuliana mentioned that her age, as well as her family history, did not suggest an added risk of breast cancer; she never thought that she needed to have early detection because the odds were in her favor. Curry expanded on this common misconception in her interview with Giuliana: "Eighty-five percent of breast cancer diagnoses are for people who don't have any prior history," and Giuliana's goal of the *Today* interview was to "give a message to women" (Curry, 2011, October 17, para. 29). Giuliana's message to her fans continued with her saying,

> I think a lot of us think we're invincible, you know. And women these days, we're busier than ever. We're multitasking, we're taking care of a million people a day and a million things a day. But we have to start putting ourselves on the to-do list.... I had a friend call me yesterday. And she said, I'm so sorry. Can I do anything for you? And I go, honestly, just don't feel sorry for me. Instead just call your doctor tomorrow, make an appointment. That's what you could do for me. You know what I mean? And I just want women out there to know that you—if you can just find it early, you will—you know, you could be OK [Curry, 2011, October 17, para. 44].

Giuliana underscored her early detection of breast cancer when she was not "due" for a mammogram. If she had not been having trouble conceiving, and if her doctor had not recommended that she have a mammogram before going through another round of IVF, she would not have known until four years later (when she was due for her first mammogram at age 40) that she had a lump that was cancerous. Notably, Giuliana's public disclosure of the circumstances surrounding her diagnosis could be deemed problematic. Mammograms pose their own risks in terms of radiation, hence, a reason for standards and protocols for their use. However, Giuliana's narrative exposes the alternative—a life saved due to early detection before the usually recommended screening date.

Bill Rancic explained in their interview with *Glamour* (Dunn, 2012) that he is proud of his wife for being brave, sharing her story, and helping other women seek early detection. He noted, "So many have written us or tweeted us, 'Hey I finally got my wife to go in for her first mammogram,' or 'got check[ed] out, thank you.' Not one or two [people] but thousands." Giuliana expanded on this conversation, mentioning that her message has already "resulted in three girls in their thirties who I know about—friends of friends—finding out they had cancer" (Dunn, 2012, para. 26). By allowing her story to be public information, Giuliana and Bill recognize the importance of their message. Their story holds the potential to prompt women to seek early detection of breast cancer through mammography screening and encourage others to overcome their struggles with cancer and/or infertility. In a flood of Facebook messages in response to Giuliana's story about her mastectomy on the *Today* show (Facebook, 2011), Twitter messages (Twitter, 2014), and comments from the *Glamour* interview (Dunn, 2012), people who do not personally know Giuliana reached out to her for support and guidance and thanked her for saving their life through early detection and promoting mammograms.

A fan of the *Glamour* article responded on March 17, 2012, saying, "I am so happy that Giuliana and Bill shared their story. I too went to get checked when I read this as I haven't since I got a lump removed ten years ago."

Multiple Facebook users responded to Giuliana and Bill's interview on *Today* with comments like Dianna's (2011, December 30): "Because of her story, my cancer was found in the early stages. She is an inspiration to all women! God Bless!" Kathy (2011, December 31) added, "Hi Giuliana, I just wanted to say thank you for your story. I've been meaning to have a Mammorgram [Mammogram] for the last six years and just hadn't done it yet. When I found out what had happened to you [I] went down a week later and had it done. I wish You and Bill the best." Rhonda (2012, April 23), another Facebook responder, noted, "Guiliana [Giuliana], you give me courage to have my yearly mamograms [mammogram] and not be afraid. I think you are a wonderful person and you deserve all the happiness in the world. God Bless you and Bill." One of just over 3 million Twitter followers, Giuliana's fan, Mylissa (2014, April 12), said, "bc [because] of you & ur [your] story I found a tumor after I watched your show I checked & found a lump. thank you! ❤" The same day, Giuliana Rancic responded to @Mylissa from her Twitter account, saying "Stay strong! Xoxo:)."

Women, either ones who have or have survived breast cancer, related to Giuliana's story and reiterated her important message about screening and prevention. Debbie (2011, December 30) posted, "Early detection ... hopefully her story will help more women get tested at an earlier time. I was diagnosed last yr. and also underwent double mastectomy, didn't want to worry about the other breast in the future. Thanks for sharing your story with the world."

Bonnie (2011, December 31) added, "you are an amazing woman!!! you chose to live, as i did. i know what you are going thru, and it isnt easy … but it does get better, and every time you get that NO CANCER report, you will celebrate. love that you are brave and sharing your diagnosis and recovery. you surely will save many women's lives for doing this."

These social media posts reveal a strong public response to Giuliana's openness about her personal health experiences with the public. Social media sites such as Facebook and Twitter provide "channels of communication with potential support providers" (High et al., 2014, p. 79). As such, responders employed social media and Giuliana's experiences to make sense of and take control of their own health care.

Stories to Form Hope

Burleson and MacGeorge (2002) explained social support as "verbal and nonverbal behavior produced with the intention of providing assistance to others perceived as needing that aid" (p. 374). Similarly, with all of Giuliana and Bill's interviews and shows being readily available on the internet, computer-mediated communication (CMC; see High et al., 2014) fosters self-disclosure from Giuliana and her fans on various social media sites. Especially with difficult health topics like breast cancer and infertility, CMC on social media sites provides a safe space for self-disclosure, a space that allows self-disclosure to occur more easily than it does in face-to-face interaction (see Tidwell & Walther, 2002). Although face-to-face interactions generally encompass more emotional support (High et al., 2014), more and more people utilize social media as a way to seek and provide means of support to people who experience similar health concerns (Davison, Pennebaker, & Dickerson, 2000). In a 2012 *Huffington Post* article, Giuliana and the editor discuss the amount of support she has received from people around the world. Giuliana explained, "I think because breast cancer touches so many people, when someone hears you have it, they just shower you with love. The one word I always saw in all the messages was strong. You're so strong, stay strong, be strong—when you hear something enough, you start believing it" ("Giuliana Rancic talks breast cancer," 2012, para. 4).

In the episode "Saving Face," (season 7, episode 7), Giuliana and the organization Bright Pink grant wishes to two "Fab-u-Wish" winners (Sizemore et al., 2014b). She heralded the strength that these women (and all women) demonstrate when going through cancer and the power that comes with sharing their stories with the world and the impact that they can have on other women experiencing cancer, asserting that "[y]ou're taking a negative experience and doing something positive. True strength really is staying strong when the whole world would forgive you if you were to fall to your knees and give up and that's true strength, not giving up."

Just like the advice that she gave these women, Giuliana's story does the same. LauraFromOurHopePlace, who read the online *Glamour* article, stated,

> Thank you for Bill & Giuliana for sharing their story of miscarriage, IVF & breast cancer. By sharing our stories we help others going thru the same situation feel less alone and give them hope.... That is exactly why we started www. OurHopePlace.com—Friends helping friends cope, hope & heal after miscarriage. Please visit if you have a loved one who has experienced miscarriage.

Likewise, Connie responded to the *Today* show report with Giuliana and Bill:

> Thank you Giuliana for sharing your story-what an amazing person you are. You truly are a fighter as well as a hero. I say this because you telling your personal story I know is helping other women to get checked etc. I wish you & all the women that have been sharing their stories the very best. You are all in my thoughts & prayers [2011, December 31].

As these posts suggest, others have benefitted as her disclosure facilitated the sharing of similar stories through online communities. Barker (2009) argued that an emotional connection between people and a cause motivates them to participate in and connect with others in online communities. For example, users of Facebook implicitly indicate support by "liking" each other's posts.

Shifting Boundaries—Private to Public

As Petronio (2002) contended, as individuals encounter new situations in their lifespan, privacy boundaries shift, and once private information may become public. Before Giuliana found out that she had breast cancer, talking to the public about early detection did not seem like information that she would necessary discuss on-air. The demands of her current health situation produced a shift in her public versus private boundary, forcing her to renegotiate these boundaries, motivating her to share her stories with others. Bute and Vik (2010) took this idea further, asserting that, with life-changing events, or "traumatic events" (such as fertility problems; p. 5), CPM permits an understanding of the way talk changes by suggesting that privacy boundaries change in response to contextual criteria.

In an interview with Health.com (Spencer, 2012), the reporter asked Giuliana a tough question: "Had you known what was coming, would you have chosen to keep any of this private [referencing starting her show, *Giuliana & Bill* prior to finding out about Giuliana's health concerns]?" Giuliana's honest answer comes as no surprise:

Had you given me a crystal ball when we were signing on to do the reality show that said, "This is what's coming up, do you want to do it?" I would've said absolutely not. You couldn't pay me enough. But, looking back, I'm so happy that I did do it. As I would question God, "Why are you doing this to me, why me?" I think God knew I was a loud-mouthed Italian girl who would get out and share my story, not tuck it under a rug [Spencer, 2012, para. 14].

Giuliana Rancic's passion to share her story and health journey extends from her will to help remove the stigma surrounding infertility (Errico, 2010) and breast cancer (Sizemore, Rott, Rancic, & Rancic, 2012a).

Her career as a television show host, actress, and executive director of her own reality television show provides Giuliana with ample opportunities to tell her stories to viewers. Allowing cameras into some of the most intimate moments of her life implicitly transforms otherwise private moments into ones available for public discourse and debate. In season 2, episode 2, "Operation Ovulation" and episode 3, "Family Matters," of *Giuliana & Bill*, the couple invited audience members along for fertility specialist appointments, egg fertilization sessions, and even moments before Bill and Giuliana do the deed in hopes of making a baby (Sizemore, Rott, Rancic, & Rancic, 2010b, 2010d). The "implications of blurring boundaries when celebrities choose to interweave their private health narratives with public discourses about health, healing, and well-being" (Beck et al., 2014, p. 244) are apparent in Giuliana's self-proclaimed social responsibility in terms of sharing her story, bringing infertility out of the shadows, and promoting early care and preventive measures (Cady, 2010, February 25; "Giuliana Rancic talks breast cancer," 2012, January 15).

When they discover that Giuliana had suffered a miscarriage in 2010, the couple said that they came forward because they did not want a stigma associated with a miscarriage. They addressed this issue further on season 3 of *Giuliana & Bill*; in episode 3, titled "A Heartbreaking Loss," Giuliana and Bill face the cameras and let them into their life during this terrible time (Sizemore, Rott, Rancic, & Rancic, 2010a).

CO-OWNERSHIP OF PRIVATE INFORMATION

Petronio's (2010) limited permeability rules explain how to control how much people outside of a marriage should know about their private information. As such, in a candid interview on January 11, 2010, with Chelsea Lately and Giuliana and Bill Rancic, the Rancics gushed about their attempts to get pregnant, and Lately joked about Bill trying to "Knock Giuliana up!" (http://www.eonline.com/shows/chelsea_lately/videos/49062/chelsea-lately-giuliana-bill, 2010). In this dynamic interview, Giuliana told Lately, "So, yes, we are trying to get preggers. But something's going on." (Giuliana snarled and laughed, referencing their inability to get pregnant). Lately joked back, stating, "What's the deal? What's wrong with your Sperm, Bill?" (The audience laughed uncontrollably). Taken off guard, Bill fired back with "Old Eggs. Old eggs over here" (Bill points at Giuliana). Giuliana and Bill treated their private matter of infertility as comical on the public television screen. Giuliana responded to Bill's "Old Eggs" comment, saying, "Ya, he calls me Old Eggs, 'OE' for short…. I'm like old eggs? What about old *sperm?*" (Emphasis given to *sperm* by Giuliana while she looked at and spoke to Bill's private area). Bill added to this comment, making sure to protect his manhood, stating, "Let me tell you; I can assure everyone there's nothing going on down here that's wrong [pointing to his private area]" (http://www.eonline.com/videos/167250/chelsea-lately-giuliana-and-bill-rancic, 2010).

Similarly to the example above from the *Chelsea Lately Show*, in the second episode of season 2, titled "Knocked-up," Giuliana and Bill made an appointment with Bill's sister's OBGYN, Dr. Sabbagha. Bill confided that he had to "provide them [the doctor] with a little deposit, if you will," referencing having to have his sperm tested to see if their fertility problems stem from him. On the way to the doctor's office, Giuliana stopped at a newsstand to get a few magazines for Bill to use to produce his sperm; she picked out *Juggs* and *Hustler* while Bill looked extremely uncomfortable with purchasing these adult magazines on camera and in public. Giuliana tried to ease the tension and told the newsstand employee about the medicinal purpose of their purchase. She continued, stating, "You know what it is? We're trying to have a baby." Eagerly, Bill tried to get Giuliana to stop talking and move away from the newsstand, which is on a busy street in downtown Chicago. Bill told Giuliana, "Honey, he doesn't care. He wants the money." She laughed back at Bill, continuing the conversation, "I want him to know so he doesn't think we're like a weird couple." She thanked the employee, and they leave, with both Giuliana and Bill expressing their embarrassment about that moment.

These examples illustrate how the couple transforms private exchanges into public ones, blurring the lines between what constitutes an intimate and emotional moment in a couples' life. Although such moments for Giuliana and Bill would otherwise be quite private, this type of information comprises what Petronio (2010) referred to as "Principle 4: Private information co-ownership and guardianship" (p. 180). When Bill allowed Giuliana to be a co-owner of this information, together, they co-negotiated the boundaries of such personal details (see Petronio, 2002). Given the public nature of their reality television show, these private boundaries are rather blurred, especially considering Petronio's (2010) limited permeability rules controlling how much people outside of a couple's marriage should know about their private, personal information. The lack of permeability rules among this private information does not limit the access to and protection of the co-owned information between Giuliana and Bill. Even more specifically, this example illustrates what Petronio (2010) termed as "socialization" occurring (p. 181). When people find themselves in an unusual situation for them (e.g., Giuliana buying adult magazines for Bill to use for a sperm analysis), they react in a way that might be contrary to the way that they might typically define privacy (Petronio, 2010). Adding another layer, through the reality show, viewers get to witness Giuliana and Bill as they co-determine what constitutes "appropriate" for interactions in terms of private practices and personal matters.

SHARING A CO-AUTHORED STORY

Health problems like infertility take a toll on both men and women. They can affect the couple as a whole, as well as affect their social circle or support system of family and friends. Research affirms that infertility takes an emotional toll on couples having trouble conceiving, with psychological effects similar to those of heart disease and cancer (Domar, Zuttermeister, & Friedman, 1993). The impact stems deeper than the individual, impacting the social well-being of the couple, resulting in social isolation, clinical depression, and a drop in job performance and life satisfaction as a result of the inability to have a child (Fidler & Bernstein, 1999). As a part of Petronio's (2010) co-ownership of private information, the Rancic couple decided to chronicle their experiences with others through advocacy efforts like public-speaking engagements.

In addition to doing interviews for the news and popular television shows like *Chelsea Lately* and the *Today* show, Giuliana and Bill also enjoy touring the country and sharing their story with communities of people who will benefit from their message. A few of these speaking engagements were included on *Giuliana & Bill*. In episode 512, Giuliana and Bill emphasized the importance of telling their story and raising awareness of breast cancer and infertility. Giuliana stated, "It's a very important mission for us [referencing speaking engagements regarding her health problems]. You know, if you can just change one life, your done. You did it."

One speaking engagement in Vail, Colorado, occurred just a month before little Duke's birth. The eager parents-to-be were excited to be in Colorado (the home of the gestational carrier, Delphine) and to spread their message at the Vail Breast Cancer Awareness Luncheon. Bill began the talk by explaining how two people make vows to God when they marry. Although a couple hopes that these vows are never tested, their vows have been—"the in sickness and in health part." Giuliana continued the story, explaining her initial reaction to the mammogram, "I wasn't due to be tested; I didn't have a lump. There is no way, I feel amazing! [Giuliana gets choked up as she continues.] I swear, it's like it never gets easy telling the story, it just brings me back to this very raw, sad place. It was just a terrible time for the two of us" (2012, July 15).

In Giuliana's efforts to share the story about her journey through breast cancer, one that she had uttered countless times on news shows and their own reality television show, she became emotional. Even though she is a celebrity, she is human, and she experiences pain and sadness. Bill stepped in and told the audience that it was hard for both of them, but "that's life" he said (episode 516). Giuliana recovered, saying,

> It's scary. I cried a lot; I bitched and moaned a lot. And just one day you go, I can try to take this negative and turn it into a positive and I encourage women to get checked because if you can find the cancer early, it's something like a over 95 percent chance that you'll be ok. I'm better now than I was before I had cancer … [applause in the crowd], thank you. I'm more than fine [2012, July 15].

On October 9, 2012, Giuliana and Bill also gave a talk at a speaking engagement for breast cancer awareness at the University of Southern Florida. This event, titled, "An Evening with Bill & Giuliana Rancic," provided an opportunity for Giuliana and Bill to discuss their journey through infertility and cancer with those in attendance (Allreadable.com, 2014b). Bill started by acknowledging that "our lives together and individually have really been what we term, an 'unplanned-plan.'" Together, they recounted their struggle to conceive and how they discovered Giuliana had breast cancer. Giuliana recalled,

> I went into get the mammogram and the doctor came in. And he goes "I'm so sorry, you have breast cancer." And I'm like, "what?" You know it was just—I became hysterical. I mean sobbing, uncontrollably. And I look at myself now and I am such a better, stronger, wiser, just all around happier person because of this major ordeal I went through [referencing cancer and IVF] [Allreadable. com, 2014b].

Giuliana stressed that cancer made her a better person because she has a different point of view on life. Even though she had multiple obstacles preventing her from having a baby, a precious little boy is in her life now, and she can claim that he helped save her life. As Bill concluded the event in Tampa, he expressed his happiness to help others:

> You know, when your plan is derailed, embrace it. Surrender to it. [Bill sighs]. Enjoy that journey. You know, when people come up and say "you know, you've

helped me go get checked" or "you saved my family's life," you know, we can't take the credit. The credit really belongs to a 14-pound little guy named Edward Duke. [Audience applauds.] Because had it not been for that guy, our story would have a much different ending. Because this little guy saved her life (pointing to Giuliana) and as a result of her strength, that little guy saved probably hundreds of other lives throughout the country and throughout the world. So, our unplanned-plan worked out pretty damn good [Allreadable.com, 2014b].

Giuliana agreed, telling Bill that she wants to do additional speaking engagements to help and encourage more women and provide them with a sense of hope through her story. Giuliana and Bill spend a lot of their time sharing their story together, as co-owners or co-authors of their reality.

Discussion

In ABC's Barbara Walters special, *Barbara Walters: Her Story*, we learn that, just like Giuliana, even Barbara experienced trouble getting pregnant, as she disclosed that she very much wanted to be a mom but after having three miscarriages, she adopted a daughter, Jacqueline (*Barbara Walters: Her Story*, 2014). As part of that special, Walters reflected on a 2004 interview with actress Diane Keaton. At age 50, Keaton decided to adopt her daughter. In her interview with Barbara Walters, Keaton explained how she was "old, too old, probably [to start a family]. But what can I do ... how could I not have this experience? How could I have gone through my life without having done this?" (*Barbara Walters: Her Story*, 2014). Like Diane Keaton, Giuliana Rancic did not want to go through life without experiencing motherhood, and, with the help of her surrogate, Delphine, Giuliana Rancic realized that dream.

Throughout this chapter, we detailed the aches and cries of Giuliana (and Bill) as they fought to add a baby into their comfortable life. As a result of that very public journey, Giuliana became a woman who promotes health and wellness through her story of her tangled web of health problems. She has served as a voice for women who battle the fight to have a baby and uses her celebrity status as a platform to educate and make more people aware of the ways in which they, too, can detect breast cancer in its early stage. Through her self-proclaimed social responsibility to use her public connections to connect with other people, she has addressed women who also suffer from infertility, miscarriages, and/or breast cancer, drawing light to those issues and urging women to continue their fight to survive. In a "Fab-u-Wish" grant by Giuliana and Bright Pink on an episode titled "Saving Face" on *Giuliana &*

Bill, Giuliana characterized her outlook on life and her journey through cancer to two women who had recently undergone breast cancer treatment while pregnant. (Both women discovered that they had breast cancer in the early stages of their pregnancies.) Giuliana stated,

> That first year was harrowing and just that idea of just always thinking about it was just daunting…. Do you ever never think about it again, of course not. But I will say as time passes, especially year two, there is such a significant difference from year one. I cannot even tell you. Like now I think about it five times a day as opposed to 100 times a day. Whereas every day I was so scared of dying now I really appreciate living [Sizemore et al., 2014b].

This excerpt underscores Giuliana's goal of encouraging these women by suggesting how their lives will sooner than later go back to normal.

Giuliana's public health narrative showcases shifting boundaries between private and public disclosure of information and indicates the power of celebrity health narratives to help others as they cope and deal with their similar health problems. As co-owner or co-author of Giuliana's story, Bill continues to co-construct the nature of their emergent journey; the difficult times appear on televisions across the world. Together, this couple travels as a team to public events, giving even more exposure to their message on overcoming health challenges.

At the beginning of season 6 of *Giuliana & Bill,* an episode titled "Rancic Rewind" reviews the life of Giuliana and Bill and the birth of their son, Duke (Sizemore, Rott, Rancic, & Rancic, 2013c). The purpose of this episode was to provide Duke with a video heirloom showcasing Giuliana and Bill's story— the good, the bad, and the ugly—in terms of how they met and the amazing journey to bring Duke into the world! The episode began by taking Duke down memory lane, telling him that Mom and Dad wanted nothing more than to have a baby together, but having him was not as easy as they thought. Bill explained to Duke that their attempt to bring him into the world brought about another difficult circumstance, Mom's breast cancer. Giuliana went on to say, "You saved my life, Duke. If we weren't trying to have you, I would never have gotten that mammogram." As discussed above, their story will continue, and it does not look like they will exit center stage anytime soon. As they attempt to have a second child, the cameras remain rolling, and Giuliana and Bill continue to share their coauthored story, encouraging women to seek early detection of breast cancer and prepare themselves now for a long journey with their family.

CHAPTER ELEVEN

Trust in Robin Roberts

The Journey of a Woman Who Breaks Her Own News

A former ESPN reporter and a current morning-show co-anchor for *Good Morning America*, Robin is most commonly known as *Reader's Digest*'s "most trusted woman on television" (Vaccariello, n.d.). In addition to being known for her trustworthiness, many likely recognize her for publically conquering both breast cancer and a blood-cell disorder known as myelodysplastic syndromes (MDS). With her experience as a news reporter under her belt, Robin took it upon herself to reveal these diagnoses on air for the whole world to see; she literally broke her own medical news on national television (see R. Roberts, 2007, August 3; 2012, June 11; 2014). After going public with each disease, she willingly allowed the cameras to roll as she battled and overcame each one. She has used her health experiences as ones that could educate and provide support for others going through similar circumstances. In her quest to survive and grow as an on-screen reporter, neither cancer nor MDS stopped her from interviewing people from Rodeo Drive to the White House. Her will to live was apparent and moving as she shared her journey to restore her health, twice, by providing the public with positive messages about early detection and treatment for her various health conditions. As she wrote in her book, *Everybody's Got Something*, she has followed her mother's advice to "make your mess your message" (2014, p. 7).

Robin Roberts—An Overview

Born in 1960 in Mississippi, Robin Roberts was the youngest of four siblings. Having two older sisters and one older brother, she came to know the role as the baby pretty well. She recalled in a *People* magazine interview that she always followed her siblings around and that she looked up to each of them (Cotliar & Jerome, 2008, October 20). Her sisters even commented that, growing up (according to Cotliar and Jerome), Robin did whatever they asked her to do; they led, and Robin followed, but her sisters admit that all changed when her career sparked, and she became the leader in their eyes.

Robin's career successes and life obstacles defined her in a new way to her sisters. She started her academic career off strong as a communication major at Southern Louisiana University (SLU). While at SLU, Robin began her life in basketball, and she could not know then that she would help shape the face of this sport for women as a point guard for the Lady Lions and later as a sports announcer. After graduating from SLU, she began working as a news announcer for a local sports network in Mississippi. ESPN hired her at the age of 29 as the host of *Sportscenter*, and she often contributed as a guest reporter on ABC's *Good Morning America* (*GMA*). Robin went from being the story as a successful basketball player, to telling other players' stories as the newscaster (R. Roberts, 2014; "Robin Roberts: Biography," 2014; see also Starpulse.com, 2014). For her work on the court and the sidelines, Roberts was inducted into the Women's Basketball Hall of Fame in 2012, and she referred to the honoree award as "freaking awesome" on *GMA* (*ABC News*, 2012, June 8).

Robin worked at ESPN for 15 years, and, in 2005, she signed on with ABC as a co-anchor for *GMA*, working alongside Diane Sawyer. Her career continued to blossom, and, throughout the years on *GMA*, her outstanding professionalism extended to her work of emotional reports including a plethora of interviews with impressive celebrities and world leaders, such as President Barack Obama and First Lady Michelle Obama (*ABC News*, 2014). In 2013, Robin Roberts was named *Reader's Digest* "most trusted woman on television" (Vaccariello, n.d., para. 10). According to Vaccariello (2013, May 7), with 56 percent of the votes in the poll, Robin surpassed Ellen DeGeneres (54 percent), her mentor and peer, Diane Sawyer (51 percent), Katie Couric (49 percent), Barbara Walters (50 percent), and Oprah Winfrey (48 percent). As Vaccariello (n.d.) noted, trust, integrity and character comprise important characteristics that a reporter must possess, and Robin exhibited those attributes when she reported on Hurricane Katrina after it devastated parts of her home state (Mississippi) and college stomping ground (Louisiana; *ABC News*, 2014) as well as on controversial issues, such as the Amanda Knox case in Italy (https://www.youtube.com/watch?v=n4hafGvxj9o).

In addition to breaking news, Robin has also grappled with reporting messages in the health arena. She has traveled all over the world with very credible leaders in efforts to improve the health status of people by educating others on prevention and early detection of various health conditions. For example, Robin journeyed to the Middle East with former First Lady Laura Bush in order to raise awareness of breast cancer among Muslim women. She also visited parts of Africa with former President Bill Clinton in an effort to publicize the AIDS crisis in those areas. In 2009, Robin ventured from the headquarters of *GMA* in New York City to the National Headquarters for the Centers for Disease Control and Prevention in Atlanta, Georgia, to give viewers a first-hand look at the Center's tracking of the H1N1 virus (i.e., swine flu; "Robin Roberts: Biography," 2014; see also Starpulse.com, 2014).

Robin Roberts has been on the forefront of the health and fitness arenas since the beginning of her career. However, her work as an advocate for health education and promotion became personal in 2007 when she discovered a lump in her breast that was, indeed, cancerous. In a letter to her fans on *ABC News*, Robin wrote,

> Never thought I'd be writing this.... I have breast cancer. It all started a few weeks ago. We had gotten the news that our dear colleague and friend Joel Siegel had passed away and we began preparing for our special tribute show for him. I did a piece about Joel's courageous battle with cancer, reporting on the way my friend had lived his life and been such a successful advocate for the importance of early cancer screenings. That very night when I went to bed, I did a self breast exam and found something that women everywhere fear: I found a lump. At first I thought, "This can't be. I am a young, healthy woman." Nevertheless, I faced my fear head on and made an appointment to see the doctor. Much as I was hoping the doctor would say it was nothing, she did a biopsy and confirmed that the lump I'd found was indeed an early form of breast cancer. Hearing the doctor say those words out loud was surreal. I will be having surgery shortly and follow-up treatment in the months to come.... To you, our viewers, please know that your thoughts and prayers very much sustain me as they always have each and every morning when I sit in the chair next to Diane and say "Good Morning America." You have always been there for me ... and I love you back [R. Roberts, 2007, August 3, para. 3–11].

In this same letter, Robin took time to credit her departed friend, Joel Siegel, saying,

> And like my good friend Joel, I can't stress enough how important it is to get screened and checked for all cancers—and to do self breast exams. I am so blessed that I found this in the early stages and the prognosis is so promising that my doctor expects me to be flying planes and hanging on to submarines in the middle of the Atlantic and scaling the Mayan Pyramids in no time in the mornings to come. Now I join the ranks of millions of Americans who are fighting this same battle each and every day. I appreciate YOUR courage and YOUR example. Thank you for showing me the way [R. Roberts, 2007, August 3, para. 11–12].

After undergoing chemotherapy and radiation to eradicate her breast cancer, Robin defied the odds and beat her triple-negative (and very aggressive form of) breast cancer (http://www.prevention.com/health/health-concerns/robin-roberts-exclusive-interview-surviving-breast-cancer).

With breast cancer in her past and a healthy life with survival in the horizon, Robin looked forward to returning to work and continuing to advance her career on *GMA*; yet, her life would change again. In 2012, Robin discovered another lump in her neck (R. Roberts, 2014; Silverstein, 2014, April 14). Robin explained in her 2014 book, *Everybody's Got Something*, that she discovered the lump while covering the 2012 Oscars; reliving in her mind what they had already gone through, her longtime partner, Amber Laign, demanded that Robin saw a doctor. As Robin wrote in her book, "I may not have even bothered to have it checked if Amber had not been there" (p. 12). Soon after the lump was tested, Robin discovered that she had a rare blood and bone-marrow disorder called myelodysplastic syndromes (MDS; Mirkinson, 2012, June 11). At the end of *GMA* on Monday, June 11, 2012, Robin announced to her fans and the world, "Sometimes treatment for cancer can lead to other serious medical issues [i.e., MDS] and that's what I'm facing right now" (Mirkinson, 2012, June 11, para. 5).

In the on-screen announcement of her diagnosis of MDS, Robin explained to her fans that she was beginning pre-treatment later that day; pre-treatment involved chemotherapy that would advance her body for her bone marrow transplant later that year (Mirkinson, 2012, June 11). Although bone marrow donors are notably scarce in the African American population (just like in the book *My Sister's Keeper* by Jodi Picoult), Robin's sister, Sally-Ann Roberts, turned out to be the perfect match that saved her life (*ABC News*, 2013, February 22; see also R. Roberts, 2012, June 11; 2014). Robin made a pledge on air to overcome MDS (*ABC News*, 2013, February 22, para. 8), and, as one of 13 of the Huffington Post's Biggest Celebrity Health Battles of 2013 (see Schocker, 2013, December 31), Robin posted the following message on her Facebook wall just a year and a half after her diagnosis and bone marrow transplant:

> At this moment I am at peace and filled with joy and gratitude. I am grateful to God, my doctors and nurses for my restored good health. I am grateful for my sister, Sally-Ann, for being my donor and giving me the gift of life. I am grateful for my entire family, my long time girlfriend, Amber, and friends as we prepare to celebrate a glorious new year together [Schocker, 2013, December 31].

Notably, she gave herself the token name of a "walking miracle' in a *People* magazine interview (Cotliar, 2014, April 16, para. 2). Robin's health struggles and journey in the public eye document her strength and desire to employ her experience to educate and inspire others. In turn, the loving support from her fans also celebrates the continuous need for her to serve the nation as a leading reporter and co-anchor of precious national and world news on *GMA* (Hater, 2013, September 20).

In order to make sense of all the feedback and support from Robin's fans, we analyzed messages posted on news sources, reports, discussion boards, and social media, and we discuss Robin's public, passionate fight to survive both deadly diseases as well as Robin's role in spreading awareness of these health conditions. In the words of Robin Roberts, "God only gives us what we can handle and that it helps to have a good sense of humor when we run smack into the absurdity of life" (2012, June 11, para. 5). To begin, though, we will provide background information on MDS and treatment options.

Background: MDS

MDS, also known as "bone marrow failure disorder," is a disorder of the bone marrow that causes an inadequate production of healthy blood cells to grow in the bone (MDS Foundation, 2014, para. 1). It can occur after some chemotherapies or radiation following cancer treatment, and, if not treated early, MDS can progress to acute myeloid leukemia (AML; MDS Foundation, 2014). Due to the vast number of individuals who undergo cancer treatment each year, putting them at risk of developing MDS over time, awareness of this disease is vital.

A bone marrow transplant constitutes a common treatment option for MDS patients. The largest survival rates from MDS (~60 percent) pertain to individuals who are fortunate enough to be able to go through high-intensity therapy. High-intensity therapy is a combination of chemotherapy and stem cell transplant (SCT; i.e., healthy bone marrow from a donor replaces the unhealthy bone marrow of the patient). Another treatment option, known as low-intensity therapy, may include a combination of immunosuppressive drugs (in lieu of SCT) and chemotherapy. Immunosuppressive drugs, unlike SCT, "counter the immune attack on the bone marrow" (Wolters Kluwer Health, 2014, para. 21).

For high-intensity therapy, attaining a bone marrow donor who is a blood relative increases the success rate of a healthy match. Furthermore, "the optimal source of stem cells is a brother or sister with a similar genetic makeup" because then they are a "matched related donor" (Wolters Kluwer Health, 2014, para. 29). Since having a sibling or a relative with matching stem cells is not always available for patients, advances in technology have improved the chance of matching unrelated donors to patients in need of a SCT. A host of celebrities and healthcare industries have sought to publicize and encourage the donation of healthy stem cells (Wolters Kluwer Health, 2014), and Robin has certainly heralded the need for stem cell donations. As she explained, "A doctor told me I had one to two years to live without a transplant" (Cotliar, 2014, April 16, para. 4).

"Woe" to "Thrive"

Rosenbaum and Rosenbaum (2011, December 31) explained that "[t]he will to live is a force within all of us to fight for survival when our lives are threatened by a disease such as cancer. Yet this force is stronger in some people than in others" (para. 2). In her public announcement that she had breast cancer, Robin Roberts (2007, August 3) said, "So in the coming months, you will probably notice that I will have my good days and my bad days, but I know I will get through it with the love and support of my family and friends (para. 8)." When faced with adversity again, with her diagnosis of MDS in 2012, Robin made an on-air pledge to overcome this deadly disease (*ABC News*, 2013, February 22). In a *People* magazine article, Robin asserted, "Yes, I am living with cancer, but don't go 'woe is me.' I don't want it. Don't need it. I'm still in the game. I don't want to say 'survivor.' I want to thrive" (Cotliar & Jerome, 2008, October, para. 7). As a direct quote from Shakespeare's *Hamlet* (Act 3, Scene 1), "O, woe is me, to have seen what I have seen, see what I see!" (see Shakespeare, 1599/2014, para. 42), "woe is me" is an outcry of sorrow and misfortune, or "to express how unhappy you are" (Cambridge Dictionaries, 2014). Robin mentioned that she did not want people to go "woe is me" or perceive her as crying out about how terrible it was that she had breast cancer; she wanted to "thrive" rather than be a "survivor."

The *Merriam-Webster Dictionary* (2014) defines the word "survivor" as "one that survives" or "one living through a time, event, or development marked by the death of others." In women, breast cancer is the second most common form of cancer and the second leading cause of death (American Cancer Society, 2014a). In 2014 alone, the American Cancer Society estimates that over 295,000 people will be diagnosed with, and 40,000 people will die from, breast cancer. Robin chose to "thrive" or, as the Merriam-Webster Dictionary (2014) defined it, "to grow vigorously" or "flourish," "to gain in wealth or possessions" or "prosper," and "to progress toward or realize a goal despite or because of circumstances." Robin wanted her fans to know that she fought to survive but only because she would thrive when faced with adversity and overcome her negative health circumstances. She sought to get healthy and flourish, and she did it in spite (and, perhaps, because) of navigating her illness narratives very much in the public eye.

Fans have certainly praised Robin's positivity and ongoing fight to thrive and survive, especially individuals with their own history of battles with cancer and/or MDS. Yet, as the following passages illustrate, exchanges between Robin and fans function as mutually beneficial and inspiring forms of social support. In response to Robin's MDS announcement, fans reached out to her with strong words of encouragement (see Roberts, 2012, June 11). Richard stated on the ABC blog area for the article, "Robin, you are an 'OVERCOMER,' you will overcome this and you have an army of Overcomers with you. You inspire me to overcome my challenges and I am with you." Likewise, sve5650 said, "Robin…. I truly wish you all the best as I will keep praying for you…. Thank you for your st[r]ong desire to keep going. You inspire more people than anyone could ever imagine. :)—Sarah." Oveykat also expressed her support to Robin on the comments area for the article online:

> Robin, You are such a motivation to all whether healthy or facing an illness. Please know that somewhere in Kentucky there is another person who will be praying for you and your family. What a wonderful thing it is that your sister can share a life continuing gift. All the best to you and her.

Furthermore, other fans expressed how Robin's story helped them to attain courage and strength in their respective personal struggles with finding a match for a bone marrow transplant, something that is instrumental in surviving MDS (MDS Foundation, 2014). Eartstarr3 wrote,

> Hang In There Robin, You WILL BEAT THIS! I Am Fighting Too, Unlike You Though, I Do Not Have A Match Yet! I Just Love Your Spirit! I Too Go To Work Daily, Treatment Weekly, Endless Blood Transfusions And Hospitalizations! Thanks For Motivating Me To Keep It Moving! I Am So Inspired By Your Strength! No Doubt That We Will Celebrate Survival And LIFE Together! We Only Have To Have FAITH The Size Of A Mustard Seed! All The Best For You And Your Family! Starr M Phipps From A Little Town In Virginia Called Lawrenceville! [2012].

Sandra, who survived breast cancer, also responded to Robin's message:

> Robin, I am praying for your total healing. You are truly an inspiration for women, of all races. I too am a breast cancer survivor. I know my faith and prayers of others help me survive. May you know how many love, and respect you. Fight like a girl!! [2012].

Mick, a fan on Twitter, wrote to Robin (2014, January 30), saying, "@Robin Roberts…. I also whooped cancer down! You were my inspiration and mentor." Notably, Robin actively responds to fellow cancer and MDS fighters, and she tweeted back with "Very happy for you … my fellow OVERCOMER! @RobinRoberts @Mickxxx" (2014, January 30). Likewise, on March 2, 2014, Robin tweeted out, "For all fellow #overcomers … this is for you. Oscars Red Carpet. #grateful http://instagram.com/p/lDw2MqKw0n/" with a picture linked to her Instagram account of her "thriving" at the Oscars, symbolic given that she found the lump on her neck that was linked to MDS at the Oscars two years earlier.

These examples indicate how both fans and Robin have used social media and the online environment (e.g., blogs for online news articles like *People* magazine or *The Hollywood Reporter*) to disclose their respective personal health stories with the world. These online outlets provide users with a space to share their courage, fears, and life experiences as a way to cope with their journey through a health problem (see Antheunis et al., 2013; High et al., 2014). Furthermore, through public spaces such as Twitter and blog forums, users can be anonymous yet invite and obtain public support regarding a plethora of topics (e.g., health-related issues, support groups, etc.). These forums enable participants to share their personal health struggles while not revealing their faces (see High et al., 2014).

Individuals can envision and treat online interactions as a type of "backstage" (see Goffman, 1959) wherein noncelebrities can expand privacy boundaries (see Petronio, 2002) at reduced risk of public face. For celebrities, such as Robin Roberts, though, interactions online can foster perceived intimacy with fans as she discloses personal information and feelings in what, for her, functions as very much a public space. Through online exchanges, Robin and her fans co-construct a dynamic as mutual cheerleaders "against" a common foe—cancer and MDS. Interactivity facilitated by social media fosters relationships that go beyond "parasocial" (see, e.g., W. J. Brown & Basil, 2010; Hartmann & Goldhoorn, 2011; Meyrowitz, 1985), likely nurturing an even more intimate (and powerful) connection between celebrity and fans (see related work by Marwick, 2013; Thackeray et al., 2013; Wheeler, 2013).

As we have detailed throughout this book, the advent of social media, coupled with the implicit expansion of privacy boundaries (see Petronio, 2002, 2004), enables fans to increasingly co-narrate celebrity health journeys through their reactions. In Robin Roberts' case, similarities in their respective situations resonated with fans and reaffirmed perspectives, but they also wrestled to reconcile different outcomes in their own lives with gratitude for Robin's miracle.

Responses to the *People* magazine article, titled "Robin Roberts Feels like She Is a 'Walking Miracle,'" included fan appreciation for the role of love and sacrifice in Robin's saga and sad acknowledgment that "love" cannot always suffice as a cure (Cotliar, 2014, April 16). DigiDoodle (2012, March) responded to the Cotliar article, stating that she was "[v]ery happy for Robin, but the header Love saved her, it is tough to read. Just lost a 32-year-old mother of two children and she was loved dearly by the community." Another fan, Lori Jan, commented on DigiDoodle's message. Lori Jan wrote,

> You took the words right out of my mouth. I lost my husband of 27 years 10 months after being diagnosed with MDS. It went into leukemia and the chemo brought his levels down so low he got pulmonary nodules. If loved saved people he would be here today because the hospital aisles were lined with family and beloved friends. I am so happy for Robin being a survivor. She is one lucky lady who beat the odds not only on being a transplant match with her sister but to beat breast cancer and MDS. No pity party for me just that MDS rest on being fortunate enough to have a donor match or beat the odds of a clinical trial. I adore you Robin and appreciate how positive you are [2012, March].

In her letter announcement to fans revealing her diagnosis with MDS (see Roberts, 2012, June 11), Robin continued her intimate (and mutually empowering) dialogue with fans, noting "When I faced breast cancer, your prayers and good wishes sustained me, gave me such hope and played a major role in my recovery. In facing this new challenge, I ask humbly for more of your prayers and love—as I will keep you in my mine and update you regularly on my condition (para. 7).

In an interview with the *Hollywood Reporter,* Robin thanked her fans for their outpouring words of encouragement, asserting that "[p]eople are going through so many things, whether it's with your heart or blood cancer or whatever. As my mom used to say, we all have something, and it was just incredible, the outpouring and support, and it became like an online community, people helping and sharing ideas. It was extremely comforting" (Zakarin, 2013, April 10, para. 6).

When asked about (see Zakarin, 2013, April 10) and reflecting on (see R. Roberts, 2012, June 11) her highest highs and lowest lows, Robin said her "proudest moment … is to be alive!" (Zakarin, 2013, April 10, para. 1). This evident and humble answer foregrounds her personal-yet-public battle with MDS and breast cancer over professional accomplishments. Interestingly, Robin received her diagnosis of MDS on the same day that *GMA* overcame their losing streak to the *Today* show, winning the morning show ratings war for the first time in 16 years (see Roberts, 2012, June 11; Zakarin, 2013, April 10). During one of the largest highs in her career (beating the *Today* show in ratings), she reached another low in her life (MDS). Furthermore, on the day that she had her bone marrow extracted for testing, she also heard exciting news in terms of her career. Robin explained,

I received word that I would interview President Obama the next day. The combination of landing the biggest interview of my career and having a drill in my back reminds me that God only gives us what we can handle and that it helps to have a good sense of humor when we run smack into the absurdity of life [R. Roberts, 2012, June 11, para. 5].

The juxtaposition between Robin's lows and highs accentuates and reinforces her will and power to thrive. Considering the words from Rosenbaum and Rosenbaum (2011, December 31) that "sometimes the biology of a cancer will dictate the course of events regardless of the patient's attitude and fighting spirit" (para. 3), it is not hard to believe that Robin's optimistic views on life and healing made it possible for her to cope with the disease and ultimately respond better to her treatment options, all while celebrating life.

The Robin Roberts Effect

As we have observed in this book thus far, celebrities such as Robin Roberts can positively affect health education and health promotion, bringing welcome (and, sometimes, rare) attention to a health condition or illness. According to Dr. Donnica Moore, M.D., as quoted in Mann's (2007, July 31) article, "I give Robin Roberts a tremendous amount of credit for going public from the beginning and using her experience to help others" (para. 5). Dr. Moore continued, arguing, "Just as we saw the 'Katie Couric effect' on the diagnosis of colon cancer, I predict that Robin Roberts' brave announcement will produce a 'Robin Roberts effect' in the increased diagnosis of breast cancer among all women" (para. 6). Mann explained the excitement behind the "Katie Couric effect": "After Couric underwent a colonoscopy on the *Today* show in March 2000, test rates jumped nationwide" (para. 7). Dr. Lichtenfeld, M.D., from the American Cancer Society, weighed in on this conversation:

> I have commented frequently about public figures facing cancer, and the special role they play in our lives. Not only do they have to deal with a serious diagnosis, but they also frequently have to cope with that diagnosis while in the public eye. Here we have someone [referencing Robin Roberts] who is very special to so many facing just that circumstance. She did so with the grace and sincerity that is so much a trademark of her "on camera" persona [2007, July 31, para. 2–3].

In response to Schocker's (2013, December 31) news article on the top 13 celebrity health battles of 2013 (one of which was Robin's), readers offered their opinions about celebrity health narratives. Donna commented, "Stars are human and suffer the same frailties as you and I, some use their celebrity to educate. This is good, I wish them all my best" (2014, January 2). Likewise,

IVFDad agreed, "It[']s great that celebrities are speaking up about the health issues, we wish them the very best of health. Is it going to take a celebrity to spread awareness on the lack of laws for IVF children and families?" (2014, January 1).

As we now detail, Robin's advocacy work for early detection of breast cancer and MDS and the public's reaction to those efforts exemplify the potential value of celebrity health narratives in terms of public dialogues about health.

TRENDING: EARLY DETECTION SAVES LIVES

Early detection of cancer falls hand-in-hand with awareness of the disease (http://www.cancer.org/cancer/breastcancer/moreinformation/breast cancerearlydetection/breast-cancer-early-detection-acs-recs-bse?doc Selected=breast-cancer-early-detection-acs-recs-clinical-breast-exam). Understanding the importance of self-breast exams and how to administer them are vital to healthy breast health as well as both the prevention and early detection of breast cancer (American Cancer Society, 2014a). Bender et al. (2011) argued that messages surrounding the promotion of healthy behaviors such as breast cancer awareness messages (BCAM; e.g., early or routine detection of breast cancer), serve as calls to action for women (or men) by encouraging and promoting positive breast health cancer awareness. Since the beginning of her diagnosis and journey through cancer survival, Robin has always been on the frontline in terms of spreading awareness of breast cancer by encouraging early detection through preventive efforts (e.g., self-breast exams, mammography, etc.; see Lichtenfeld, 2007, July 31; R. Roberts, 2007, August 3). Because many of the news reports on the Internet include links to social media sites like Twitter and Facebook, the reach of health promotion efforts expands when high-profile celebrity spokespersons with personal experience (i.e., Robin Roberts) spread messages such as BCAM, especially when they interact with followers on social media sites (e.g., ~733K Twitter followers and ~481K Facebook followers; see Thackeray et al., 2013).

Such promotion ultimately aids in engaging followers in a conversation about breast cancer that has the potential to influence their decision to seek preventive, lifesaving behaviors (Thackeray et al., 2013). In the case of Robin Roberts, fans actively recognize that she has made a difference in their lives as well as in the lives of others by encouraging healthy preventive behaviors. In a tweet on Twitter, @4everdetermined writes, "@RobinRoberts Thank u 4 being an inspiration from a early breast cancer survivor!" (2014, May 3).

Robin quickly responded, saying, "Beautiful! @4everdetermined" (2014), affirming her support for the act of early detection.

Ellen, a woman who responded to the American Cancer Society announcement by Dr. Lichtenfeld (2007, July 31), wrote about what Robin's work meant to her:

> Dear Dr. L, In a day and age when "heros/heroines" for young people are questionable, Robin Roberts is stellar!! Not just a wonderful athlete, not just a competent tv personality, but someone who is one of the best models of healthly [healthy], holy and wholesome living. Robin is not just "grace," but "Amazing Grace." I, along with you and thousands of other viewers will keep her in our prayers—not just on Friday when she has her surgery, but in the days, weeks and months ahead. God writes straight with crooked lines—Robin has already demonstrated that she will be an advocate for early detection [2007, August 1].

Mirroring Ellen's point that Robin's awareness encourages life-saving preventive efforts, a fan named Jones La-La recorded his opinion to Cotliar's (2014, April 16) article, noting, "I would rather see stories about her than many of the celebs that *People* features. She is a class act and a great example of keeping a positive attitude and pushing through hard times." Anonymous Guest also responded to Cotliar's article, echoing Jones La-La's response, "Cancer is an ongoing battle—I am a survivor of almost 8 years, and have also had struggles, surgeries, etc., related to this horrible disease. She is an inspiration, and I would rather see her on the cover of *People* than someone like the Kardashians, The Bachelor alumni, or some celebrity who can't handle their fame without alcohol or drugs."

These fans stress the importance of having positive celebrities, such as Robin, who, when faced with adversity, use their status to endorse healthy behaviors that can ultimately save lives. Furthermore, these messages reiterate that a meaningful connection with others and a common health-related cause foster mutual support both online (e.g., blog, discussion board, etc.) and face-to-face in a support group (Barker, 2009).

In addition to Robin's inspirational interviews and supportive and inter-active immediacy through social media, she has also actively employed her work on *GMA* as a platform for advocacy. To spread awareness of breast cancer (in hopes of encouraging early detection through preventive efforts such as self-breast exams and mammography), *GMA* kicked off October's Breast Cancer Awareness Month with a bang. Co-host Amy Robach agreed to do the first-ever, live on-screen mammogram (see Robach, 2013, November 11), with a stunning outcome and initiating yet another public health saga as we detail in our final chapter.

Breaking News: MDS Awareness on the Rise

In addition to Robin's successful efforts to promote awareness of and promotion for early detection of breast cancer, she also employs her celebrity status to educate the public about MDS and highlight the importance of organ donations, specifically in the form of bone marrow (see R. Roberts, 2012, June 11).

Robin's fans commend her on her ability to bring awareness to such devastating disease. When she disclosed her MDS diagnosis (see R. Roberts, 2012, June 11), fans poured in their support and appreciation for her work. As Jupitercheryl stated in the blog area for the online article, "Robin thank you for letting people know about this disease. Most people have never heard of it. I was diagnosed in November of last year and I am trying medication first before a transplant. I sure hope it works. I hope to be as strong and brave as you have been" (2013, May).

Likewise, Andeesue credited Roberts with informing her about the disease:

> [I was] recently diagnosed with MDS and must thank Robin for bringing awareness to this disease. I luckily found the website of the Aplastic Anemia and MDS Foundation that gave me so much information. Still, this journey is so scary with a bone marrow transplant as the only cure, and there are so many risks. Reading the *Parade* magazine featuring her in March, I thought, oh my- I'm experiencing the same symptoms Robin described ... sure enough, the bone marrow biopsy confirmed. I so appreciate the bravery and grace that Robin has demonstrated, and will look toward her model as one to learn from [2013, October].

In addition to raising awareness of the diseases, Robin also dedicates considerable time to discussing the importance of organ donation, specifically in the form of bone marrow donation (see Cotliar, 2014, April 16; R. Roberts, 2012, June 11; Zakarin, 2013, April 10). For example, she interacts with fans through Twitter about her own life-saving transplant. @Timothyxxxxx tweeted @RobinRoberts (2014, March 21), "Today's day +100 from my bone marrow transplant!" Robin responded, saying, "Such an important milestone. Very happy for you Tim, yay!! @Timothyxxxxx." In a response to @Nataliexxxxxxx's tweet (2014, March 26), "@RobinRoberts my nephew just received his bone marrow transplant from his sister they are 3 & 5! GO MIGHTY MACK!," Robin returned the tweet, saying, "YES! XO! @Nataliexxxxxxx." She is a celebrity who works hard to respond to important Tweets surrounding survival of MDS, providing her fellow fans with the social support that they need to continue fighting their disease (see High et al.,2014; Lichtenfeld, 2007, July 31; Mann, 2007, July 31).

Robin's announcement to the public about her diagnosis with MDS on June 11, 2012, stressed the need for bone marrow donors to help save lives through SCT. Roberts wrote:

> Today, I will start what is known as pre-treatment—chemotherapy in advance of a bone marrow transplant later this year. Bone marrow donors are scarce and particularly for African-American women. I am very fortunate to have a sister who is an excellent match, and this greatly improves my chances for a cure. As you know from my recent interview with Mark Zuckerberg, organ donation is vitally important. Many people don't realize they can be bone marrow donors. I encourage everyone to sign up on a donor registry like bethematch.org [2012, para. 4].

On the same day that Robin went public with her illness, she provided her audience members with an action step for how they can make a difference in organ donation by contacting bethematch.org. As a response to her message, another "Robin Roberts effect" occurred when bethematch.org "experienced an 1,800 percent spike in bone marrow donors" on June 11, 2012 (see Vaccariello, n.d.), affirming that Robin Roberts affected her audience, just as Katie Couric did regarding colon cancer screening (see Mann, 2007, July 31).

A Twitter conversation between Robin and @momaryxx also exemplified Robin's positive effect on promoting MDS treatment. @momaryxx tweeted @RobinRoberts and @BeTheMatch on May 2014, saying "Have you seen this? LOVE this story about the Ohio State baseball team: http://cbsprt.co/Buck eyesCancer." Robin endorsed this tweet by re-tweeting the story on her Twitter wall and responding with "XO" to @momary95. In the report from the Ohio State baseball team, readers learn that a member of the team was diagnosed with a blood disorder, and survival required an SCT. In a response to his diagnosis, the player's teammates banded together and got tested to see if any of them could be a match to save his life. This story constitutes a beautiful example of a support system rallying together to help find a cure for someone with MDS. Further, through her network of followers on Twitter, Robin attracted even more public attention to it, underscoring Robin's commitment as an activist for promoting awareness of stem cell donation for MDS patients.

In her public statement about MDS (see Roberts, 2012, June 11), Robin encouraged her readers to become organ donors. A fan named sve5650 also responded to Robin's announcement:

> Robin, because of your story and how brave you are everyday; I have made it my own duty to help my cousin find his match. He was also diagnosed with MDS. I got our family together and we just did the Be The One Run in Columbus, Ohio at the end of July. We were able to raise over DOUBLE our goal! It was such a great experiance [experience]. I truly wish you all the best as I will keep praying for you, please pray for my cousin as he started his chemo last week.

Thank you for your st[r]ong desire to keep going. You inspire more people than anyone could ever imagine. :)—Sarah [2012].

As we have indicated, fans praise Robin on her ability to spread awareness of the importance of bone marrow donors for a healthy transplant in an MDS patient. Although she has provided the public with information on MDS and the need for donors (see Cotliar, 2014, April 16; R. Roberts, 2012, June 11), some voice even higher expectations. CF responded to the *People* magazine article (Cotliar, 2014, April 16) by challenging Robin's contributions and, implicitly, fulfillment of implied social responsibility:

> She [Robin] actually hasn't said enough about her experience. Being a blood cancer survivor myself, I wish she would really let people know the truth about how hard it really is and how she was lucky to have a related donor. There is only a 25 percent chance tha[t] you will have a related donor. More often than not they have to go to the international bone marrow registry to find a donor. 5 out of 10 patients in need of a none [bone] marrow transplant. NEVER find a match. And die because of this. So I personally wish she would talk more about it, to educate people and let people know we need more donors. My only chance to survive was finding a non related donor. I was one of the lucky ones. I am. 1.5 years post transplant. Too many people are misinformed about what being a donor really is all about. It is not a horrific procedure like it was years ago. She has an audience that I don't have and the ability to really make people listen and understand and she doesn't. That's great she has support but pay it forward and use her experience to inform and potential save someone else's life just by educating people.

Borrowing from Fisher (1984, 1985a, 1987a), Roberts' narrative did not ring true or do justice to the master narrative of struggling to obtain a donor, given that her story "beat" the odds and became an exception to the rule. On the other hand, a responder to Silverstein's (2014, April 14) article about Robin's upcoming memoir, disagreed with CF. Arthur argued:

> Back in the days when a celebrity had cancer I would say they want publicity. I have been diagnosed with MDS and now I want to say a big THANK YOU Robin because in following you I feel that I might have a chance too. I have no siblings but I have faith. Robin it helps you discussing the disease and it helps knowing you beat it [2014, April].

These opposing opinions expose expectations that celebrities *should* engage in public discourse about personal health-related matters, and they also reveal the complexities of such involvement. In spite of emphasizing her unique physical attributes (youth and fitness) as well as good fortunate at identifying a donor so quickly, does Robin's exceptionally positive narrative spark false hope or downplay risks or alternate realities (and inevitabilities)? Robin admitted that "if you Google MDS, you may find some scary stuff, including statistics that my doctors insist don't apply to me. They say I'm younger and fitter than most people who confront this disease and will be cured" (R. Roberts, 2012, June 11, para. 3). She acknowledged "scary stuff" that falls hand-in-hand with being diagnosed with and the treatment options for MDS; she noted that her situation may be relevant to a particular population of people. Does her position as a celebrity require her to uncover seemingly daunting statistics on survival? Does her celebrity status make her a credible source for claims beyond her own personal journey?

Certainly, the extent to which celebrity advocates must go beyond their individual health narratives to claim medical knowledge remains murky and, perhaps, contingent on the specific celebrity and even types of external audiences. As Dr. Lichtenfeld (2007, July 31) commented in his report on the American Cancer Society website, "Celebrities represent all of us, especially when they share some of their most personal life events. Few have done so with such grace. Robin, we wish you well" (para. 26). Robin continues to show her journey through breast cancer and MDS recoveries on a public stage, but engaging in a public conversation with the world about her health issues makes her vulnerable to attacks in the media. That vulnerability has not silenced Robin or hindered her from attempting to make a difference in the lives of others.

When Robin Roberts addresses the public about one of her health issues, in effect, she offers a huge (plus free and endorsed) public service announcement (see Mann, 2007, July 31). Just as with the "Katie Couric effect" with colon cancer screenings through colonoscopy (see Mann, 2007, July 31), Robin Roberts has initiated a "Robin Roberts effect" on women (and men) with increased diagnosis of breast cancer through mammography screenings, exemplified on screen with colleague Amy Robach.

As this chapter has detailed, a celebrity health narrative holds the potential to motivate and encourage the adoption of healthy, routine, preventable behaviors, such as the "Robin Roberts effect" on seeking a mammogram, evaluating a lump, or becoming an organ donor. If a celebrity has a passion for either advocating for early detection of a disease or condition or promoting helping find a cure, and they have the reach through social media to share their messages with thousands or even millions of viewers, the potential *effect* that it could have on that disease or condition is incredible.

Discussion

Robin Roberts did not want to be perceived by others as someone who was suffering from breast cancer or MDS; she wanted the world to see her thrive as she overcame some of life's largest obstacles, health issues. As a reporter, Robin has experience with cameras following her, and she continued to allow them to roll even when she began to experience new, seemingly less ideal life circumstances; in those moments, privacy boundaries shifted, and what many might construe and treat as private information (e.g., health conditions) became collaboratively co-constructed as public (see Petronio, 2002).

Moreover, Robin actively capitalized on her celebrity status as a way to increase awareness of, education on, and early detection of breast cancer and MDS. Fans generously communicated support for Robin as she navigated through her illnesses. Those relationships fostered a dynamic of mutual trust and concern, establishing a fertile context for the "Robin Roberts effect" to occur (see Vaccariello, 2013).

Notably, in addition to trusting Robin enough to seek health preventive treatments like mammograms, fans must identify with a celebrity in order to make life changes (see Mann, 2007, July 31). Vaccariello (n.d.) quoted Elayne Rapping, a pop-culture expert from the University at Buffalo, as asserting that "people identify with those who can recover from adversity" (para. 1). As Robin wrote in her book, "As my mom always said, everybody's got something" (2014, p. 49). She showed the world that, just like her, they could overcome a life-threatening disease by simply learning about it in its beginning stages (for related work on identification, see Burke (1950/1969). Learning about breast cancer in the beginning stages statistically enhances survival rates for women (National Breast Cancer Foundation, 2012, para. 2). Having a donor for SCT increases her rate of survival by 60 percent (Wolters Kluwer Health, 2014, para. 21). With the power of these two statistics alone, Robin employed her celebrity status to encourage mammograms and organ donation (see Lichtenfeld, 2007, July 31; Mann, 2007, July 31). Because Robin brought these issues to light through candid and intimate disclosures, she expanded her privacy boundaries, embracing others as now part of her emergent journey (see Petronio, 2002; Vaccariello, n.d.).

CHAPTER TWELVE

She Turns the World Around with Their Smiles

Mary Tyler Moore Takes Kids to Congress

Mary Tyler Moore charmed the world in her CBS television series, the *Mary Tyler Moore Show*. The theme song to the show, "Love Is All Around," beautifully captured her one-of-a-kind spirit of optimism and possibility, and with the toss of her hat, she reassured us that we're "gonna make it after all." Near the beginning of her work on this now classic and legendary series, at the age of 33, Mary was diagnosed with type 1 diabetes, and, eventually, she embraced her role as a celebrity advocate working to make sure that all of those living with diabetes do, in fact, have a chance to make it. Mary currently serves as the International Chairman of the Juvenile Diabetes Research Foundation (JDRF), formerly the Juvenile Diabetes Foundation (JDF), using her celebrity profile in a variety of capacities to help raise awareness of the disease and increase funding for research. For example, with the JDRF's Children's Congress event, she accompanies more than 100 children living with type 1 diabetes to Washington, D.C., to meet face-to-face with members of Congress. JDRF dubbed her "The Magnificent Mary," and she has referred to these children as her "heroes" ("The Magnificent Mary," 2000, Summer).

Within this chapter, guided by narrative, aesthetic, and pragmatic theoretical sensibilities, we attend to Mary Tyler Moore's use of her celebrity status to create a platform from which hundreds of young voices have also been granted the opportunity to share their own personal experiences in an effort to advocate for research funding that will lead to better treatments, prevention, and, hopefully, a cure for type 1 diabetes. In the process, their willingness to tell their stories has inspired a personal approach to advocacy that highlights vulnerability and creativity, while fostering social support among children and families affected by type 1 diabetes who are trying to live fully and purposefully despite the odds set against them. As this chapter will detail, Mary Tyler Moore's journey exemplifies a unique and powerful spirit of partnering and co-authoring emergent public health narratives, especially as she has mobilized and empowered others who also struggle with the illness (and whose voices might otherwise never have had a chance to be heard).

Type 1 Diabetes: An Invisible Illness Demands Attention

Type 1 diabetes (T1D), often referred to as juvenile diabetes, is most commonly diagnosed in children and young adults. The American Diabetes Association (2013) explained,

> A diagnosis of type 1 diabetes means your pancreas is no longer capable of producing insulin. Through multiple daily injections with insulin pens or syringes or an insulin pump, it will be up to you to monitor your blood glucose levels and appropriately administer your insulin [para. 3].

Further, proper management of the disease involves constant attention to exercise and nutrition, and often requires significant emotional and instrumental support from family, friends, and others living with the disease. Notably, unlike type 2 diabetes, this disease is not preventable; individuals who suffer from this chronic illness do not "do" anything that causes them to be at risk (such as poor diet or lack of exercise). Unfortunately, the disease currently has no cure and cannot be reversed (American Diabetes Association, 2013).

People living with T1D, or those who take care of individuals with the disease, must work every day to keep blood sugar levels as close to normal as possible. Low (hypoglycemia) and high (hyperglycemia) blood sugar episodes are not simply unpleasant experiences when they occur, but they also contribute to long-term complications of the disease, as it develops gradually throughout the life course. Disabling and life-threatening complications that arise as an effect of poorly controlled diabetes include heart and blood vessel disease, nerve damage, kidney damage, eye damage, foot damage, skin conditions, osteoporosis, and brain problems (CNN Health, 2013).

Doctors consider T1D to be an invisible chronic illness, due to its ever present symptoms and the ongoing monitoring required for those people living with the disease—people who otherwise appear to be healthy and unmarked by illness. Mary Tyler Moore's journey after her diagnosis provides a vivid example of the invisibility of this disease. *The Mary Tyler Moore Show* debuted in 1970, the year following Mary's diagnosis. The show aired for seven years, and it has been referred to as "amongst the finest television programs ever produced in America" (IMDB, 2014f). While excelling so brilliantly on the screen, Mary admitted to feeling like she was "failing miserably on a personal level," because, as she wrote, she "tried to make [diabetes] the last thing on [her] mind, without neglecting the basics" (Moore, 2009, p. 36).

The Cost of Separating the Personal and the Public

For the duration of *The Mary Tyler Moore Show*, she kept her struggle with diabetes private, testing blood sugar and managing insulin levels between filming scenes. In her book *Growing Up Again* she explained, "I wasn't keeping it a secret exactly" (Moore, 2009, p. 116), but she acknowledged fearing that widespread knowledge of her illness would have a negative effect on the public's perception of her, as well as their understanding of T1D. Clearly, she prioritized managing her career and public image. No part of her desired sympathy from fans—she did not want them to begin seeing a disease instead of a person, nor did she want them to feel bad for her. Instead, she desired for viewers to simply enjoy her artistry and contributions to television and film.

Further, in all of her attempts to continue acting, she did not want to project a misconceived image of the disease as one that does not take a toll on the individuals living with the illness. Mary did not want the public to see the active, healthy, optimistic, and unstoppable "Mary" on-screen and naively assume the polished, fictional picture to be a realistic glimpse of a person living with T1D (Moore, 2009). These fears were valid. The public was not privy to the behind the scenes footage that included the hypoglycemic episodes that she suffered after skipping snacks and engaging in the increased physical activity demanded by her role as an actress. As Mary detailed for readers in *Growing Up Again*, the reality of her situation was not one that remained invisible at all times:

> One [episode] that stands out in my memory happened during one of our Monday-morning meetings, when the cast would assemble to read through that week's script. On this particular Monday we had a guest director, so this was an important opportunity to get to know one another as we found the jokes and added to them, as well. I'd felt a bit jittery as I'd driven to work, but I didn't know what could account for it. Certainly I wasn't nervous about meeting the new director (well, yes, a bit); certainly I had had enough to eat (well, I was on a diet to lose a few pounds gained on vacation and was familiar with the vague light-headedness that goes along with hunger). But the truth was, I was relatively

new to the signs of the carnival ride awaiting me. So that morning, unbeknownst to me, I was being swept off my feet by hypoglycemia—low blood sugar....

As the cast and crew introduced themselves to the new guy, I felt my voice wavering. I remember the unsure faces of my dear friends as they tried to make sense of the apparition who used to be Mary. I began crying while trying to explain what it was: "It's my diabetes. No, my diet. I didn't recognize it. It's not your fault." I jabbered on in an attempt to will the now-terrifying feeling away.

At some point our producer, Allan Burns, grabbed my hair, pulled my head back, and began to pour orange juice down my throat. He'd had the presence of mind to call my doctor. It worked. In ten minutes I could feel myself returning to normal [Moore, 2009, pp. 14–15].

Following her description of the episode above, Mary recalled the horror she felt years later when she learned that the guest director had suggested to others that the horrific event was caused by her addiction to diet pills. When fellow actress Cloris Leachman expressed confusion about the event and asked, "What does diabetes have to do with acting so strangely anyway?!" (Moore, 2009, p. 15), Mary realized a great need for public education about the disease and its symptoms.

Mary was also surprised when the Juvenile Diabetes Foundation (JDF, now JDRF) asked her to star in a couple of television public service announcements requesting donations. Mary noted that, at this point, "The spots said nothing about my also being a diabetic. I felt virtuous and yet protected from public scrutiny of my disease" (Moore, 2009, p. 115). These commercials enabled her to contribute to the societal education about the disease and join the effort to raise funds for research aimed at finding a cure—both goals for which she was passionate, given her personal experience.

At the time, Mary continued to conceal the private reality of living with T1D. She used her charm and charisma to advance the JDF mission while maintaining an illusory distance from the disease—she was not yet prepared to accept the vulnerability that inevitably accompanied her public announcement of illness. However, a short time later, she received an invitation that, if accepted, would unveil her secret health narrative and launch a lifetime of public health advocacy through personal testimony. In 1984, 15 years after Mary received her diabetes diagnosis, Gloria Pennington, JDF executive director, asked her to make a decision about "owning diabetes" (Moore, 2009, p. 115) in a public fashion:

Mary, would you consider becoming the international chairman of JDF? We've done some testing on how people feel about you, and apparently they trust you. You are a diabetic and they believe what you say and admire how you've conducted your life. The board of directors has met and unanimously agreed you're the right person.

Intrigued, yet hesitant, Mary considered the request—one founded upon the emotional connection that she had created with individuals she had never met, individuals who apparently admired the way she lived her life. In *Growing Up Again*, though, Mary wrote of her extreme frustration with herself for the ways in which her lifestyle habits were likely responsible for many of the diabetic complications that she had experienced. Deterioration of her body—neuropathy, vision problems, peripheral artery disease, struggles with balance—was most likely influenced by her smoking, drinking, indulging in sweets, and not testing blood sugar. She admitted, "I excelled as a professional ... [but] I feared I was failing miserably on a personal level" (Moore, 2009, p. 36).

Admittedly, she was not perfect. However, what good could come of making that fact a publicly acknowledged one? Could her story, her disease, her personal struggle possibly make a positive influence in the quest to find a cure? Upon reflection, Mary remembered her own "lifesaver," Betty Ford, whose willingness to share her struggle with alcoholism comprised an integral component in Mary's recovery her own alcohol addiction. Mary wrote, "Despite what [Betty] described as pit-of-the-stomach fear, she shattered her protective shield of privacy and bravely took her situation to the public" (Moore, 2009, p. 67). Betty's health narrative, and the "brutal honesty" with which she told it, allowed Mary to "grow emotionally ... [it] transformed my life" (p. 67). In light of those recollections, Mary accepted Gloria Pennington's invitation and officially joined the JDF team as the international chairman. In retrospect, after years of worrying about her public image, the possible professional cost of admitting her illness, and the responsibility of being an image of diabetes for the world to see, she remembered finally thinking, "'The hell with it,' and [she's] proud of the work [she has] done" (Moore, 1995, p. 137).

According to Brene Brown (2012), vulnerability—such as that displayed by Mary Tyler Moore's willingness to go public with her illness and invite others into the intimate details of her life—"is the birthplace of love, belonging, joy, courage, empathy, and creativity. It is the source of hope, empathy, accountability, and authenticity" (p. 34). Vulnerability welcomes risk and emotional exposure. At its best, it also creates an environment that engenders identification, connection, community, and support. Indeed, Mary's public announcement of her illness and integration into the JDF advocacy team transformed the way the public understood the disease—others living with the illness identified with Mary in a new way; those who admired her learned about and connected with the disease in a way that meaningfully mattered to them, and her education and fundraising efforts drew noteworthy attention to the cause in ways that otherwise may have been unattainable. Her face, widely recognized as one of America's most loved on-screen sweethearts, now serves as the smile associated with hope of and active pursuit for a cure for T1D (Hingley, 1995, November–December, p. 66). Her voice, one that captured a nationwide audience's attention with charming variations of "Oh, Rob" on the *Dick Van Dyke Show*, now narrates the story of a complex illness.

The Work of Stories

> Stories animate human life; that is their work. Stories work with people, for people, and always stories work *on* people, affecting what people are able to see as real, as possible, and as worth doing or best avoided. What is it about stories—what are their particularities—that enable them to work as they do? More than mere curiosity is at stake in this question, because human life depends on the stories we tell: the sense of self that those stories impart, the relationships constructed around shared stories, and the sense of purpose that stories both propose and foreclose [Frank, 2010, p. 3].

Mary Tyler Moore's commitment to advocacy initiated a new public conversation about T1D. In a *CBS News* (2009, June 23) story titled *Mary's Mission: Moore Raises Awareness, Funds for Diabetes*, a news anchor, in reference to her book, *Growing Up Again*, asked Mary to explain how she had grown throughout her journey with diabetes. She replied, "I was talking primarily about my attitude toward dealing with diabetes. It's a tremendous burden; it affects you emotionally as well as physically. And that's why I wrote the book." Mary's advocacy work has brought her face-to-face with countless others living with the emotional and physical challenges imposed by the disease. When she speaks with these individuals, she reminds them, and herself in turn, "You truly have to make the very best of what you've got" (DiEdwardo, 2009, December 28, para. 19). Actively taking her own advice for more than 40 years, Moore has continued to share her story because, as she wrote, "It is what I have to give" (Moore, 2009, p. 2).

As Frank (2010) suggested, this gift of a personal narrative does important work. By willingly sharing her narrative account of illness, Mary Tyler Moore has brought relevance and urgency to a health issue in need of attention. Although she admitted, "It took me years and years to get to the point where I could announce to the world, 'I am Mary Tyler Moore, and I have diabetes'" (Moore, 2009, p. 115), once she did confide her story, incredible things happened. As Hingley (1995, November/December) described, Mary's public acknowledgment of her life experience with this chronic disease has transformed her into "a symbol of hope to others in the process" (p. 38).

Moore's advocacy efforts educated the public about the intricacies of the illness and the ongoing challenges imposed upon those living with the disease, or as *Good Morning America* (2009, March 31) articulated in Diane Sawyer's introduction of Mary,

> Off-screen surround of needles, glucose, testing tapes, fear of careening numbers, the assault of diabetes on eyesight ... and yet, she has said, "If only wonderful things happen to us, how do we grow? How do we ever know how brave we really are?"

In addition to her autobiographies that detailed accounts of her experiences of life as a diabetic (see Moore 1995, 2009), Mary prioritized explaining the daily responsibilities and ever present risks of life as a diabetic in widely publicized interviews with popular media outlets, some of which include CNN (2002, May 8; 2005, July 1), *USA Today* (Marcus, 2009, March 22), *Good Morning America* (2009, March 31), and the *Saturday Evening Post* (Hingley, 1995; Miller, 2005, November–December).

Not Just My Story, but Ours

Although Mary Tyler Moore's decision to disclose her personal health narrative served as an important step in JDRF fundraising efforts, which made incredible advances in advocacy on behalf of individuals living with diabetes, it would not be the final one. After actively fulfilling the duties of her role as the JDRF international chairman—filming public service announcements, appearing before Congress to request the passage of bills that would provide further funding for research, and persuading CEOs to commit large corporate donations to the cause—she realized that part of the discourse about T1D was still missing. Mary recognized that her story was a partial one. She was only one person living with the disease in a nation where nearly 2 million individuals are diagnosed each year (JDRF, 2014h). Further, as someone diagnosed at the age of 33, her experience differed from a child diagnosed with the disease today. Those children's voices deserved to be heard too, and Moore embraced an idea posed by a young JDF volunteer in 1999. She initiated a program to spotlight children and inform members of Congress about the impact that the disease has on their daily lives.

CHILDREN'S CONGRESS IS BORN

Tommy Solo, an 8-year-old JDRF volunteer from Boston living with T1D, was frustrated by the lack of a cure for his illness, and he wanted to do something about it. After overhearing adult volunteers discuss their upcoming trip to Washington, D.C., he suggested that kids should go, too, "because no one knows better what it's like to live with type 1 diabetes than kids who have it" (JDRF, 2014a, para. 2). Since its inception, eight biannual Children's Congress events have taken place every other summer. The event has evolved into an elaborate week-long experience for children, their parents, members of Congress, and other key federal policymakers that involves:

> Hill visits to respective offices, a legislative hearing about continued T1D research funding, a town hall style event with JDFR celebrity advocates, and of course, the important opportunity for JDRF's delegates and their families to build relationship within the T1D community itself. Additionally, the relationships built between T1D advocates and their Members of Congress are meant to last, as advocates help remind Congressional Members the importance of uninterrupted federal funding for Type 1 research through the Special Diabetes Program (SDP), at the National Institutes of Health (NIH), and beyond [JDRF, 2014c, para. 3].

As JDRF international chairman, Mary decided to capitalize upon Solo's creative idea that would interject otherwise muted voices into public and political conversations about diabetes. Children's Congress became a space where individuals and families living with the disease were able to add their personal experiences to the larger public narrative of T1D. Child delegates Mollie and Jackie told Mary,

> We were just kids, and it was overwhelming to be there walking the hall of Congress with you, Mary. It was. And meeting a lot of other kids who had diabetes meant so much. When I was first diagnosed there was no one for me to talk to. I didn't know anyone else who had diabetes. When Jackie and I finally came to the Children's Congress there were a hundred kids with diabetes and so many adults. The government officials that we spoke to really cared about what we had to say [Moore, 2009, p. 121].

In addition to the cultivation of a platform from which children's stories could be shared, Mary also recognized the opportunity to use this event as a way to educate and inspire the youth delegates who joined the JDRF advocacy efforts. Thus, Children's Congress has welcomed many other celebrities to join in a variety of capacities as "celebrity advocates" because of their ability to draw the public's attention and "serve as role models or ambassadors for the children" (Symetra Tour, 2014, para. 4). Following Mary's lead, these celebrities have integrated their personal accounts of T1D to support the JDRF mission and the children and families affected by the disease. Some of the celebrity advocates whom Mary has accompanied on Capitol Hill include Sugar Ray Leonard (retired boxing legend), Ray Allen (NBA All-Star), Nick

Jonas (singer, *Jonas Brothers*), Kevin Kline (Academy Award–winning actor), Charlie Kimball (racecar driver), Nat Strand (*Amazing Race* contestant), Sam Talbot (semi-finalist on Bravo's *Top Chef*), Mary Mouser (actress), Crystal Bowersox (*American Idol* season 9 runner-up), Nicole Johnson (Miss America 1999), Jean Smart (Emmy-winning actress), Gary Hall, Jr. (Olympic multi-medal-winning Hall of Fame swimmer), and Carling Coffing (LPGA tour player) (Cairns Pastor, 2009, June 24; JDRF, 2001, June 19; JDRF, 2009, June 22; JDRF, 2011, June 13; JDRF, 2013; Symetra Tour, 2014).

Stefany Shaheen, Children's Congress 2011 Chair mother, posted in a blog following the event that she was "struck by the energy between each special guest and every Children's Congress delegate. The connectedness created in these events was clearly mutually beneficial and greatly appreciated by all" (AllisonN, 2011, July 20, para. 14). One of the special moments at Children's Congress 2011 was a Town Hall event.

> U.S. Supreme Court Justice Sonia Sotomayor [spoke] for the first time since her appointment about having type 1 diabetes. The 150 delegates sat on the floor around Justice Sotomayor, creating an intimate storytelling-like atmosphere in which she proceeded to tell them about her diagnosis as a child, her personal challenges, the improvements in technology, and more. She looked the children in the eyes, and spoke in a slow, clear, sweet voice that seemed to hold each one of them warmly. She answered their questions, like whether diabetes gets easier as an adult, and how it affects her job, and each response was candid, genuine, and positive [AllisonN, 2011, July 20, para. 11].

Because of Children's Congress events, individuals diagnosed with T1D have been given (and co-constructed as) co-fighters, people who understand their struggle, partners in survival, teammates in the fight against the threat of not having a cure. Mary Tyler Moore and her fellow celebrity advocates "each have a unique story of perseverance, dedication, and strength that … inspire our delegates and their families, and provide a positive example in the fight against this disease" (JDRF, 2011, June 13, para. 4). Parents of Children's Congress delegates shared that "the whole experience was overwhelming, inspiring and emotional…. It makes me want to get more involved. It was impressive to see the power of JDRF and [children] have on making a difference" (Bhargava, 2009, July 11, para. 30).

The stories actively performed work—working *with* people, working *for* people, and working *on* people. Their emergent collective health narrative fostered meaningful relationships, allowed possibilities for their lives and their hope for a cure to take shape, gave them a sense of purpose. Notably, this effort extended the emphasis on personal narratives that have been an integral component to raising $1.7 billion dollars for diabetes research to cure, treat, and prevent the disease since the inception of JDF in 1970 (JDRF, 2014h). As Rock (2003) noted, "Stories about specific individuals and face-to-face contact" (p. 225) are significant and substantial knowledge-building opportunities that hold the potential to affect political decision-making. As we consider the impact of these stories, we recall Frank's (2010) question regarding the particularities of stories that enable them to have such significant influence. For, quite literally in this case, as he noted, "human life depends on the stories" that individuals co-author.

2009 Children's Congress Hearing

Nine a.m. Wednesday, June 24, 2009. Members of the Senate Committee on Homeland Security and Governmental Affairs filed through aisles to fill their seats on Capitol Hill. For the hearing that morning entitled *Type 1 Diabetes Research: Real Progress and Real Hope for a Cure*, Senator Susan Collins and Senator Joseph Lieberman invited "expert witnesses to testify on the merits of the proposal" (U.S. Senate Committee on Homeland Security & Governmental Affairs, 2013, para. 3). The list of "experts" to testify on behalf of the proposal to sustain robust federal funding for diabetes research included Ms. Mary Tyler Moore, international chairman of the Juvenile Diabetes Research Foundation; Griffin P. Rodgers, M. D., director of the National Institute of Diabetes and Digestive and Kidney Disease at the National Institutes of Health; Sugar Ray Leonard, retired professional boxer; Nicholas J. Jonas, singer, songwriter, and actor; 11-year-old Hannah Ryder from Cumberland, Maine; 13-year-old J. Patrick Lacher II, from South Glastonbury, Connecticut; 16-year-old Asa Kelly, from Charlotte, North Carolina; and Ellen Gould from Nashville, Tennessee, a mother of four children, ages 17, 12, 10, and 5, all of whom have type 1 diabetes. In addition, 150 delegates between the ages of 4 and 17 from every state in the nation and a few others from around the world joined these experts in their efforts to help Congress "better understand just what it is like to have diabetes, how serious it is, and how important it is that we all work together to try to find a cure" (U. S. Senate Hearing 111–908, 2009, June 24, para. 3).

In her address to Congressional members, Mary Tyler Moore asserted,

As JDRF's International Chairman, I am actually just one volunteer in an army of determined moms, dads, children, loved ones, and friends personally affected by diabetes. We are not sitting back waiting for the cure. These children before you have built lemonade stands, created walk teams, held bake sales, and organized car washes. Most importantly, they have spoken out about their lives with diabetes and shown, by their courage and hard work, that they can accomplish anything—including being an important part of finding their own cures.

Overall, JDRF's efforts have enabled us to contribute over $1.3 billion to diabetes research since our founding in 1970 and over $150 million last year alone. But curing diabetes is an enormous task. We cannot do it alone. And that is why we are here.... As their Chairman and "oldest delegate," I am proud to be leading our 2009 Children's Congress Delegates in their efforts this week. As we have started to do in this special hearing, today our goal is to persuade our Senators and Representatives to also make a promise. We hope you will "promise to remember us" when you vote on the Special Diabetes Program and other important issues that affect all of us with diabetes [U. S. Senate Hearing 111–908, 2009, June 24, para. 83, 91–93].

Mary's address was followed by personal testimonies from all of the experts who joined her at the podium. Each of them contributed to the collective story of T1D in powerful ways as their young voices described life with diabetes as a child and the critical need for research efforts to find better treatment options, preventive measures, and, hopefully, a cure.

A Co-created Narrative Portrait Contributes to Knowledgeable Advocacy

In her book *Growing Up Again*, for which all proceeds are donated to JDRF to advance research to find a cure, Mary noted that "after many years of interaction with Congress," she has "come to understand better the difference between the political hug and knowledgeable advocacy" (Moore, 2009, p. 118). She recognizes the Children's Congress program as an integral component to the successes of JDRF's knowledge-based advocacy that integrates firsthand accounts of individuals' experiences as they live with T1D. This effort personalizes advocacy efforts and connects Congressional debates to the details of lived experience of those whose lives are affected daily by congressional decisions.

The children's testimonies constitute a work of art in that they "embrace diverse modes of sensing and expressing lived realities" (Harter, 2013, p. 4), inviting listeners to acknowledge the vulnerabilities that comprise their lives and enlarging possibilities for empathy and edifying response. The whole idea serves as a beautiful application of artful, pragmatic sensibilities through use of narrative to "encourage the sort of absorptive, engaged attention to the rich present that is so often lost in today's fragmented world" (Stroud, 2011, p. 11), an especially useful tool when considering the context of Congress members' jam-packed schedules, lengthy lists of causes begging their attention, and stress of daily responsibilities.

"The young delegates' stories, told in their own words, are often more powerful than almost any other type of legislator education" (JDRF, 2014d, para. 9). The inclusion of children sharing their own journeys, frustrations, daily challenges, and hopeful anticipation of a cure exemplifies invitational rhetoric, an approach to public dialogue that seeks to engage multiple perspectives in discussion so that everyone "gains a greater understanding of the issue in its subtlety, richness, and complexity" (Foss & Griffin, 1995, p. 5). The aesthetic qualities of their storytelling performances, from advocacy videos and scrapbooks to face-to-face conversations with representatives and legislators and public testimony at Congressional hearings, provide an intimate portrait, demand attention, and transform daily political issues into weighty decisions that will directly affect children's lives and their families in profound ways. Charon (2005) suggested that such creative forms of narrative hold the potential to open dialogue in more life-affirming ways. The cultivation of aesthetic, embodied experiences for Congressional members to witness these children's lives, families, and stories is knowledge-producing and emotionally charged in ways that would not be achieved void the presence of Children's Congress participants. In fact, as Mary Tyler Moore emphasized, "Of all our [JDRF] members, it is our children who possess our most eloquent and persuasive voices" (Moore, 2007, Summer, p. 4).

From a narrative perspective, we recognize our lives as a trajectory of once-occurring moments (Bakhtin, 1981). Some of these moments comprise what Kermode (1966/2000) called impression points, or particular moments that, for one reason or another, are full of significant meaning. For children living with type 1 diabetes, as well as for their families, a diagnosis of this life-long illness certainly serves as a life-altering impression point. Fortunately, thanks to programs such as Children's Congress (and many other advocacy and fundraising opportunities which can be explored at www.jdrf. org/get-involved), children and families are able to, as Mary Tyler Moore said it best, "make the very best of what [they've] got" (DiEdwardo, 2009, December 28, para. 19) by providing policymakers with firsthand accounts of what it is like to live with diabetes as a child.

As these children and families meet in mutual effort to advocate for research funding, they also create connections with others who share similar experiences and build communities of social support—another meaningful impression point in their journey. As Platt, the Children's Congress 2013 Chair Family, contended,

> The primary role of JDRF Children's Congress delegates is a powerful one—to deliver our important messages to our country's leaders. Equally important, however, is your experience building relationships and forming friendships with your fellow delegates and their families. Prepare to be transformed by your Children's Congress experience! [2013, para. 2].

Our lives are characterized by countless aesthetic, embodied storied performances, such as Children's Congress, that contribute to the ongoing development of self, meaning-making, and purpose—they are transformative (James, 1981; Kermode 1966/2000). Rather than be defined and isolated by their diagnosis that currently has no cure, these advocates unite together to collectively give voice to the need for better treatment options, possible prevention measures, and ultimately a cure for type 1 diabetes. John, a child delegate at Children's Congress 2005, explained,

> We (the Children's Congress) represent a group of individuals who face a life threatening disease on a daily basis.... And our strength, determination, and hope to realize a cure should not only educate others, but inspire them to act and walk beside us in our quest for a cure [JDRF, 2005, June 20, para. 8].

The Children's Congress participants' stories "humanize the experience of illness" and allow them to reclaim agency through their testimony (Ellis & Bochner, 2000, p. 749). Arianna, a 13-year-old Children's Congress 2003 delegate, echoed this goal in anticipation of the event—" I am looking forward to putting a face on all our stories and telling our Congressmen about what it's like to live with diabetes" (JDRF, 2003, June 21, para. 5). As Chair Rik Bonness, former NFL player and father of the Children's Congress 2003 Chair Family, explained to delegates during the opening banquet, "As we break from our circle of hope, we know our dream of a cure will also come true. Over the next three days, Congress will see in our children's eyes and hear in our children's voices the best humanity has to offer, conveying the passion of JDRF—the passion that will ensure our victory over type 1 diabetes" (JDRF, 2003, June 21, para. 3). Children's Congress participants have the opportunity to "re-author" and shape the momentum of their lives in purposeful directions with every new telling of their stories (White & Epston, 1990, p. 82).

Mary Tyler Moore's celebrity status created a platform from which young advocates have been able to contribute to an ongoing co-created narrative portrait of life with type 1 diabetes. Each of their narrative accounts poetically joins with others' individual experiences in remarkable ways, building a more complete picture of the disease and the daily challenges that it poses for those diagnosed. As Dewey (1934/1980) suggested, these qualities of their narrative performances provide "a clarified, coherent, and intensified or 'impassioned' experience" (p. 303) for all involved. We now turn our attention in response to Frank's (2010) question about the particularities of stories—the aesthetic qualities that lure our attention, stir our emotion, invite us into edifying relationship with others, and beg our response.

CHILDREN'S CONTRIBUTIONS TO THEIR
CO-CREATED NARRATIVE OF TYPE 1 DIABETES

As children share their unique stories, they create *aligning moments* and *narrative jolts*, described by Sharf et al. (2011) as "an experience of genuine shared understanding" (p. 46), which encourages thoughtful reflection of others' perspectives, stirs curiosity, and entices to purposeful action. When we consider these moments in the context of eight Children's Congress events with 100–150 children attending each, we begin to see the impact that these young advocates have made.

For the Children's Congress 2013, nearly 1,500 children and teenagers applied for the opportunity to share their stories with Congress. A JDRF volunteer-based committee selected 150 participants, a group of Children's Congress delegates comprised of representatives from every state, the District of Columbia and six other countries (JDRF, 2014d). One of these delegates, Avery, referred to as "Sweets" by her mother, lives in Ohio. Their blog, titled "The Princess and the Pump" (2013, July 8), showcases a darling Precious Moments quality photograph of the seven-year-old dressed in hot pink with her light brunette curls falling over her shoulder and her blue eyes sparkling as well as a description about what she did to prepare for her advocacy adventure. In addition to her mother's explanation of what was in store for them in Washington, D.C., the blog highlights Avery's handwritten letters to the Congressional representatives with whom she would meet at the Children's Congress event. To assist her in telling her personal story of life with T1D, she also created a scrapbook to give to the representatives and senators to help them understand what living with the disease is like for her. This young girl, accompanied by her big dreams of one day being a teacher, a doctor, and a pop star, has taken her advocacy role seriously, welcoming any opportunity to tell her story—she has been featured on local media channels and on Ohio State Representative Jean Schmidt's website (JDRF, 2014e).

Tristin, Michigan native who was diagnosed with T1D at the age of 2, also served as a 2013 advocate. This 10-year-old boy (well known at home for his love of art, playing guitar, and basketball) captivated the selection committee with a video that he made and submitted with his "powerful and well-written application" (Haroldson, 2013, June 21, para. 2). In his video, as he sat next to a table full of the diabetes supplies upon which his life depends, he shared his heartfelt desire

> to be a normal kid—to know what it is like to be able to eat whatever I want whenever I want and not need to take insulin…. A cure is important because I don't want to be hooked to a machine that keeps me alive for the rest of my

life.... Special Diabetes Program means so much to me and my family. My great aunt was diagnosed at 10 with Type 1 and my family saw her struggle every day living with the disease before finally dying from complications of diabetes— two weeks before I was diagnosed. Thankfully today, there is better care and options for people with diabetes and most of that is credited to the JDRF and the Special Diabetes Program.... Please make my dream of life without diabetes a possibility. A cure is something to believe in [JDRF, 2014g].

In addition to the scrapbooks, videos, and letters that these children bring with them to Children's Congress, they also bring their smiles, young voices, caretaking parents, hopeful optimism, and genuine desire to contribute to finding a cure. Each year, a handful of advocates accompany Mary Tyler Moore to the podium during the congressional hearing and give a brief testimony before countless congressional members, families, and fellow child advocates. In 2009, Hannah testified about the complexities that constituted her daily life:

Three years ago my life changed forever when I was diagnosed with type 1 diabetes. After being in the hospital for 4 days, I hoped that I was cured when I got home. But I soon figured out that this was not going away when my parents kept checking my blood sugar, giving me shots, and measuring all my food. Everyone kept asking me how I was feeling. Before I could go back to school or play on a sports team, we had to meet with all of the nurses, teachers, and coaches, and anyone else that my parents thought could help keep me safe.

Sometimes I do not like all the attention, but I know it is the attention that is going to keep me safe, and it is the attention like this that is going to help find a cure.

Diabetes not only affects me physically, it affects me emotionally as well. Sometimes I get mad, especially when people say things like I am lucky I missed a class because my blood sugar got too low. Or I get sad when people eat some of my favorite foods and say how good they are, and I cannot eat them because I have celiac, which a lot of people with type 1 diabetes have, too.

But I feel happy to have family and friends that help me out, like my walk team, Hannah's Heroes. This year my team did a bunch of fundraisers. We walked in the Diabetes Walk. We had a yard sale with all of the stuff my family does not use. We had a bake sale and a lemonade stand. So far, we have raised over $5,000. I hope that we raised enough money with our team, and I hope that Congress gives scientists the rest of the money that they need because I really do not want other kids to get diabetes [U. S. Senate Hearing 111–908, 2009, June 24, para. 157–160].

Children's Congress provides a forum for such inspirational and powerful narratives as well as a vehicle for making a positive difference in a variety of ways using their creativity and capitalizing on their personalities. For instance, seven-year-old Andrew, another 2013 delegate, crafted a video that included his own illustrations of life with diabetes. His narration of his diabetes story, detailed with his white pages filled with colored marker drawings, captured the young eager tone of his voice:

> Hi, my name is Andrew. I got diagnosed when I was only 23 months old. I look like this. My mom, she takes care of me all day long, except for when I'm at school. This is my dad. He is a dentist. He checks my blood sugar in the middle of the night and sometimes at three in the morning, so my mom can get some sleep. This is my twin brother, Nick. He does not have Type I diabetes. I'm lucky to have diabetes because I get to get out of school for doctors' appointments and I get to eat candy. Sometimes you're super high, sometimes you're super low. It's like being on a roller coaster all day. If there was a cure for diabetes, I would never have to check my blood sugar, or give myself insulin, or count my carbs and then I'll get to play outside all day. Please support diabetes research and say yes to funding this Special Diabetes Program [JDRF, 2014f].

In addition to his work as a Children's Congress advocate, he and his twin brother decided to write a children's book to help kids better understand the disease, while also using the book project as a way to raise money to advance T1D research.

Austin, a 2013 delegate from California, shared his passion for T1D advocacy in a video that he created of himself while holding a basketball at his side in the court in his driveway. His spunky spirit was evident when he joked, "My mom said to speak from the heart, but I told her I would speak from the pancreas" (JDRF, 2014b). His video and trip to Washington marked just the beginning of his contributions, though, as the experience sparked a desire to serve as a JDRF youth ambassador by mentoring newly diagnosed children looking for support and speaking to a variety of audiences to educate them about the disease.

As Bakhtin (1981) proposed, emergent personal narratives exist in concert with other stories, and all hold the potential to do significant work (Frank, 2010), even those of children. In the case of Children's Congress, though, that potential would have remained untapped without Mary Tyler Moore, a well-loved celebrity willing to shift the spotlight from herself to reflect on the bright faces of her young counterparts. She paved a way for their voices to be heard, their challenges acknowledged, and their hopes pursued. At the Children's Congress 2007 (U.S. Senate Hearing 110–316, 2007, June 19), Senator Collins' concluding remarks testified to the importance of JDRF, Mary Tyler Moore, celebrity advocates, and child delegates in achieving these outcomes:

> All of you have asked that I remember you, and I just wanted to say to all the children who are here today that I promise to remember each and every one of you and to work for the funding that will produce better treatments, but most importantly, that will point the way to a cure.

So thank you so much for coming all the way from your home States to be with us today. You remind us of what this is all about, and you inspire us to continue to fight for the money for diabetes research. So thank you so much for being here today.

I want to thank JDRF for doing just a wonderful job and Mary Tyler Moore, who is such an inspiring international chairman and who has helped advance the public's understanding of this terrible disease....

Thank you all for teaching us so much today, for putting a human face, such wonderful human faces, on this disease and for inspiring us to fight for a cure. Thank you [para. 279–281].

Beyond the immediate impact that these children make at the Children's Congress events, considerable press coverage of the event ensures that millions around the globe learn about their daily battles and need for a cure. In fact, Mary Tyler Moore stated that Tommy Solo's idea and the 1999 Children's Congress event achieved "the most national attention that [had] ever been paid to the children and adults who live with the daily burden of the disease" (JDRF, 2013, April 30, para. 3). This mediated circulation of their efforts still continues in incredible fashion today:

In 2011, Children's Congress generated 294 print stories (print and online), 117 television stories, and 3,548 radio station airings throughout the country, including national outlets and outlets in designated legislative priority areas. Print reached 9.2 million impressions, online stories reached 13 million impressions, and broadcast numbers (TV and radio) reached 7 million viewers and listeners [JDRF, 2014a, para. 3].

Media outlets write feature articles about their local delegates; the children pursue new opportunities to educate the public and raise funds; parents and kids alike blog about their time in D.C., and the JDRF highlights photographs, videos, and details of their efforts on their website. Although the direct target audience of Children's Congress includes the governmental decision-makers, officials constitute just a small, although incredibly important, portion of the individuals invited to learn more about life with T1D from the perspective of a child and join the cause to raise funds for a cure.

As we have discussed throughout this chapter, Mary Tyler Moore's personal, yet public, account of her T1D elevated the potential for such personal narratives to transform public and political dialogues about T1D. Her story has served as a springboard from which others could reveal details of their respective life journeys, and the public and government have responded generously. To date, the collective narrative of these individuals has contributed to JDRF's standing as the "largest charitable supporter of T1D research ... sponsoring $520 million in scientific research in 17 countries"—one reason JDRF was named by *Forbes* magazine as "one of its five All-Star charities" for its "efficiency and effectiveness" (JDRF, 2013, September 25, para. 11). JDRF (2013, September 25, para. 9) attributes much of its success to Mary's active involvement in "supporting the organization's mission with a willingness to share her personal story of type 1 diabetes (T1D) publicly." JDRF upholds Mary as a "magnificent" member of their team ("The Magnificent Mary," 2000, Summer) because of her unique ability to motivate continued personal advocacy with her "frequent visits to Capitol Hill, Congressional testimony, and highly visible public service campaigns [which] have strengthened JDRF's research and advocacy efforts on behalf of people with T1D" (JDRF, 2013, September 25, para. 9).

Mary Tyler Moore has earned countless awards in her lifetime for her numerous roles in entertainment, philanthropy, and advocacy. One such prominent recognition was the 2011 Screen Actor's Guild Life Achievement Award, for which it was written:

> Moore has been the JDRF's International Chairman since 1984. She has also chaired JDRF's biennial Children's Congress since its inception in 1999 … Moore has been at the vanguard of JDRF's visit on Capitol Hill, testifying before the House and Senate on behalf of increased National Institutes of Health (NIH) funding for Type 1 diabetes, which affects as many as 3 million children and adults. Moore and her husband, Dr. S. Robert Levine, have been generous supporters of JDRF's research programs and in 2003 established JDRF's "Excellence in Clinical Research Award" in recognition of outstanding diabetes researchers. She herself was honored by JDRF in 2007 with its Humanitarian of the Year Award [Screen Actor's Guild, 2011, September 8, para. 15].

Vanguard, she is. Mary has now chaired eight Children's Congress events, served as the opening testimony for each of these Senate hearings, and invited other celebrities to join with the youth delegates in the telling of their own stories of life with T1D and the necessity for finding better treatments, prevention measures, and a cure.

Conclusion

After spending years "agoniz[ing] about going public about her disease," Mary explained that she "called on [her] own common sense and realized it was an opportunity to help an enormous number of people" (DiEdwardo, 2009, December 28, para. 4). She chose to share her story and, along the way, learned to use her celebrity status as a platform for others to do the same. Although smaller in stature than most who roam our nation's Capitol, some of the most engaging individuals who have accepted Mary's invitation to advocate for T1D research using their personal health narratives are between the ages of 4 and 17. Mary admitted that, when the idea for Children's Congress was presented to her in 1999, she was "unprepared for the enormous impact this event had: on Congressional representatives, members of the present administration, the public ... and on me!" ("The Magnificent Mary," 2000, Summer, para. 2).

The presence of these children, in all their innocence and maturity, disrupts patriarchal approaches to politics. The aesthetic qualities of their storied performances—their personal health narratives—transcend traditional text-based, statistical persuasive appeals and instead foster meaningful storytelling occasions that unite congressional members, celebrities, children, and families in their shared humanity. These young advocates do much more than ask for funding; they ask people to understand, to be willing to look at life from their perspective, to hope for a cure with them. They engage in what Harter and Rawlins (2011) articulated as the *worlding of possibilities*—the imaginative pursuit of creating better realities; in their case, it is a reality in which suffering from T1D is diminished and a cure might be discovered. As Mary Tyler Moore has taught them, they are trying to turn the world around with more than their smiles—they are making a positive difference with their testimonies, their voices, their videos, their scrapbooks, their laughter, and the strength that they demonstrate in their vulnerability.

CHAPTER THIRTEEN

Continuing the Conversation

As we mentioned in our chapter on Robin Roberts, Amy Robach, Robin's co-host on *Good Morning America*, knew the importance of early detection, but, although she was 40 years old and due for her first mammogram, she had not yet made the time to call her doctor and set the appointment. In her report with *ABC News* (2013, November 11), Amy admitted putting off getting a mammogram because she considered it to be "virtually impossible that I would have cancer" (para. 6); she had little family history, was healthy, exercised, and ate right. Ironically, she sat daily beside a woman who had worked for nearly six years to dispel just that misconception, urging all women to get checked, regardless of family history and lifestyle choices, given that 80 percent of women have no risk other than having breasts (see Mann, 2007, July 31, para. 10; Robach, 2013, November 11).

As part of Breast Cancer Awareness Month, Robin urged Amy to agree to having the first on-air mammogram on *Good Morning America*, telling her that, even if she saved one life, it would be worth it. With Robin's words of encouragement, coupled with Amy's desire to support her friend and co-worker by helping to promote this important cause, she consented, announcing on *ABC News*, "On Oct. 1, I had my first mammogram in front of millions of people" (Robach, 2013, November 11, para. 8), joining other celebrities who have undergone live testing on national television to encourage viewers to do the same. Katie Couric famously had a live colonoscopy on the *Today* show in March of 2000 to encourage screening for colon cancer after the death of her husband from the disease (see, for example, Balzora, 2013, July 8). Only a month after Robach's mammography, viewers watched Al Roker and Matt Lauer obtain prostate exams, also live on the *Today* show (Stump, 2013, November 7). As Balzora wrote regarding Couric's colonoscopy, Katie "demystified the procedure so that others could understand the ins and outs not only of her insides, but also about the importance of the screening procedure itself. And it worked—beautifully" (para. 9).

However, unlike Katie Couric, Matt Lauer, or Al Roker, Amy's on-air

203

exam did not simply provide important information about a medical screening to viewers—she learned that she had breast cancer. Robach shared, "The doctors told me bluntly: 'That mammogram just saved your life'" (2013, November 11, para. 14). Robach thanked Robin for giving her the confidence to get her exam (Nelson, 2014, March 21), as she explained, if "several producers and even Robin Roberts herself hadn't convinced me that doing this on live television would save lives, I would never have been able to save my own" (Robach, 2013, November 11, para. 7).

Amy faced the difficult news and well of emotions that followed in the limelight, as she observed, "For the past 20 years, sadly, a large part of my job deals in tragedy—other peoples' tragedies—but never my own" (Robach, 2013, November 11, para. 4). She continued, "I can only hope my story will ... inspire every woman who hears it to get a mammogram, to take a self exam. No excuses. It is the difference between life and death" (Robach, 2013, November 11, para. 16).

Robach's testimony underscores the importance of early detection for saving lives as well as illustrates the power of celebrity health narratives. By commemorating Breast Cancer Awareness Month with a nationally broadcast mammogram, Robach unexpectedly set her own personal-yet-public health narrative in motion, implicitly contributing to broader conversations about breast cancer awareness, all extending from an intimate physical exam. Robach emphasized, "I did not want to do the mammogram in front of 5 million people.... It felt a little too personal" (Cotliar, 2013, December 16, p. 66). However, as Robach also acknowledged, as someone in the public eye every weekday on *Good Morning America*, "If you have a platform, you can change someone's life.... You almost feel like you have to" (Cotliar, 2013, December 16, p. 66).

Robin and Amy continue to draw attention to the value of early detection and their cancer sagas, sharing raw, candid accounts of what would have been otherwise private moments of their respective journeys (see Taibi, C., 2014, January 25; 2014, April 25; Tuck, 2014, May 21). For example, Robach allowed cameras to roll as a hair stylist cut her hair (before she lost it due to cancer treatments), and she tweeted pictures during chemo sessions (Taibi, 2014, April 25). Robach "hopes her decision will inspire bravery in other patients fighting against cancer" (Taibi, 2014, April 25, para. 5). Tuck heralded Robach as part of a next generation of breast cancer advocates:

> While the stigma of breast cancer seemingly dissipated when famous women like Happy Rockefeller and Betty Ford exposed their personal battles, the addition of social media has only increased exposure. Perhaps it was these pioneers who made it possible for women to fight cancer in public, but it's women like

[Samantha] Harris, Robach, and [Angelina] Jolie who will encourage people to advocate for their own health and be more aware of risks [para 8].

Fans weighed in on Amy's diagnosis, buttressing Robin's ongoing promotion of breast health. Nancy responded to the *People* magazine article by Nelson (2014, March 21), saying, "She [Amy] is one very lucky woman. Had she not decided to have that mammogram … we might be reading a different story about Amy. Wise decision. All the best to you Amy!" Likewise, Maggie also commented on the *People* magazine article, "I love Robin and I am not surprised at all that she is supporting Amy." Rose responded to Amy's announcement about her recent diagnosis of breast cancer (see Robach, 2013, November 11):

> My Dear "Sister" Amy, I, too am facing a mastectomy on November 22. On September 25, 2013, I had surgery to "remove" a renal cell carcinoma; other than knowing I would have to undergo tests every 6 months, I felt cancer free. Out of the clear blue, a little something showed up on a chest x-ray, which led to a cat scan, which led to an ultrasound and mammogram, which led to biopsies, which led to a diagnosis of invasive ductal carcinoma. I have watched Robin and now you, go through this journey with such grace and positivity, something I fear I am lacking at this moment. I will remember you and your loved ones in my prayers. Please know you have an "army" of cancer warriors standing beside you.

A Few Key Threads

We began this chapter with an interesting case—Amy Robach's health saga began when it did because of (a) the influence of another celebrity who has battled with cancer and now promotes screening and early detection and (b) the possibility of using her own celebrity status to bring attention about mammography to her audience members even before she knew that the screening would unveil a hidden and growing cancer. However, Robach's narrative echoes familiar threads of other similar stories that we have recounted throughout this book—a celebrity receives a life-altering, personal diagnosis about an illness or injury, decides to confide that intimate information to others in the general public, and, in so doing, engages in important advocacy work while also receiving expressions of support, advice, and encouragement from fans, followers, and casual onlookers.

In this book, we have highlighted instances of celebrity health narratives that prompt compassion and identification and those that spark indignation and outrage. We have discussed celebrities, like Robach, who disclosed their diagnoses right away and others who delayed, for a plethora of reasons, ranging from sick relatives to concern about stigma that could hurt chances at a part in a movie or place on the field. We have mentioned celebrities who work tirelessly to raise awareness and encourage early detection, and we have highlighted others who campaign for research dollars, establish foundations, and lobby Congress. These famed individuals have spanned a wide range of ages, wrestling in the glare of the public eye with illnesses (both visible and not readily apparent) and injuries (from career to life-threatening).

As we close this book, we discuss two themes that we believe resonate throughout this volume and that certainly merit future examination. First, the increasing prevalence of social media poses challenges for celebrities in terms of negotiating privacy boundaries and contesting "ownership" of personal health narratives. Second, we reflect on broader social and medical implications of celebrity health narratives, especially regarding health advocacy, education, and public policy.

Co-ownership of Public-yet-Private Health Narratives

By virtue of divulging private details about personal health journeys in traditional and/or social media, famous individuals implicitly broaden the scope of others who know about their respective health situations and, by virtue of expanding privacy boundaries, invite those others to become co-owners of the emergent narrative (for related arguments, see Petronio, 2000, 2002, 2004, 2013). Social media has cultivated a culture of blurring private and public boundaries, as celebrities routinely take to Twitter, Facebook, YouTube, Instagram, blogs, etc. (see, e.g., High et al., 2014; Marwick, 2013; Thackeray et al., 2013). Through those snapshots from their lives (and plugs for their movies, teams, music, etc.), they have fostered perceptions of intimacy and, to some extent, relationships (for work on parasocial interactions, see Hartmann & Goldhoorn, 2011; Kassing & Sanderson, 2009; E. Lee & Jang, 2013; Meyrowitz, 1985; Ramasubramanian & Kornfield, 2012; Savage & Spence, 2014; Sood & Rogers, 2001).

The prevalence of celebrity interaction through social media, in general, and about personal health issues, in particular, has prompted expectations, among some onlookers, that celebrities hold moral and social obligations for disclosure. Catherine Zeta-Jones experienced backlash when she tried to shift away from being "the poster child" for bipolar disorder. Critics bashed Paula Deen for delaying her disclosure with type 2 diabetes. Associations that advocate for various medical conditions seem almost giddy when a celebrity reveals a personally devastating diagnosis that can bring a familiar face to their respective cause.

Yet, ethically and morally, do celebrities need to disclose personal health information, simply because they pursue careers such as acting or athletics? We think of Dana Reeve, for example, who battled actively and passionately for spinal injury research funding on behalf of her husband, Christopher Reeve, but, a short time after Christopher's death due to complications from his injuries, she stayed very quiet about her subsequent lung cancer diagnosis, opting to pass away out of the public eye. To what extent should celebrities embrace being "the poster child" in the public eye while they struggle personally with treatments, options, and physical implications of a given condition? Answers to these questions, like the emergent health narratives themselves, constitute complex, multifaceted, and quite individualized contributions to public dialogues about health.

For Brooke Burke-Charvet, Kim Kardashian, and Robin Roberts, public responses by fans and followers on Facebook and Twitter have tended to be overwhelmingly positive and supportive, and we were struck by the spirit of reciprocity that emerged as fans/followers and celebrities engage in chatter-like exchanges. Yet, as we have realized through this research, emergent private-yet-public health narratives become increasingly complicated and fractured as more and more individuals learn about a celebrity illness or injury and, with the ease of a tweet or post on a Facebook wall, comment, commiserate, and sometimes critique what would otherwise be very personal choices. Onlookers feel empowered to "judge" a celebrity's body and speculate on potential eating disorders. Certainly, Paula Deen faced very vocal resistance as she sought to advance a particular version of her own journey with type 2 diabetes.

When celebrity health narratives don't quite "ring true" (see Fisher, 1984, 1985a, 1987a), onlookers do not hesitate to chime in and dispute the emergent narrative. For example, one person posted the following comment about Amy Robach on an online discussion board for individuals with breast cancer:

> I hardly ever watch tv in the mornings, but today (of all days!) I turned on Good Morning America while I had my breakfast. Amy Robach finished chemo yesterday and they were all celebrating her victory with her.
>
> She didn't lose her hair, or her eyebrows, or her eyelashes. She's at work all bright and chipper the DAY after her final (8th) chemo. I'm so jealous and pissed off I could spit. She becoming an advocate for early detection. Yeah, thanks. Because Komen et al. SO need another voice shouting out that message, don't they?
>
> But the kicker ... her statement that so touched her and she needed to share on air—"tough times don't last, but tough people do".

UGH! F you Amy Robach. Here's a newsflash for you. Tough people die every day from cancer … tougher people than I hope you will ever need to be [2014, April 25].

Another individual echoed those sentiments, arguing,

I'm brave, I'm tough, I'm strong, I lost my hair and I was told I'd beat cancer but It came back with a vengeance just a few years later. No one is safe from occurrences but these celebrities just make it seem so easy to deal with cancer!!! I think they are missing the big picture; too many people still dies every year from this horrible disease. If people aren't made aware of the truth there will never be enough research to find the CURE. I wish someone one day will finally speak up and go out to the media and let people know what is really going on [2014, April 25].

Notably, Robach's journey will always be uniquely her own—whatever has happened or will transpire with her body. Her physical frame has and must endure the treatments, and she has and will have her own personal physical, emotional, social, and spiritual responses. Yet, as she shares details with others, they have (and often embrace) opportunities to respond (and, sometimes, contest) the broader public narrative as enacted in the spotlight of media attention (for related arguments, see, for, e.g., Bamberg & Andrews, 2004; Harter, 2009, 2013). As the two individuals note above (with their identities and that of the specific online forum intentionally preserved in respect to their health circumstances), onlookers challenge celebrity health narratives not necessarily to be unkind to a given person but rather to pointedly observe that illness doesn't always unfold for others in the same way, and, as such, those comments also powerfully contribute to and impact the public dialogue about life with a particular illness.

The second person above expressed frustration that the "real story" has not yet been told. Of course, a celebrity's journey constitutes only one type of health experience. Arthur Ashe acknowledged that he did not encounter the same type of discrimination as others with HIV/AIDS. Certainly, celebrity access to medical and financial resources might well differ from people in different vocations and socioeconomic situations. Further, "ordinary" people do not usually get invited to speak before Congress or give interviews to the press about the challenges of life with a particular ailment. Celebrities such as Michael J. Fox, Michael Zaslow, Jim Valvano, Robin Roberts, Mary Tyler Moore, and Christopher Reeve have openly recognized that celebrity status opened doors for advocacy and awareness efforts that would not have otherwise been cracked, if they were not famous. Michael J. Fox (2002) noted that others in the Parkinson's community, who don't have his claim to fame, "tell me, over and over, … if I get a shot in front of a microphone—I should start talking. So here I am" (p. 252–253), with a chance to tell at least part of "the" story. As we detail in the next section, celebrity health narratives serve an important purpose of sparking conversation online, face-to-face, and even in the halls of Congress.

Implications of Celebrity Health Narratives

The Couric effect. The Goody effect. The Roberts effect. A plethora of foundations, books, press, and publicity. In some ways, it's difficult to bring this book to a close. As Christie (lead author of this book) was in the very final stages of editing the last few chapters, she stepped away from the computer to go to Walmart for some more Diet Coke and a Father's Day card for her husband. While standing in the 20-items-or-less check-out aisle (behind someone who clearly had a few more than 20 items), she spotted the most recent *People* magazine with Angelina Jolie on the cover. Instinctively, she picked it up and plopped it down on the counter—after 17 years of data collection, buying anything that looks potentially useful might be a tough habit to break. She paused and carefully placed the magazine back on the shelf. Although tempting to continue our research, it's time to get out of the field, but, absolutely, conversations about this intriguing topic will endure, especially as we reflect on implications of the ever expanding list of celebrities who blur private and public boundaries about intimate health issues.

Indeed, even as we have been working on finalizing the book, more celebrities joined the ranks of individuals who choose to confide health issues with individuals beyond their close social circles. For example, in May 2014, actor Hugh Jackman posted a picture of his bandaged nose on Instagram and revealed his bout with skin cancer. According to Blaustein (2014, May 12, para. 1) "Hugh Jackman just revealed last week his second bout with cancer, now he's explaining why he is pleading with people to wear sunscreen and get checked out." Blaustein (2014, May 12, para. 2) quoted Jackman:

> "We are all human, this happened to me, I didn't wear sun screen when I was a kid," he told ABC News at the "X-Men: Days of Future Past" premiere over the weekend. "I don't want kids to be as stupid as me and maybe they'll listen to Wolverine more than they'll listen to teachers at school."

By posting the photo on Instagram and acknowledging the reason for the bandage, Jackman introduced his own story as a lesson for others (especially children) to use sunscreen. Throughout all of the celebrity health narratives, we identified two clear sub-themes about this form of health activism—they function as sources of encouragement and support and, like Jackman's photo and brief comments, bring vital attention to an important cause.

As we have documented throughout this book, celebrity health narratives can prompt expressions of support and comfort, both to and from fans and celebrities (see chapters on Brooke Burke-Charvet, Kim Kardashian, Giuliana Rancic, and Robin Roberts). As we mentioned in the chapter about Catherine Zeta-Jones and bipolar disorder, Patty Duke has written about her struggles with manic depression, and the following comments about her books underscore the power of celebrity health narratives to serve as a source of information and inspiration, especially to others who silently suffer from potentially stigmatizing conditions. On December 26, 2000, Karla wrote that Patty Duke "helped to break the stereotypes that go along with mental illness…. I thank her for that, and for helping me to finally get a name to what was wrong with me all my life!" In an August 25, 1999, online review of Patty Duke's book about manic depression, one fan, Suzy, wrote,

> I read this book about 10 years ago, and it began a healing process in my own life…. And a MUST after reading Patty Duke's (Anna) autobiography is to read her sequel which gives even more encouragement that those of us with any mental disorder are "not freaks" but can live healthy, functional lives and be of great help to our whole society.

Our book was well into production when we learned the shocking news that Robin Williams, a beloved and celebrated comedian and actor, passed away at age 63 on August 11, 2014 (Dennis et al., 2014, August 25). Sadly, we realized that we should insert a few words about him and this loss in our final reflections on celebrity health (and death) narratives. Williams had been very open about his decades-long struggle with addiction (Aitkenhead, 2010, September 19); however, Williams' stunning suicide sparked an outpouring of calls (by fellow celebrities and fans on Facebook) for our society to invest vastly more attention and resources to mental health issues, given that Williams struggled for years with depression (Huffington, 2014, August 18; Wetli, 2014, August 12)—a condition further complicated by his recent diagnosis with Parkinson's disease. As Wetli asserted, "His untimely death is tragically ironic because it illuminates our culture's overwhelming failure in dealing with mental illness and illustrates the harsh stigma that surrounds depression and substance abuse" (para. 5). Williams' widow, Susan Schneider, noted, "It is our hope in the wake of Robin's tragic passing that others will find the strength to seek the care and support they need to treat whatever battles they are facing so they may feel less afraid" (Dillon, 2014, August 20, para. 7).

Beyond comfort and encouragement for individuals, this volume has provided numerous examples of celebrities with a quest to raise awareness and money for research. Michael J. Fox, Christopher Reeve, and Mary Tyler Moore have all addressed Congress about the need for stem cell research, and all three have also testified on behalf of the need for funding for their respective conditions (Parkinson's disease, spinal cord injuries, and type 1 diabetes). Others who have testified before Congress include:

> cancer (Gene Wilder, Katie Couric, Bob Dole, Jill Eikenberry, Rod Carew, Lynda Carter, Geraldine Ferraro, and Lance Armstrong), Alzheimer's disease (Nancy Reagan, Maureen Reagan, and Angie Dickinson), kidney disease (Gary Coleman), Down syndrome (Christopher Burke), arthritis and musculoskeletal and skin disease (Hugh Downs), Crohn's disease (Mary Ann Mobley), and AIDS (Elizabeth Taylor) [Beck et al., 2014, p. 251].

Moreover, the list of foundations that have been initiated by celebrities encompasses the Muhammad Ali Parkinson Center as well as

> the Leeza Gibbons Memory Foundation, Jimmy V Foundation, ZazAngels, the Elizabeth Glaser Pediatric AIDS Foundation, the Lance Armstrong Foundation, the Michael J. Fox Foundation for Parkinson's Research, the Larry King Cardiac Foundation, the National Colorectal Cancer Research Alliance (founded by Katie Couric, Lilly Tartikoff, and the Entertainment Industry Foundation), and the Christopher and Dana Reeve Foundation [Beck et al., 2014, p. 251].

Clearly, these celebrities and many others have transformed their own personal health-related challenges into opportunities for giving voice on behalf of others who lack the same entryway into the public eye and the halls of Congress. As we close this book, we commend these efforts but also wonder about long-term policy decisions that might be impacted by this "disease of the week" approach. How can advocacy groups partner with stakeholders on Capitol Hill for research funding? Moreover, how should money be allocated for research on the array of illnesses and injuries that plague individuals across the world? In what ways should we prioritize monetary allocations, educational efforts, and awareness campaigns? These very moral and ethical questions should guide future conversations about celebrity health narratives as integral aspects of public dialogues about health.

Although complicated and occasionally controversial, celebrity health narratives, at the very least, draw important attention to various types of human suffering, struggles, and stories of success. We herald the sacrifice that celebrities make as they yield some of their privacy to attract attention, promote understanding, and, ideally, prevent future health situations for others by sharing their health narratives with us. We believe that the last few lines of "For Good," a song from the hit Broadway musical *Wicked*, capture the essence of celebrity health narratives for both famous and not so famous individuals who co-tell the emergent public story of a health condition. In the musical, the characters reflect on whether or not they have been affected by each other positively or negatively, ultimately deciding that their relationship has been not only positive but also lasting. Although we could also continue to debate the valuable and problematic aspects of celebrity health narratives, based on our data set, we affirm their impact on unfolding public dialogues about health endures in important and influential ways: "I do believe I have been changed for the better. Because I knew you. Because I knew you. I have been changed for good."

References

Abcarian, R. (2013, May 21). Angelina Jolie's courageous act will save women's lives. *Los Angeles Times*. Retrieved from http://articles.latimes.com/2013/may/21/local/la-me-abcarian-angelina-20130521.

ABC News. (2007, August 3). ABC's Robin Roberts: "I have breast cancer." *ABC News*. Retrieved from http://abcnews.go.com/GMA/CancerPreventionAndTreatment/abcs-robin-roberts-breast-cancer/print?id=3430554.

ABC News. (2011, August 8). Kardashian family empire: Day in the lives of the Kim, Kourtney, and Khloe Kardashian [Video file]. Retrieved from http://www.youtube.com/watch?v=GJOxkvandwA.

ABC News. (2012, June 8). Women's basketball hall of fame inducts Robin Roberts. *ABC News*. Retrieved from http://abcnews.go.com/GMA/video/womens-basketball-hall-fame-inducts-robin-roberts-16524077.

ABC News. (2013, February 22). Robin Roberts' journey: Inside her courageous fight against MDS. *ABC News*. Retrieved from http://abcnews.go.com/Health/robin-roberts-journey-inside-courageous-fight-mds/story?id=18562093#disqus_thread.

ABC News. (2014). Robin Roberts. *ABC News*. Retrieved from http://abcnews.go.com/Author/Robin_Roberts.

"About Scott Hamilton." (2014, June 3). Cleveland Clinic. Retrieved from http://www.clevelandclinic.org/cancer/scottcares/scott/about.asp.

"Actress Colleen Zenk Pinter partners with the Oral Cancer Foundation to raise public…" (2007, November 30). Reuters. Retrieved from http://www.reuters.com/article/2007/11/30/idUS6739+30-Nov-2007+PRN20071130.

Adams, M. (2013, May 16). EXPOSED: Angelina Jolie part of a clever corporate scheme to protect billions in BRCA gene patents, influence Supreme Court decision (opinion). Retrieved from http://www.naturalnews.com/040365_Angelina_Jolie_gene_patents_Supreme_Court_decis.

Adler, J., M. Hager, J. Gordon, E. Yoffe, P. Yang, L. Beachy. (1991, November 18). Magic's message: A beloved superstar's HIV infection stuns the world—and energizes the battle against AIDS. *Newsweek*, 58–64.

Agne, R. R., T. L. Thompson, and L. P. Cusella (2000). Stigma in the line of face: Self-disclosure of patients' HIV status to health care providers. *Journal of Applied Communication Research, 28*(3), 235–261.

Aitkenhead, D. (2010, September 19). Robin Williams: "I was shameful, did stuff that caused disgust—that's hard to recover from." Retrieved from http://www.theguardian.com/film/2010/sep/20/robin-williams-worlds-greatest-dad-alcohol.

Allin, O. (2011, July 25). Kim Kardashian opens up about psoriasis on reality show. Retrieved from http://www.ontheredcarpet.com/Kim-Kardashian-opens-up-about-psoriasis-on-reality-show/8270668.

Allison, N. (2011, July 20). *Mom at the Helm of the JDRF Children's Congress* [Blog]. Retrieved from http://www.diabetesmine.com/2011/07/mom-at-the-helm-of-the-jdrf-childrens-congress.html.

Allreadable.com. (2014a). Season 6, Episode 5, Baby on the Loose. Retrieved from http://www.allreadable.com/vid/baby-on-the-loose-522794.html.

Allreadable.com. (2014b). Season 5, Episode 21, Holy Baby. *Readable*. Retrieved from http://www.allreadable.com/vid/holy-baby!-1050211.html.

Al-Samarrie, N. (2012, October). Paula Deen: Cooking up a new life with diabetes. *Diabetes Health, 21*(5), 27–29.

Altman, I., and D. A. Taylor. (1973). *Social penetration: The development of interpersonal relationships*. New York: Holt, Rinehart, & Winston.

American Cancer Society. (2014a). Breast cancer overview. Retrieved from http://www.cancer.org/cancer/breastcancer/overviewguide/breast-cancer-overview-key-statistics.

American Cancer Society. (2014b). Thyroid cancer. Retrieved from http://www.cancer.org/cancer/thyroidcancer/.

American Diabetes Association. (2013). *Type 1 diabetes*. Retrieved from http://www.diabetes.org/living-with-diabetes/recently-diagnosed/living-with-type-1-diabetes.html.

American Diabetes Association. (2014). Statistics about diabetes. Retrieved from http://www.diabetes.org/diabetes-basics/statistics/?loc=db-slabnav.

"Angelina Jolie's aunt dies of breast cancer." (2013, May 27). BBC News. Retrieved from www.bbc.co.uknews/world-us-canada-22677972.

Antheunis, M. L., K. Tates, and T. E. Nieboer. (2013). Patients' and health professionals' use social media in health care: Motives, barriers and expectations. *Patient Education and Counseling, 92*, 426–431. doi:10.1016/j.pec.2013.06.020.

"Applause, applause: A sampling of viewer comments on Michael Zaslow's return to daytime TV on *One Life to Live*." (1999, April 12). Retrieved from http://www.america.net/~gwp/usmz/zaznotes.html.

Arnowitz, L. (2013, June 27). Paula Deen's show ratings down before Food Network dismissal. Fox News. Retrieved from http://foxnews.com/entertainment/2013/06/27/paula-deen-show-struggled-with-ratin…

Aronson, J. (1994). A pragmatic view of thematic analysis. *The Qualitative Report, 2*(1). Retrieved from http://www.nova.edu/ssss/QR/BackIssues/QR2–1/aronson.html.

Atkins-Sayre, W., and A. Q. Stokes. (2014). Crafting the cornbread nation: The Southern foodways alliance and Southern identity. *Southern Communication Journal, 79*(2), 77–93. doi: 1080/1041794X.2013.861010.

Austin, R. (2012). Pencil-like thin icons of feminity in the Indian media. *Global Media Journal, 3*, 1–8.

Baek, Y. M., Y. Bae, and H. Jang. (2013). Social and parasocial relationships on social network sites and their differential relationships with users' psychological well-being. *Cyberpsychology, Behavior, and Social Networking, 16*, 512–517. doi: 10.1089/cyber.2012.0510.

Baker, K. C. (2011, April 21). Jane Pauley: Catherine Zeta-Jones makes the world safer for people with bipolar disorder. *People*. Retrieved from http://people.com/people/article/0,,20483525,00.html.

Bakhtin, M. M. (1981). *The dialogic imagination: Four essays*. (C. Emerson and M. Holquist, Trans.). Austin: University of Texas Press.

Balter-Reitz, S., and S. Keller. (2005). Censoring thinspiration: The debate over pro-anorexic web sites. *Free Speech Yearbook, 42*, 79–90.

Balzora, S. (2013, July 8). How Katie Couric continues to influence the colonoscopy debate. Retrieved from http://www.kevinmd.com/blog/2013/07/katie-couric-continues-influence-colonoscopy-debate.html.

Bamberg, M. (2012). Why narrative? *Narrative Inquiry, 22*, 202–210. doi: 10.1075/ni.22.1.16bam.

Bamberg, M., and M. Andrews. (Eds.). (2004). *Considering counter-narratives: Narrating, resisting, making sense*. Amsterdam, The Netherlands: John Benjamins.

Bannon, J. (1993, April 29). Jim Valvano. *USA Today*, 1C.

Barker, V. (2009). Older adolescents' motivations for social network site use: The influence of gender, group identity, and collective self-esteem. *Cyberpsychology & Behavior, 12*, 209–213. doi: 10.1089/cpb.2008.0228.

Baylis, S. C. (2013, October 03). Giuliana Rancic after cancer: More junk food & less exercise. *People*. Retrieved from http://www.people.com/people/article/0,,20740818,00.html.

Baym, N. (2010). *Personal connections in the digital age*. Cambridge, England: Polity.

Beagan, G. (2012, July 1). Soap opera actress from Stuart is cancer survivor. Retrieved from http://tcpalm.com/news/2012/jul/01/soap-opera-actress-from-stuart-is-cancer-heroine/.

Beamon, K. (2012). "I'm a baller": Athletic identity foreclosure among African-American former student-athletes. *Journal of African American Studies, 16*, 195–208. doi: 10.1007/s12111-012-92-11-8.

Beck, C. S. (2001). *Communicating for better health: A guide through the medical mazes*. Boston: Allyn & Bacon.

Beck, C. S. (2005). Personal stories and public activism: The implications of Michael J. Fox's public health narrative for policy and perspectives. In E. Ray (Ed.), *Case studies in health communication* (pp. 335–345). Mahwah, NJ: Erlbaum.

Beck, C. S. (2012). Intersecting narratives: Enjoying daytime drama as viewers (and actors) experience the days of their lives. *Communication Studies, 63*, 152–171. doi: 10.1080/10510974.2011.638413.

Beck, C. S., S. Aubuchon, T. McKenna, S. Ruhl, and N. Simmons. (2014). Blurring personal health and public priorities: An analysis of celebrity health narratives in the public sphere. *Health Communication*, 1–13. doi: 10.1080/10410236.2012.741668.

Bell, K. (2011). "A delicious way to help save lives": Race, commodification, and celebrity in Product (RED). *Journal of International and Intercultural Communication, 4*, 163–180. doi: 10.1080/17513057.2011.569972.

Bender, J. L., M. C. Jimenez-Marroquin, and A. R. Jadad. (2011). Seeking support on Facebook: A content analysis of breast cancer groups. *Journal of Medical Internet Research, 13*, e16. doi:10.2196/jmir.1560.

Berezow, A. (2013, December 11). Are repeated concussions really killing NFL football players? *Forbes*. Retrieved from http://www.forbes.com/sites/alexberezow/2013/12/11/are-repeated-concussions-really-killing…

Berger, J. (1985, October 3). Rock Hudson, screen idol, dies at 59. *Science*. Retrieved from http://partners.nytimes.com/library/national/science/aids/100385sci-aids.html.

Bergstrom, R. L., and C. Neighbors. (2006). Body image disturbance and the social norms approach: An integrative review of the literature. *Journal of Social and Clinical Psychology, 25,* 975–1000. doi: 10.1521/jscp.2006.25.9.975.

Bhargava, J. (2009, July 11). Fairway girl urges Congress to help find a cure for diabetes. *Kansas City Star*. Retrieved from http://infoweb.newsbank.com.proxy.library.ohiou.edu/iw…

Billhartz, C. (2002, March 5). "Ana" and "Mia" on the Web and out of control. *St. Louis Post-Dispatch*, E1.

Billings, A. C., M. L. Butterworth, and P. D. Turman. (2012). *Communication and sport: Surveying the field*. Thousand Oaks, CA: Sage.

Blacklow, J. (2013, July 22). Catherine Zeta-Jones says Michael Douglas' cancer was a "trigger" for her bipolar disorder. *Yahoo! Celebrity*. Retrieved from http://celebrity.yahoo.com/blogs/celeb-news/catherine-zeta-jones-says-michael-douglas-cancer-trigger-020040250.html.

Blaustein, D., with N. Rothman. (2014, May 12). Hugh Jackman opens up about battle with skin cancer. *ABC News*. Retrieved from http://abcnews.go.com/Entertainment/hugh-jackman-talks-battle-skin-cancer/story?id=23682657.

Bochner, A. P. (2014). *Coming to narrative: A personal history of paradigm change in the human sciences*. Walnut Creek, CA: Left Coast Press.

Booth, P. (2010). *Digital fandom: New media studies*. New York: Peter Lang.

Boren, C. (2014, February 18). Move over, Barbie, the *Sports Illustrated* swimsuit issue is here. *Washington Post*. Retrieved from http://www.washingtonpost.com/blogs/eaerly-lead/wp/2014/02/18/move-over-barbie-the-sp…

Botta, R. A. (1999). Television images and adolescent girls' body image disturbance. *Journal of Communication, 49*(2), 22–41.

Boyatzis, R. (1998). *Transforming qualitative information: Thematic analysis and code development*. Thousand Oaks, CA: Sage.

Boyle, R., and R. Haynes. (2000). *Power play: Sport, the media and popular culture*. Harlow, England: Pearson.

BrightPink.org. (2014). BrightPink. Retrieved from http://www.brightpink.org/.

Brock, B. L. (Eds.). (1999). *Kenneth Burke and the 21st century*. Albany: State University of New York Press.

Brook, S. (2007, January 22). Keira Knightley takes action against Mail. *The Guardian*. Retrieved from http://www.theguardian.com/media/2007/jan/22/dailymail.pressand publishing.

Brookes, R. (2002). *Representing sports*. London: Oxford University Press.

Brown, B. (2012). *Daring greatly: How the courage to be vulnerable transforms the way we live, love, parent, and lead*. New York: Gotham Books.

Brown, B., and M. Baranowski. (1996). Searching for the Magic Johnson effect: AIDS, adolescents, and celebrity disclosure. *Adolescence, 31,* 253–265.

Brown, W. J., and M. Basil. (1995). Media celebrities and public health: Responses to "Magic" Johnson's HIV disclosure and its impact on AIDS risk and high-risk behaviors. *Health Communication, 7,* 345–370. doi: 10.1207/s15327027hc0704_4.

Brown, W. J., and M. D. Basil. (2010). Parasocial interaction and identification: Social change processes for effective health interventions. *Health Communication, 25,* 601–602. doi: 10.1080/10410236.2010.496830.

Brown, W. J., M. D. Basil, and M. Bocarnea. (2003a). Social influence of an international celebrity: Responses to the death of Princess Diana. *Journal of Communication, 534,* 587–605.

Brown, W. J., M. D. Basil, and M. Bocarnea. (2003b). The influence of famous athletes on health beliefs and practices: Mark McGwire, child abuse prevention, and adrostenedione. *Journal of Health Communication, 8,* 41–57.

Brown, W. J., and M. De Matviuk. (2010). Sports celebrities and public health: Diego Maradona's influence on drug use prevention. *Journal of Health Communication, 15,* 358–373. doi: 10.1080/10810730903460575.

Brunsdon, C. (2000). *The feminist, the housewife, and the soap opera*. Oxford, England: Clarendon Press.

Bryant, J., and R. G. Cummins. (2010). The effects of outcome of mediated and live sporting events on sports fans' self- and social identities. In H. L. Hundley and A. C. Billings (Eds.), *Examining identity in sports media* (pp. 217–238). Thousand Oaks, CA: Sage.

Burke, E. (2006). Feminine visions: Anorexia and contagion in pop discourse. *Feminist Media Studies, 6,* 315–330. doi: 10.1080/1468 0770600802066.

Burke, K. (1950/1969). *A rhetoric of motives*. Berkeley: University of California Press.

Burke, M. (2012, December 7). Average player

salaries in the four major American sports leagues. *Forbes.* http://www.forbes.com/sites/monteburke/2012/12/07/average-player-salaries-in-the-four-major-american-sports-leagues/.

Burke-Charvet, B. (2012, November 8). Cancer. Me? Retrieved from http://www.modern mom.com/98795a8a-3b3e-11e3-be8a-bc764e04a41e.html.

Burke-Charvet, B. (2013, February 4). Joining hands and hearts on world cancer day. Retrieved from http://www.modernmom.com/c072f5b4-3b3e-11e3-be8a-bc764e04a41e.html.

Burke-Charvet, B. (2014). Ultrasound, Biopsy and Fear. Retrieved from http://www.modern mom.com/ea3823f2-3b3d-11e3-be8a-bc764e04a41e.html.

Burleson, B. R., and E. L. MacGeorge. (2002). Supportive communication. In M. L. Knapp and J. A. Daly (Eds.), *Handbook of interpersonal communication* (3rd ed., pp. 374–424). Thousand Oaks, CA: Sage.

Buscemi, R. (2014). Television as a trattoria: Constructing the woman in the kitchen on Italian food shows. *European Journal of Communication, 29,* 304–318. doi: 10.1177/026732 3114523147.

Bute, J. J., and T. A. Vik. (2010). Privacy management as unfinished business: Shifting boundaries in the context of infertility. *Communication Studies, 61,* 1–20. doi: 10.1080/105 10970903405997.

Cady, J. (2010, February 25). Giuliana & Bill Rancic share in vitro struggle. Retrieved from http://www.eonline.com/news/168892/giuliana-bill-rancic-share-in-vitro-struggle.

Cairns Pastor, C. (2009, June 24). Odessa youngster meets Obama during diabetes event. *Tampa Tribune.* Retrieved from http://tbo.com/carrollwood/odessa-youngster-meets-obama-during-diabetes-event-100590.

Cambridge Dictionaries. (2014). Cambridge dictionaries online. *Cambridge University Press.* Retrieved from http://dictionary.cambridge.org/us/dictionary/british/woe-is-me.

Carless, D., and K. Douglas. (2013a). "In the boat" but "selling myself short": Stories, narratives, and identity development in elite sport. *The Sport Psychologist, 27,* 27–39.

Carless, D., and K. Douglas. (2013b). Living, resisting, and playing the part of athlete: Narrative tensions in elite sport. *Psychology of Sport and Exercise,* 14, 701–708.

Carlyle, E. (2012, July 18). Paula Deen: Diabetes diagnosis hasn't dented her earnings. *Forbes.* Retrieved from http://www.forbes.com.

Casey, M., M. Allen, T. Emmers-Sommer, E. Sahlstein, D. DeGooyer, A. Winters, et al. (2003). When a celebrity contracts a disease: The example of Earvin "Magic" Johnson's announcement. *Journal of Health Communica-*

tion, 8, 249–266. doi: 10/080/10810730390 196471.

"Catherine Zeta-Jones: I don't want to be the 'poster child' for bipolar disorder." (2012, December 8). *US Magazine.* Retrieved from http://www.usmagazine.com.

CBS News. (2009, June 23). Mary Tyler Moore's mission [*The Early Show*]. *CBS News.* Retrieved from http://www.cbsnews.com/videos/mary-tyler-moores-mission/.

CBS This Morning. (1992, August 28). Retrieved from http://www.contentville.com/efull/trans …sp?PRT=199208280700cbs&CT=TVTran script.

"Celebs react to Michael Jackson's death." (2009, June 26). *US Magazine.* Retrieved from http://www.usmagazine.com/celebrity-news/news/celebs-react-to-michael-jacksons-death-2009266.

Chan, S. (2008, January 28). The death of Heath Ledger. *New York Times.* Retrieved from http://cityroom.blogs.nytimes.com/2008/01/22/actor-heath-ledger-is-found-dead/?_php=true&_type=blogs&_r=0.

Chang, S. (2012, November 15). Keira Knightley slams anorexia talk: Eating disorder rumors hurt my feelings. *Examiner.* Retrieved from http://www.examiner.com/article/keira-knightley-slams-anorexia-talk-but-admits-the-rumors-made-her-insecure.

Chang, S. (2014, February 3). Keira Knightley reveals family anorexia history: Mom and grandma were anorexic. Retrieved from http://www.examiner.com/article/keira-knightley-reveals-family-history-of-anorexia-diet-and-workout-plan.

"Charita Bauer." (2013, March 19). Wikipedia. Retrieved from http://en.wikipedia.org/wiki/Charita_Bauer.

Charon, R. (2005). Narrative medicine: Attention, representation, affiliation. *Narrative, 13,* 261–270.

Charon, R. (2009a). Narrative medicine as witness for the self-telling body. *Journal of Applied Communication Research, 37,* 118–131. doi: 10.1080/00909880902792248.

Charon, R. (2009b). The polis of a discursive narrative medicine. *Journal of Applied Communication Research, 37,* 196–201.

Childs, D. (2009, June 27). Farrah Fawcett's anal cancer: Fighting the stigma. *ABC News.* Retrieved from http://abcnews.go.com/Health/story?id=7939402&page=1#.UHcUWK4jYSE.

Chou, W. S., Y. M. Hunt, E. B. Beckjord, R. P. Moser, and B. W. Hesse. (2009). Social media use in the United States: Implications for health communication. *Journal of Medical Internet Research,11*(4), 48. Retrieved online from http://www.jmir.org/2009/4/e48/doi:10.2196/jmir.1249.

Chua-Eoan, H., S. Wulf, J. Kluger, C. Redman,

and D. Van Biema. (1997, September 8). Diana 1961–1997: Death of a princess. *Time*. Retrieved from http://www.time.com/time/magazine/article/0,9171,986949,00.html.

Chung, C. (1991, December 11). *Face to Face with Connie Chung: Special program/interview: Magic Johnson discusses revealing he has HIV virus*. Retrieved from http://www.contentville.com/efull/trans...sp?PRT=199112112200cbs&CT=TVTranscript.

Cinoğlu, H., and Y. Arikan. (2012). Self, identity, and identity formation: From the perspectives of three major theories. *International Journal of Human Sciences, 9* (2), 1,114–1,131.

Clark, L., and M. Tiggemann. (2006). Appearance culture in nine- to 12-year-old girls: Media and peer influences on body dissatisfaction. *Social Development, 15*, 628–643. doi:10.1111/j.1467–9507.2006.00361.x.

Clarke, H. (2012, January 17). Novo Nordisk partners with Paula Deen and sons, Bobby and Jamie Deen, on national diabetes initiative. *PR Newswire U.S.* Retrieved from http://www.bloomberg.com/apps/news?pid=newsarchive&sid=aKCtvr4zwDAI.

Cleveland Clinic. (2014). Diseases and conditions: Thyroid Disease. Retrieved from http://my.clevelandclinic.org/disorders/hyperthyroidism/hic_.

CNN. (2002, May 8). Interview with Mary Tyler Moore [*Larry King Live*]. Retrieved from http://transcripts.cnn.com/TRANSCRIPTS/0205/08/lkl.00.html.

CNN. (2005, July 1). Interview with Mary Tyler Moore [*Larry King Live*]. Retrieved from http://transcripts.cnn.com/TRANSCRIPTS/0507/01/lkl.01.html.

CNN Health. (2013). *Type 1 diabetes in children*. CNN. Retrieved from http://www.cnn.com/HEALTH/library/type-1-diabetes-in-children/DS00931.html.

Cohen, S. B. (2006). Media exposure and the subsequent effects on body dissatisfaction, disordered eating, and drive for thinness: A review of the current research. *Mind Matters: The Wesleyan Journal of Psychology, 1*, 57–71.

Cole, C. E. (2010). Problematizing therapeutic assumptions about narratives: A case study of storytelling events in a post-conflict context. *Health Communication, 25*, 650–660. doi: 10.1080/10410236.2010.521905.

Collins, J. M. (2004, November-December). Nurturing destruction: Eating disorders online. *Off Our Backs*, 20–22.

Conley, M. (2012, January 18). Anthony Bourdain slams Paula Deen for diabetes-drug partnership. Retrieved from http://abcnews.go.com.

"Controversy of the week: Jolie: A powerful message about breasts and cancer." (2013, May 31). *The Week, 13* (619), 4.

Cooper, J., with L. Harrison. (2012). *Not young, still restless*. New York: HarperCollins.

Cotliar, S. (2013, December 16). Amy Robach's breast cancer battle: "I have a lot to fight for." *People, 80*(25), 64–67.

Cotliar, S. (2014, April 16). Robin Roberts feels like she's a "walking miracle." *People Magazine*. Retrieved from http://people.com/people/article/O,,20807339,00.html.

Cotliar, S., and R. Jerome. (2008, October 20). Breast cancer survivor Robin Roberts and her sisters the power of three. *People Magazine, 70*(16). Retrieved from http://www.people.com/people/archive/article/0,,20238177,00.html.

Cotliar, S., and M. Tauber. (2011, May 2). Her private struggle. *People, 75*(17), 52–56.

Cotterill, S. (2012). *Team psychology in sports: Theory and practice*. London: Routledge.

Coyle, J. (n.d.). News of Jackson's death first spread online. *ABC News*. Retrieved from http://abcnews.go.com/Technology/story?id=7938705&page=1&singlePage=true.

Craig, B. (2012, April). Soap opera actress an amputee, like her character. Retrieved from http://www.healio.com/orthotics-prosthetics/prosthetics/news/print/o-and-p-business-news/%7BOc61f3a-6b46–47bo\O-9135-c2860817d3c3%7D/soap-opera-actress-an-amputee-like-her-character.

Cram, P., A. M. Fendrick, J. Inadomi, M. Cowen, D. Carpenter, and S. Vijan. (2003). The impact of a celebrity promotional campaign on the use of colon cancer screening. *Archives of Internal Medicine, 163*, 1,601–1,605.

Crane, M. (2001, April 10). Spielman is fighting recurrence of disease. *Columbus Dispatch*, 130(283), A1.

Curry, A. (2011, October 17). *The Today Show*: E!'s Giuliana Rancic reveals she has breast cancer. Retrieved from http://www.today.com/video/today/44928433#44928433.

Cushion, C., and R. Jones. (2014). A Bourdieusian analysis of cultural reproduction: Socialisation and the "hidden curriculum" in professional football. *Sport, Education, and Society, 19* (3), 276–298. doi: 10.1080/13573322.2012.666966.

Daily Dish. (2012, December 7). Catherine Zeta-Jones: "Stop asking me about bipolar diagnosis." Retrieved from http://blogs.sfgate.com/dailydish.

Darman, J., and L. H. Teslik. (2006). In Missouri, the Fox effect. *Newsweek, 148*(19), 41–42. Retrieved from http://web.ebscohost.com/ehost/detail?vid=4&hid=105&sid=cfe2a1fb-aa8a-462b-ba67–90.

Davies, L., and H. G. Welch. (2006). Increasing incidence of thyroid cancer in the United States, 1973–2002. *Journal of the American Medical Association, 295*, 2,164–2,167. doi:10.1001/jama.295.18.2164.

Davison, K. P., J. W. Pennebaker, and S. S. Dickerson. (2000). Who talks? The social psychology of illness support groups. *American Psychologist, 55,* 205–217.

Dean, P. (n.d.). Diabetes in a new light. Retrieved from http://www.pauladeen.com/article_view/diabetes_in_a_new_light/.

De Block, L. (2012). Entertainment education and social change: Evaluating a children's soap opera in Kenya. *International Journal of Educational Development, 32,* 608–614. doi: 10.1016/j.ijedudev.2011.09.005.

DeFina, A., and A. Georgakopoulou. (2008). Analysing narratives as practices. *Qualitative Research, 8,* 379–387. doi: 10.1177/146879410 6093634.

De Graaf, A., H. Hoeken, J. Sanders, and J. W. J. Beentjes. (2012). Identification as a mechanism of narrative persuasion. *Communication Research, 39,* 802–823. doi: 10.1177/0093650 211408594.

Dennis, A., K. Coyne, T. Fowler, P. Gomez, M. Green, S. Helling, et al. (2014, August 25). 1951–2014 Robin Williams (cover story). *People.* Retrieved from http://web.b.ebscohost.com/ehost/delivery?sid=da2e6649–7dd5–4815–8eb4-cc5db459df86…

Derlega, V. J., B. A. Winstead, and K. Greene. (2008). Self-disclosure and starting a close relationship. In S. Sprecher, A. Wensel, and J. Harvey (Eds.), *Handbook of relationship beginnings* (pp. 153–174). New York: Psychology Press.

Dewey, J. (1934/1980). *Art as experience.* New York: Penguin Group.

"Diabetes has not slowed down 15-year-old Nick Jonas!" (2008, April-May). *Diabetes Health.* Retrieved from www.DiabetesHealth.com.

DiEdwardo, J. A. (2009, December 28). Mary Tyler Moore: Making a difference in the fight against type 1 diabetes. *Success.* Retrieved from http://www.success.com/article/mary-tyler-moore-making-a-difference-in-the-fight-against-type-1-diabetes.

Dillon, N. (2012, December 7). Catherine Zeta-Jones is "sick" of talking about her bipolar disorder: "I never wanted to be the poster child for this." *New York Daily News.* Retrieved from http://www.nydailynews.com/entertainment/gossip/catherine-zeta-jones-sick-talking-bi-polar-article-1.1215661.

Dillon, N. (2013, May 22). Brad Pitt and Angelina Jolie covered their tracks to keep double mastectomy surgeries secret. Retrieved from http://www.nydailynews.comentertainment/gossip/pitt-jolie-covered-tracks-article-1.1351.

Dillon, N. (2014, August 20) Robin Williams' ashes scattered in San Francisco Bay: report. Retrieved from http://www.nydailynews.com/entertainment/gossip/robin-williams-ashes-scattered-san-francisco-bay-article-1.1911219#ixzz3B2heyuxa.

"Di's private battle: The princess' struggle with bulimia brings a puzzling disease out of the shadows" (1992, August 8). *People Magazine.* Retrieved from http://www.people.com/people/archive/article/0,,20113238,00.html.

Domar, A. D., P. C. Zuttermeister, and R. Friedman. (1993). The psychological impact of infertility: A comparison with patients with other medical conditions. *Journal of Psychosomatic Obstetrics & Gynecology, 12,* 45–52.

Dowell, B. (2007, May 24). Mail pays out over anorexia story. *The Guardian.* Retrieved from http://www.theguardian.com/media/2007/may/24/dailymail.pressandpublishing.

Dravecky, D., with T. Stafford. (1990). *Comeback.* Grand Rapids, MI: Zondervan.

Dravecky, D., and J. Dravecky. (1992). *When you can't come back: A story of courage and grace.* Grand Rapids, MI: Zondervan.

Drugs.com. (2014). Drug-related deaths—notable celebrities. Retrieved from http://www.drugs.com/celebrity_deaths.html.

Dube, R. (2011, April 14). Zeta-Jones may help dispel stigma of bipolar disorder. MSNBC. Retrieved from http://today.msnbc.msn.com/id/42589427/ns/today-today?health/t/zeta-jones-may-help-dispel-stigma-bipolar-disorder.

Duggan, M., and A. Smith. (2013, December 30). Social media update 2013. *Pew Research Internet Project.* Retrieved from http://www.pewinternet.org/2013/12/30/social-media-update-2013/.

Duke, A. (2009, September 4). Michael Jackson reaches his "final resting place." *CNN.com/entertainment.* Retrieved from http://www.cnn.com/2009/SHOWBIZ/Music/09/04/jackson.burial/index.html.

Duke, A., and T. Leopold. (2014, April 7). Legendary actor Mickey Rooney dies at 93. *CNN Entertainment.* Retrieved from http://www.cnn.com/2014/04/07/showbiz/mickey-rooney-obit/.

Duke, P. (1987). *Call me Anna: The autobiography of Patty Duke.* New York: Bantam Books.

Duke, P. (1992). *A brilliant madness: Living with manic depression.* New York: Bantam Books.

Dunlop, S., M. Wakefield, and Y. Kashima. (2010). Pathways to persuasion: Cognitive and experiential responses to health-promoting mass media messages. *Communication Research, 37,* 133–164. doi: 10.1177/0093650209 351912.

Dunn, S. (2012). Diary of a mastectomy: Giuliana and Bill Rancic. *Glamour Health & Diet.* Retrieved from http://www.glamour.com/health-fitness/2012/03/glamour-exclusive-interview-giuliana-rancic-bill-rancic-diary-of-a-mastectomy.

Du Pre, A. (2014). *Communicating about health: Current issues and perspectives* (4th ed.). New York: Oxford.

Earnheardt, A. C., and P. M. Haridakis. (2009). An examination of fan-athlete interaction: Freedom, parasocial interaction, and identification. *Ohio Communication Journal, 47,* 27–53.

Earnheardt, A. C., P. M. Haridakis, and B. S. Hugenberg (Eds.). (2012). *Sports fans, identity, and socialization: Exploring the fandemonium.* Lanham, MD: Lexington Books.

"Eating disorder statistics." (2014). National Association of Anorexia Nervosa and Associated Disorders. Retrieved from http://www.anad.org/get-information/about-eating-disorders/eating-disorders-statistics/.

Editorial Board. (2013, May 15). Our view: Angelina Jolie, breast cancer fighter. *USA Today,* 8A.

Editorial Board (2013, May 17). Angelina Jolie's disclosures. *New York Times.* Retrieved from http://www.nytimes.com/2013/05/18/opinion/angelina-jolies-disclosure.html.

Eggermont, S., K. Beullens, and J. Van den Bulck. (2005). Television viewing and adolescent females' body dissatisfaction: The mediating role of opposite sex expectations. *Communications: The European Journal of Communication Research, 30*(3), 343–357. doi:10.1515/comm.2005.30.3.343.

Ekberg, A. (2009, June 25). Farrah Fawcett, Michael Jackson, and other celebrities that died on the same day. Retrieved from http://voices.yahoo.com/farrah-fawcett-michael-jackson-other-celebrities-3673748.html?cat=2.

Elliott, J. (2009, March 22). The Jade Goody effect on screening. *BBC News.* Retrieved from news.bbc.co.uk/2/hi/health/7925685.stm.

Ellis, C. S., and A. P. Bochner. (2000). Autoethnography, personal narrative, reflexivity: Researcher as subject. In N. K. Denzin and Y. S. Lincoln (Eds.), *Handbook of qualitative research* (2nd ed., pp. 733–768). Thousand Oaks, CA: Sage.

"Emmy-winner Zaslow dies." (1998, December 29). *Soap Opera Digest, 23*(52), 4.

EOL. (2010, September 30). Giuliana Rancic opens up about her miscarriage. EOnline. Retrieved from http://www.eonline.com/shows/e_news/news/203375/giuliana-rancic-opens-up-about-her-miscarriage.

Errico, M. (2010, Sept. 30). Bill and Giuliana Rancic: We had a miscarriage. Retrieved from http://www.eonline.com/news/203222/bill-and-giuliana-rancic-we-had-a-miscarriage.

Espejo, R. (Ed.). (2009). *Can celebrities change the world?* Detroit, MI: Greenhaven Press.

Etherington, K. (2006). Understanding drug misuse and changing identities: A life story approach. *Drugs: Education, Prevention & Policy, 13,* 233–245. doi:10.1080/09687630500537555.

Evans, E. (2011). *Transmedia television: Audiences, new media, and daily life.* New York: Routledge.

Facebook.com. (2014). Brooke Burke-Charvet. Retrieved from https://www.facebook.com/pages/Brooke-Burke/261925180496418.

Fainaru-Wada, M., and S. Fainaru. (2013). *League of denial: The NFL, concussions, and the battle for truth.* New York: Crown Archetype.

Fallon, A. (2011, April 13). Catherine Zeta-Jones checks into clinic for bipolar disorder treatment. *The Guardian.* Retrieved from http://www.guardian.co.uk.

"Famous faces of eating disorders learn about those who dealt with eating disorders in the public limelight." (2011, July 6). *Healthline.* Retrieved from http://www.healthline.com/health-slideshow/celebrities-with-eating-disorders#1.

"'Farrah's Story'—Video of Cancer Documentary Now Available Online." (2009, May 16). Retrieved from http://careaware.wordpress.com/2009/05/16/%E2%80%9Cfarrah%E2%80%99s-story%E2%80%9D-video-of-cancer-documentary-now-available-online/.

Feyerick, D., S. Chun, M. Susana, and E. Pontz. (2008, January 22). Actor Heath Ledger dies at age 28. CNN. Retrieved from http://www.cnn.com/2008/SHOWBIZ/Movies/01/22/heath.ledger.dead/.

Fidler, A. T., and J. Bernstein. (1999). Infertility: From a personal to a public health problem. *Public Health Reports, 114,* 494–511.

Fisher, W. R. (1984). Narration as a human communication paradigm: The case of public moral argument. *Communication Monographs, 51*(1), 1–22.

Fisher, W. R. (1985a). The narrative paradigm: An elaboration. *Communication Monographs, 52*(4), 347–367.

Fisher, W. R. (1985b). The narrative paradigm: In the beginning. *Journal of Communication, 35,* 74–89. doi: 10.1111/j.1460–2466.1985.tb02974.x.

Fisher, W. R. (1987a). *Human communication as narration: Toward a philosophy of reason, value, and action.* Columbia: University of South Carolina Press.

Fisher, W. R. (1987b). Technical logic, rhetorical logic, and narrative rationality. *Argumentation, 1,* 3–21.

Fisher, W. R. (1989). Clarifying the narrative paradigm. *Communication Monographs, 56* (1), 55–58.

Fisher, W. R. (1994). Narrative rationality and

the logic of scientific discourse. *Argumentation, 8,* 21–32.

"Follow the script: Sofia Vegara and her story." (2014). Retrieved from http://www.followthe-scriptcampaign.com/.

Ford, J. A., and L. Blumenstein. (2013). Self-control and substance use among college students. *Journal of Drug Issues, 43*(1), 56–68. doi:10.1177/0022042612462216.

Ford, S., A. De Kosnik, and C. L. Harrington. (2011a). Introduction: The crisis of daytime drama and what it means. In S. Ford, A. De Kosnik, and C. L. Harrington (Eds.), *The survival of soap opera: Transformations for a new media era* (pp. 3–21). Jackson: University of Mississippi Press.

Ford, S., A. De Kosnik, and C. L. Harrington. (Eds.). (2011b). *The survival of soap opera: Transformations for a new media era.* Jackson: University of Mississippi Press.

ForeverLoyaltyMgmt. (2011, December 17). Barbara Walters vs. The Kardashians [Video file]. Retrieved from http://www.youtube.com/watch?v=6sK1JfbENUs#at=484.

Foss, S. K., and C. L. Griffin. (1995). Beyond persuasion: A proposal for an invitational rhetoric. *Communication Monographs, 62,* 2–18.

Foundation for a Drug Free World. (2014). The truth about prescription drug abuse. Retrieved from http://www.drugfreeworld.org/drugfacts/prescription-drugs.html.

"4 celebrities die in one week: Michael Jackson, Farrah Fawcett, Billy Mays, and Ed McMahon." (2009, June 28). Retrieved from http://www.humblelibertarian.com/2009/06/4-celebrities-die-in-one-week-michael.html.

Fox, M. J. (2002). *Lucky man: A memoir.* New York: Hyperion.

FoxNews.com. (2014). Celebrities with thyroid disorders. *Fox News.* Retrieved from http://www.foxnews.com/slideshow/health/2011/01/25/celebrities-thyroid-disorders/#slide=10.

Frank, A. W. (2010) *Letting stories breathe: A socio-narratology.* Chicago: University of Chicago Press.

Freydkin, D. (2005, June 8). The two sides of Angelina Jolie. *USA Today.* Retrieved from http://usatoday30.usatoday.com/life/people/2005-06-07-angelina-jolie_x.htm?csp=34.

Fulton, E., with D. Atholl, and M. Cherkinian. (1995). *As my world still turns: The uncensored memoirs of American's soap opera queen.* New York: Birch Lane Press.

Furlong, M. (2011, August 19). The top 10 biggest Kardashian family TMI moments on tv. Retrieved from http://www.aoltv.com/2011/08/19/biggest-kardashian-family-tmi-moments.

Garfinkel, H. (1967). *Studies in ethnomethodology.* New York: Prentice-Hall.

Gauntlett, D. (2011). *Making is connecting: The social meaning of creativity, from DIY and knitting to YouTube and Web 2.0.* Cambridge, England: Polity.

Geddie, B., and B. Walters. (Executive producers) (2014). Barbara Walters: Her Story. *Barbara Walters Special.* ABC Broadcasting.

"General information." (n.d.). National Eating Disorders Association. Retrieved from http://www.nationaleatingdisorders.org/general-information.

Gennis, S. (2013, May 10). The Young and the Restless plans tribute to Jeanne Cooper. *TV Guide.* Retrieved from http://www.tvguide.com/news/young-restless-jeanne-cooper-tribute-1065318.aspx.

Gergen, K. (1991). *The saturated self: Dilemmas of identity in contemporary life.* New York: Basic Books.

Gergen, K. (1994). *Realities and relationships: Soundings in social construction.* Cambridge, MA: Harvard University Press.

Gerosa, M. (1999, November). In sickness. *Ladies' Home Journal, 116*(11), 182, 238–240.

Gesser-Edelsburg, A., and R. Endevelt. (2011). An entertainment-education study of stereotypes and prejudice against fat women: An evaluation of *Fat Pig. Health Education Journal, 70*(4), 374–382. doi: 10.1177/0017896911414043.

Gibbs, J. T., and D. Fuery. (1994). Mental health and well-being of black women: Toward strategies of empowerment. *American Journal of Community Psychology, 22,* 559–82.

Gicas, P. (2012, December 7). Catherine Zeta-Jones "sick of talking about" bipolar disorder. *E! Entertainment Television.* Retrieved from http://www.eonline.com.

"Giuliana Rancic talks breast cancer recovery in 'Michigan Avenue.'" (2012, January 15). *Huffington Post.* Retrieved from http://www.huffingtonpost.com/2012/01/15/giuliana-rancic-breast-cancer-recovery_n_1207389.html.

Goffman, E. (1959). *The presentation of self in everyday life.* Garden City, NY: Doubleday Anchor Books.

Goffman, E. (1963). *Stigma: Notes on the management of spoiled identity.* Englewood Cliffs, NJ: Prentice-Hall.

Goffman, E. (1967). *Interaction ritual.* New York: Pantheon Books.

Goffman, E. (1976). *Gender advertisements.* New York: Harper & Row.

Goldberg, D. (2013). Mild traumatic brain injury, the National Football League, and the manufacture of doubt: An ethical, legal, and historical analysis. *The Journal of Legal Medicine, 34,* 157–191.

Goncalves, K. (2013). "Cooking lunch, that's Swiss": Constructing hybrid identities based on socio-cultural practices. *Multilingua, 32,* 527–547. doi: 10.1515/multi-2013-0026.

Goodman, D. (2009, June 26). Michael Jackson overshadows Farrah Fawcett on a sad day. Reuters. Retrieved from http://blogs.reuters.com/fanfare/2009/06/26/michael-jackson-overshadows-farrah-fawcett-on-a-sad-day/.

Good Morning America. (2009, March 31). America's sweetheart returns. ABC News. Retrieved from http://abcnews.go.com/GMA/video?id=7216347.

Good Morning America. (2012, December 7). Zeta-Jones "Never wanted to be the poster child" for bi-polar. ABC News. Retrieved from http://abcnews.go.com/GMA/video/catherine-zeta-jones-bipolar-wanted-poster-child-gma–17902860.

Gorgan, E. (2012, November 14). Keira Knightley talks anorexia, having a cleavage no one wants to see. Softpedia. Retrieved from http://news.softpedia.com/news/Keira-Knightley-Talks-Anorexia-Having-a-Cleavage-No-One-Wants-to-See-306959.shtml.

Gossipcop. (2012, December 7). Catherine Zeta-Jones gets annoyed on GMA: I'm "sick" of bipolar disorder talk. Retrieved from http://www.gossipcop.com.

Grabe, S., L. Ward, and J. Hyde. (2008). The role of the media in body image concerns among women: A meta-analysis of experimental and correlational studies. Psychological Bulletin, 134, 460–476. doi:10.1037/0033–2909.134.3.460.

Gray, J., C. Sandvoss, and C. L. Harrington (Eds.). (2007). Fandom: Identities and communities in a mediated world. New York, NY: New York University Press.

Green, M. C., and T. C. Brock. (2000). The role of transportation in the persuasiveness of public narratives. Journal of Personality and Social Psychology, 79, 700–721. doi: 10.1037//0022–3514.79.5.701.

Gring-Pemble, L. M. (2001). "Are we going to now govern by anecdote?": Rhetorical constructions of welfare recipients in Congressional hearings, debates, and legislation, 1992–1996. Quarterly Journal of Speech, 87(4), 341–365.

Groesz, L. M., M. P. Levine, and S. K. Murnen. (2002). The effect of experimental presentation of thin media images on body satisfaction: A meta-analytic review. International Journal of Eating Disorders, 31(1), 1–16.

Grogan, S. (1999). Body image: Understanding body dissatisfaction in men, women and children. London: Routledge.

"Guiding Light star talks about her weight loss surgery." (2008, September 30). Huffington Post. Retrieved from http://www.huffingtonpost.com2008/09/30/guiding-light-star-talks_n_130479.html.

"Guiding Light star weighs in on weight-loss story" (2008, May 28). TV Guide. Retrieved from http://www.tvguide.com/soaps/guiding-light-star-10094.aspx.

Guttman, N. (1997). Ethical dilemmas in health campaigns. Health Communication, 9, 155–190.

Guttman, N. (2000). Public health communication interventions: Values and ethical dilemmas. Thousand Oaks, CA: Sage.

Hadhazy, A. (2011, November 7). How Has Magic Johnson Survived 20 Years with HIV? Retrieved from http://www.livescience.com/16909-magic-johnson-hiv-aids-anniversary.html.

Hamilton, S. (1997, September 8). Fighting heart. People, pp. 99–107.

Hamm, L. (2012, July 9). Paula Deen: "It's not easy to lose weight!" People, 78(2), 46–51.

Hamm, L., A. Chiu, A. Fogle, K. Mascia, and H. Prabhakar. (2012, January 30). Paula Deen's diabetes diagnosis: One meal at a time. People, 77(4), 73–75.

Haroldson, T. (2013, June 21). Vicksburg youth selected to attend type 1 diabetes conference in Washington D. C. MLive. Retrieved from http://www.mlive.com/news/kalamazoo/index.ssf/2013/06/vicksburg_youth_selected_to_at.html.

Harrington, C. L., and D. Bielby. (1995). Soap fans: Pursuing pleasures and making meaning in everyday life. Philadelphia, PA: Temple University Press.

Harris, J. (2009). Television viewing and unhealthy diet: Implications for children and media intervention. Health Communication, 24, 660–673.

Harris, J. (2013). Sport, celebrity, and the meaning of style. In P. Pedersen (Ed.), Routledge handbook of sport communication (pp. 388–397). London: Routledge.

Harrison, K. (2000). The body electric: Thin-ideal media and eating disorders in adolescents. Journal of Communication, 50(3), 119–143.

Hart, B., P. Sainsbury, and S. Short. (1998). Whose dying? A sociological critique of the "good death." Mortality, 3, 65–77. doi:10.1080/713685884.

Harter, L. M. (2009). Narratives as dialogic, contested, and aesthetic performances. Journal of Applied Communication Research, 37, 140–150. doi: 10.1080/00909880902792255.

Harter, L. M. (2013). The work of art. Qualitative Communication Research, 2, 1–11.

Harter, L. M., and A. P. Bochner. (2009). Healing through stories: A special issue on narrative medicine. Journal of Applied Communication Research, 37, 113–117.

Harter, L. M., P. M. Japp, and C. S. Beck (Eds.). (2005). Narratives, health, and healing: Communication theory, research, and practice. Mahwah, NJ: Erlbaum.

Harter, L. M., and W. K. Rawlins. (2011). The worlding of possibilities in a collaborative art studio: Organizing embodied differences with aesthetic and dialogic sensibilities. In D. K. Mumby (Ed.), *Reframing difference in organizational studies: Research, pedagogy, practice* (pp. 267–289). Thousand Oaks, CA: Sage.

Harter, L. M., J. A. Scott, D. R. Novak, M. Leeman, and J. F. Morris. (2006). Freedom through flight: Performing a counter-narrative of disability. *Journal of Applied Communication Research, 34,* 3–29. doi: 10.1080/00909880500 420192.

Hartmann, T., and C. Goldhoorn. (2011). Horton and Wohl revisited: Exploring viewers' experience of parasocial interaction. *Journal of Communication, 61,* 1,104–1,121. doi: 10.1111/j.1460–2466.2011.01595.x.

Hass, N. (2012, December). No time for secrets. *InStyle, 19*(13), 431–441.

Hastings, J. (2009, January). The truth about the thyroid: Sometimes you can blame your weight on your glands. *O, The Oprah Magazine.* Retrieved from http://www.oprah.com/health/The-Truth-About-the-Thyroid-and-Weight-Gain.

Hater, H. (2013, September 20). Robin Roberts celebrates one year anniversary of bone marrow transplant. *The Hollywood Gossip.* Retrieved from http://www.thehollywoodgossip.com/2013/09/robin-roberts-celebrates-one-year-anniversary-of-bone-marrow-tra/.

Hayes, B., and S. Seaforth Hayes. (2005). *Like sands through the hourglass.* New York: New American Library.

Haythorn, R. (2013, Oct 19). Peyton Manning walks the talk at his namesake children's hospital. Retrieved from http://www.theindychannel.com/news/local-news/peyton-manning-walks-the-talk-at-his-namesake-childrens-hospital.

Hayward, J. (1997). *Consuming pleasures: Active audiences and serial fictions from Dickens to soap opera.* Lexington: University of Kentucky Press.

Health Media Ventures. (2014). Bipolar celebrities: Does it make them more creative? Retrieved from http://www.health.com.

Heffernan, V. (2008, May 25). The medium: Narrow minded. *New York Times.*

Henderson, N. (2013, November 10–16). Facing a new opponent. *American Profile,* pp. 4–8.

Herrman, A. R., and K. E. Tenzek. (2011, November). *Gender differences in peer influence on body image dissatisfaction: A meta-analytic review.* Presented at the annual meeting of the National Communication Association, New Orleans, LA.

Herrman, A. R., and K. E. Tenzek. (2014, April). *Expressions of uncertainty: An examination of a pro-ana website.* Presented at the annual

meeting of the Central States Communication Association, Minneapolis, MN.

Herzog, B. (2013, June 18). Gunnar Esiason is winning at the game of life. *Newsday.* Retrieved from http://www.newsday.com/sports/columnists/bob-herzog/gunnar-esiason-is-winning-at-the-game-of-life-1.5516776.

Hewitt, B., L. Wright, L. Stambler, R. Jones, and A. Brooks. (1994, November 21). Into the twilight. *People, 42*(21), 60–63.

High, A. C., A. Oeldorf-Hirsch, and S. Bellur. (2014). Misery rarely gets company: The influence of emotional bandwidth on supportive communication on Facebook. *Computers in Human Behavior, 34,* 79–88. doi.org/10.1016/j.chb.2014.01.037.

Hilden, H., and M. Honkasalo. (2006). Unethical bunglers or humane professionals? Discussions in the media of end-of-life treatment decisions. *Communication & Medicine 3*(2),125–134 doi 10.1515/CAM.2006.

Hills, M. (2002). *Fan cultures.* New York: Routledge.

Hilton, S., and K. Hunt. (2010). Coverage of Jade Goody's cervical cancer in UK newspapers: A missed opportunity for health promotion? *BMC Public Health, 10,* 368–376.

Hingley, A. T. (1995, November/December). Mary Tyler Moore: After all. *Saturday Evening Post, 267,* 38.

Hinsey, C. (2011). *Afternoon delight: Why soaps still matter.* Santa Monica, CA: 4th Street Media.

Hobson, D. (2003). *Soap opera.* Cambridge, England: Polity.

Holland, P. G. (2013). The most dangerous woman in America: Paula Deen's ethical issues. *Journal of the International Academy for Case Studies, 19,* 79–83.

Holland, S., and D. Novak. (2013). "Food changed my life": The Chef Jeff project and the politics of rehabilitative cooking. *Critical Studies in Media Communication, 30,* 34–51. doi: 10.1080/15295036.2012.693939.

Hollander, D. (1993). Publicity about Magic Johnson may have led some to reduce their risky behavior, request HIV testing. *Family Planning Perspectives, 25,* 192–196.

"Hollywood icon Rock Hudson dies of AIDS." (1985, October 2). Retrieved from http://www.history.com/this-day-in-history/hollywood-icon-rock-hudson-dies-of-aids.

Holmstrom, A. J. (2004). The effects of the media on body image: A meta-analysis. *Journal of Broadcasting & Electronic Media, 48,* 196–217.

Horner, A., and A. Keane (Eds.). (2000). *Body matters: Feminism, textuality, corporeality.* Manchester, England: Manchester University Press.

Houck, D. W. (2006). Sporting bodies. In A. A. Raney and J. Bryant (Eds.), *Handbook of* sports and media (pp. 543–558). Mahwah, NJ: Erlbaum.

Houston, T., A. Cherrington, H. Coley, K. Robinson, J. Trobaugh, J. Williams, et al. (2011). The art and science of patient story-telling: Harnessing narrative communication for behavioral interventions: The ACCE project. *Journal of Health Communication, 16,* 686–698. doi: 10.1080/10810730.2011.551997.

Howard, J. (1996, May 16). The Carew nobody knew. *Sports Illustrated, 84,* 76.

Howard, J. V. (2012, November 27). V's voice: Where were you? From Jamie. Jimmy V. Foundation. Retrieved from http://www.jimmyv.org/2012/11/where-were-you/.

Howard, J. V. (2013, May 16). About us: Jim Valvano 1946–1993. Jimmy V. Foundation. Retrieved from http://www.jimmyv.org/about-us/remembering-jim/jim-valvano-1946–1993/

HSN. (2012, October 12). Exclusive interview: Giuliana Rancic talks about her struggles with breast cancer and pregnancy. Retrieved from https://www.youtube.com/watch?v=nim2KAgf8sQ.

Huffington, A. (2014, August 18). Robin Williams, connectedness and the need to end the stigma around mental illness. Retrieved from: http://www.huffingtonpost.com/arianna-huffington/robin-williams-mental-illness_b_56884.

Huffpost Celebrity. (2012, December 12). Catherine Zeta-Jones' bipolar disorder: Actress talks mental health. *Huffington Post.* Retrieved from http://www.huffingtonpost.com.

Hugenberg, L. W., P. M. Haridakis, and A. C. Earnheardt (Eds.). (2008). *Sports mania: Essays on fandom and the media in the 21st century.* Jefferson, NC: McFarland.

Hundley, H. L., and A. C. Billings (Eds.). (2010). *Examining identity in sports media.* Thousand Oaks, CA: Sage.

Hutchins, B., and D. Rowe. (2012). *Sport beyond television: The Internet, digital media and the rise of networked media sport.* New York: Routledge.

Ibroscheva, E. (2013). Selling the post-communist female body: Portrayals of women and gender in Bulgarian advertising. *Feminist Media Studies, 13*(3), 443–462. doi: 10.1080/14680777.2012.708515.

IMDB. (2014a). Brooke Burke-Charvet. Retrieved from http://www.imdb.com/name/nm1036361/?ref_=nv_sr_1.

IMDB. (2014b). *Catherine Zeta-Jones.* Retrieved from http://www.imdb.com/name/nm0001876/.

IMDB. (2014c). Giuliana & Bill. Retrieved from http://www.imdb.com/title/tt1484626/?ref_=tt_ov_inf.

IMDB. (2014d). Heath Ledger. Retrieved from http://www.imdb.com/name/nm0005132/?ref_=nv_sr_1.

IMDB. (2014e). Keira Knightley. Retrieved from http://www.imdb.com/name/nm0461136/?ref_=nv_sr_1.

IMDB. (2014f). *Mary Tyler Moore: Biography.* Retrieved from http://www.imdb.com/name/nm0001546/bio.

IMDB. (2014g). Michael Jackson. Retrieved from http://www.imdb.com/name/nm0001391/?ref_=fn_al_nm_1.

IMDB. (2014h). Philip Seymour Hoffman. Retrieved from http://www.imdb.com/name/nm0000450/?ref_=fn_al_nm_1.

IMDB. (2014i). Philip Seymour Hoffman. *Biography, Trivia.* Retrieved from http://www.imdb.com/name/nm0000450/bio?ref_=nm_ov_bio_sm.

IMDB. (2014j). Whitney Houston. Retrieved from http://www.imdb.com/name/nm0001365/?ref_=fn_al_nm_1.

InnerBody.com. (2013). InnerBody: Thyroid gland. Retrieved from http://www.innerbody.com/image_dige01/endo04.html#full-description.

International Bipolar Foundation. (2014). Causes of bipolar disorder. Retrieved from http://ibpf.org/.

Jackson, N. (2013). *Slow getting up: A story of NFL survival from the bottom of the pile.* New York: HarperCollins.

James, W. (1981). *Pragmatism.* Indianapolis, IN: Hackett.

JDRF. (2001, June 19). *200 children with diabetes from across America head to D. C. for Children's Congress 2001.* Retrieved from http://islet.org/forum021/messages/18580.htm.

JDRF. (2003, June 21). *200 children with diabetes from across America arrive in Washington, D. C., for Children's Congress 2003* [Press release]. Retrieved from http://www.thefreelibrary.com/200+Children+with+Diabetes+from+Across+America+Arrive+in+Washington...-a0103892443.

JDRF. (2005, June 20). *Three Georgians head to Washington, D. C., as Georgia delegate for Children's Congress 2005* [Press release]. Retrieved from http://www.prnewswire.com/news-releases/three-georgians-head-to-washington-dc-as-georgia-delegate-for-childrens-congress-2005-54735582.html.

JDRF. (2009, June 22). *150 children, celebrities with type 1 diabetes converge on Capitol Hill for JDRF's Children's Congress 2009: Kid delegates meet elected officials, testify at Senate hearing, and urge legislators to request fund research* [Press release]. Retrieved from http://jdrf.org/press-releases/150-nbsp-children-celebrities-with-type-1-diabetes-converge-on-capitol-hill-for-jdrf-s-children-s-congress-2009/.

JDRF. (2011, June 13). *JDRF announces celebrity advocates and town hall panelists for Children's*

Congress 2011 [Press release]. Retrieved from http://jdrf.org/press-releases/jdrf-announces-celebrity-advocates-and-town-hall-panelists-for-children-s-congress-2011/.

JDRF. (2013, April 30). *Children's Congress 2013 welcome message from Mary Tyler Moore, JDRF International Chairman* [Blog]. Retrieved from http://cc.jdrf.org/2013/04/30/childrens-congress-2013-welcome-message-from-mary-tyler-moore-jdrf-international-chairman/.

JDRF. (2013, September 25). *JDRF honors researchers whose insights on early Type 1 Diabetes development have set the stage for disease prevention in children* [Press release]. *PR Newswire.*

JDRF. (2013). *Our special friends.* Retrieved from http://cc.jdrf.org/our-special-friends/.

JDRF. (2014a). *About JDRF Children's Congress.* Retrieved from http://cc.jdrf.org/about-jdrf-childrens-congress/.

JDRF. (2014b). *California, CC 2013: Austin.* Retrieved from http://cc.jdrf.org/delegates/austin/.

JDRF. (2014c). *Children's Congress.* Retrieved from http://advocacy.jdrf.org/our-programs/childrens-congress/.

JDRF. (2014d). *JDRF announces delegates for its 2013 Children's Congress* [Press release]. Retrieved from http://jdrf.org/press-releases/jdrf-announces-delegates-for-its-2013-childrens-congress/.

JDRF. (2014e) *Ohio, CC 2013: Avery.* Retrieved from http://cc.jdrf.org/delegates/avery-2/.

JDRF. (2014f). *Michigan, CC 2013: Andrew.* Retrieved from http://cc.jdrf.org/delegates/andrew-2/.

JDRF. (2014g). *Michigan, CC 2013: Tristin.* Retrieved from http://cc.jdrf.org/delegates/tristin/.

JDRF. (2014h). *Research Funding Facts.* Retrieved from https://jdrf.org/about-jdrf/fact-sheets/research-funding-facts/.

Jenkins, H. (2006). *Convergence culture: Where old and new media collide.* New York: New York University Press.

Jenkins, H., S. Ford, and J. Green (2013). *Spreadable media: Creating value and meaning in a networked culture.* New York: New York University Press.

Jenkins, S. (2012, June). Well done, coach. *Athlon Sports,* pp. 8–9.

Jensen, R. E. (2005). The eating disordered lifestyle: Imagetexts and the performance of similitude. *Argumentation & Advocacy, 42,* 1–18.

Jessen, M. (2007, May 2). Keira Knightley "devastated" by anorexia rumors. *People.* Retrieved from http://www.people.com/people/article/0,,20037486,00.html.

Jin, S. (2013). Peeling back the multiple layers of

Twitter's private disclosure onion: The roles of virtual identity discrepancy and personality traits in communication privacy management on Twitter. *New Media & Society, 15,* 813–833. doi:10.1177/1461444812471814.

Johnson, C. (2012, December 7). Bipolar Catherine Zeta-Jones insists she is "not a victim" and is "sick" of talking about mental condition. *Dailymail.* Retrieved from http://www.dailymail.co.uk.

Johnson, E. (2013, April 20). Carrie Fisher talks about mental illness and career. *Herald Tribune.* Retrieved from http://health.heraldtribute.com/2013/04/20/14065.

Johnson, Z. (2012, November 13). Keira Knightley poses topless, addresses anorexia rumors. *Us Weekly.* Retrieved from http://www.usmagazine.com/celebrity-body/news/keira-knightley-poses-.

Jolie, A. (2013, May 14). My medical choice. *New York Times.* Retrieved from http://www.nytimes.com/2013/05/14/opinion/my-medical-choice.html.

Jose-Miller, A. B., J. W. Boyden, and K. A. Frey. (2007). Infertility. *American Academy of Family Medicine,75,* 849–856.

Jury, L. (2007, January 23). Knightley sues "Daily Mail" for suggesting she has anorexia. *The Independent.* Retrieved from http://www.independent.co.uk/news/uk/crime/knightley-sues-daily-mail-for-suggesting-she-has-anorexia-433320.html.

Kackman, M., M. Binfield, M. Payne, A. Perlman, and B. Sebok (Eds.). (2011). *Flow TV: Television in the age of media convergence.* New York: Routledge.

Kalb, C., P. Wingert, and D. Foote. (2000). Stars, money, and medical crusades. *Newsweek, 135* (21), 58–61. Retrieved from http://web.ebscohost.com/ehost/detail?vid=4&hid=105&sid=cfe2a1fb-aa8a-462b-ba67-90...

Kaldhusdal, T., and M. Bernhagen. (2011). *Consider the conversation, a documentary on a taboo subject.* Jefferson, WI: Burning Hay Wagon Productions.

Kalichman, S., and T. Hunter. (1992). The disclosure of celebrity HIV infection: Its effect on public attitudes. *American Journal of Public Health, 82,* 1,374–1,376.

Kassing, J. W. (2013). For the cure, the kids, and the cause: Practicing advocacy through communication and sport. In P. Pedersen (Ed.), *Routledge handbook of sport communication* (pp. 431–440). London: Routledge.

Kassing, J. W., and J. Sanderson. (2009). "You're the kind of guy that we all want for a drinking buddy": Expressions of parasocial interaction on Floydlandis.com. *Western Journal of Communication, 73,* 182–203. doi: 10.1080/10570310902856063.

Kaufman, D. (2012, December 10). Catherine

Zeta-Jones, please don't stop talking about bipolar disorder! *iVillage*. Retrieved from http://www.ivillage.com.

Keeley, M., and J. Koenig Kellas. (2005). Constructing life and death through final conversation narratives. In L. M. Harter, P. M. Japp, and C. S. Beck (Eds.) *Narratives, health, and healing: Communication theory, research, and practice* (pp. 365–390). Mahwah, NJ: Erlbaum.

"Keira Knightley disappointed by weight accusations and 'droopy' boobs." (2012, November 13). *Inquisitr*. Retrieved from http://www.inquisitr.com/397746/keira-knightley-dis appointed-by-weight-accusations-and-droopy-boobs/.

"Keira Knightley wins anorexia libel claim against British tabloid." (2007, May 25). *Fox-News*. Retrieved from http://www.foxnews.com/story/2007/05/25/keira-knightley-wins-anorexia-libel-claim-against-british-tabloid/.

"Keira Knightley wins damages over weight slur." (2007, May 24). *Reuters*. Retrieved from http://www.reuters.com/article/2007/05/24/us-britain-knightley-idUSL2437024920070524.

Kennedy, M., V. Beck, and V. Freimuth. (2008). Entertainment education and HIV prevention. In T. Edgar, S. Noar, and V. Freimuth (Eds.), *Communication perspectives on HIV/AIDS for the 21st century* (pp. 253–276). New York: Erlbaum.

Kennedy, M., A. O'Leary, V. Beck, K. Pollard, and P. Simpson. (2004). Increases in calls to the CDC National STD and AIDS Hotline following AIDS-related episodes in a soap opera. *Journal of Communication, 54*, 287–301.

Kermode, F. (1966/2000). *The sense of an ending: Studies in the theory of fiction*. New York: Oxford University Press.

Kerr, Z. Y., S. W. Marshall, H. P. Harding Jr., and K. M. Guskiewicz. (2012). Nine-year risk of depression diagnosis increases with increasing self-reported concussions in retired professional football players. *The American Journal of Sports Medicine, 40*, 2,206–2,212.

Kim, H. S., C. A. Bigman, A. E. Leader, C. Lerman, and J. N. Cappella. (2012). Narrative health communication and behavior change: The influence of exemplars in the news on intention to quit smoking. *Journal of Communication, 62*, 473–492. doi: 10.1111.j.1460–2466.2012.01644.x.

"Kim Kardashian shows off her heart shaped psoriasis." (2011, August 15). *The Huffington Post*. Retrieved from http://www.huffingtonpost.com/2011/08/15/kim-kardashian-shows-off-heart-shaped-psoriasis_n_927408.html?#s330417title=Kim_Kardashian_

King, P. (2010, November 1). Concussions: The hits that are changing football. *Sports Illustrated, 11* (3), 34–40.

Kirkova, D. (2013, July 21). "I look back and I can't believe the strength he had": Catherine Zeta Jones opens up about her husband's battle with cancer, and her own wrestle with bipolar disorder. *Dailymail*. Retrieved from http://www.dailymail.co.uk/femail/article-2372304/Catherine-Zeta-Jones-bipolar-disorder-husband-Michael-Douglas-cancer-battle.html.

Kisken, T. (2012, January 21). Deep-fried butter lathers debate over Paula Deen's diabetes. *Venture County Star*. Retrieved from http://www.vcstar.com.

Klein, B. (2011). Entertaining ideas: Social issues in entertainment television. *Media, Culture, & Society, 33*, 905–921. doi: 10/1177/01634437 11411008.

Klein, B. (2012). Entertainment-education for the media saturated: Audience perspectives on social issues in entertainment programming. *European Journal of Cultural Studies, 16*, 43–57. doi: 10.1177/1367549412457482.

"Knightley talks breasts, anorexic rumors and marriage." (2012, November 13). *FoxNews*. Retrieved from http://www.foxnews.com/enter tainment/2012/11/13/keira-knightley-talks-breasts-anorexic-rumors-and-marriage/.

"Knightley wins over weight slur." (2007, May 24). *The Sydney Morning Herald*. Retrieved from http://www.smh.com.au/news/people/knightley-wins-over-weight-slur/2007/05/25/1179601642401.html.

Knobloch-Westerwick, S., and J. Crane. (2012). A losing battle: effects of prolonged exposure to thin-ideal images on dieting and body satisfaction. *Communication Research, 39*(1), 79–102. doi: 10.1177/0093650211400596.

Kontos, P., and W. Martin. (2013). Embodiment and dementia: Exploring critical narratives of selfhood, surveillance, and dementia care. *Dementia, 12*, 288–302. doi: 10.1177/1413012 13479787.

Kreis, A. (2013, May 16). "V's voice" (2013). Jimmy V. Foundation. Retrieved from http://www.jimmyv.org/2013/05/where-we-started-where-we-are-and-where-we-want-to-b…

Kroll, D. J. (2007, October 28). Colleen Zenk Pinter diagnosed with oral cancer. Retrieved from http://soapcentral.com/atwt/new/2007/1029-zenkpinter.php.

"The Krispy Kreme Burger." (2008, June 9). *New York Times*. Retrieved from http://laughlines.blogs.nytimes.com/2008/06/09/the-krispy-kreme-burger/?_php=true&_type=blogs&_r=0.

Kruger, J., A. Park, K. Pickert, S. Schrobsdorff, A. Sifferlin, and L. Rothman. (2013, May 27). The Angelina effect. *Time, 181*, 28–34.

Kubic, K. N., and R. M. Chory. (2007). Exposure to television makeover programs and perceptions of self. *Communication Research Reports, 24*, 283–291.

Lalvani, P. (2011). Constructing the (m)other: Dominant and contested narratives on mothering a child with Down syndrome. *Narrative Inquiry, 21,* 276–293. doi: 10.1075/ni.21.2.06lal.

Lane, R., A. N. Miller, C. Brown, and N. Vilar. (2013). An examination of the narrative persuasion with epilogue through the lens of the Elaboration Likelihood Model. *Communication Quarterly, 61,* 431–445. doi: 10.1080/01463 373.2013.799510.

Lang, S. (1997, September 1). Utter dismay. *People.* Retrieved from http://www.people.com/people/article/0,,20123055,00.html.

Larkey, L., and M. Hecht. (2010). A model of effects of narrative as culture-centric health promotion. *Journal of Health Communication, 15,* 114–135. doi: 10.1080/10810730903528017.

Lately, C. (2010, January 11). Chelsea Lately: Giuliana and Bill Rancic. Retrieved from http://www.eonline.com/videos/167250/chelsea-lately-giuliana-and-bill-rancic.

Ledger-Enquirer. (2012, January 17). *Paula Deen confirms that she has type 2 diabetes.* Retrieved from http://www.ledger-enquirer.com/2012/01/17/1896487_paula-deen-confirms-that-she-has.html.

"Ledger's death caused by accidental overdose." (2008, February 6). Retrieved from http://wwww.cnn.com/2008/SHOWBIZ/Movies/02/06/heath.ledger/index.html?_s=PM%253 Cimg%2520class=.

Lee, A. (2012, January 17). Paula Deen launches "Diabetes in a New Light" online program. *Reality TV Magazine.* Retrieved from http://realitytvmagazine.sheknows.com/2012/01/17/paula-deen-launches-diabetes-in-a-new-light-online-program/.

Lee, E. (2014, April 16). Catherine Zeta-Jones and Michael Douglas walk first red carpet together since separating in August 2013. *US Magazine.* Retrieved from http://www.usmag azine.com/celebrity-news/news/catherine-zeta-jones-michael-douglas-reunite-on-first-red-carpet-2014164.

Lee, E., and J. Jang. (2013). Not so imaginary interpersonal contact with public figures on social network sites: How affiliative tendency moderates its effects. *Communication Research, 40,* 27–51. doi: 10.1177/0093650211431579.

Lee, J. K., M. L. Hecht, M. Miller-Day, and E. Elek. (2011). Evaluating mediated perception of narrative health messages: The perception of Narrative Performance Scale. *Communication Methods and Measures, 5,* 126–145. doi: 10.1080/19312458.2011.568374.

Leerhsen, C., D. Foote, J. Gordon, E. Yoffe, F. Washington, V. Smith, et al. (1991, November 18). Magic's message. *Newsweek, 118,* 58–62.

Le Miere, J. (2012, February 24). Paula Deen to cut the fat: Food Network star to serve lighter dishes after diabetes diagnosis. *International Business Times.* Retrieved from http://www.ibtimes.com/paula-deen-cut-fat-food-network-star-serve-lighter-dishes-after-diabetes-diagnosis-415950.

Lerner, B. H. (2006). *When illness goes public: Celebrity patients and how we look at medicine.* Baltimore, MD: Johns Hopkins Press.

"Letters." (1993, October 11). *Sports Illustrated,* p. 8.

Levitt, S., and J. Wagner. (1994, January 31). Weight & see. *People, 41*(4), 50–54.

Lewis-Boothman, D., and D. Shira. (2011, June 23). Missy Elliott: My battle with Graves' disease. *People.* Retrieved from http://www.people.com/people/article/0,,20505206,00.html.

Lichtenfeld, J. L. (2007, July 31). Robin Roberts: The journey begins. *American Cancer Society, Incorporated.* Retrieved from http://www.cancer.org/aboutus/drlensblog/post/2007/07/31/robin-roberts-the-journey-begins.aspx.

Lin, J. C. (2014, February 3). Celebrities react to Philip Seymour Hoffman's death on Twitter. *Time.* Retrieved from http://time.com/3789/celebrities-react-to-philip-seymour-hoffmans-death-on-twitter/.

Lindlof, T., and B. Taylor. (2011). *Qualitative communication research methods* (3rd ed.). Los Angeles: Sage.

Link, B. G., and J. C. Phelan. (2006). Stigma and its public health implications. *Lancet, 367* (9509), 528–529. doi: 10.1016/S0140–6736(06) 68184–1.

Lipp, A. (2011). Stigma in abortion care: Application to a grounded theory study. *Contemporary Nurse: A Journal for the Australian Nursing Profession, 37*(2), 115–123.

Lipton, M., and C. Wang. (1998, June 1). A life to live. *People, 49*(21), 83–86.

Lipton, M., and C. Wang. (1998, December 21). One life to give. *People, 50*(23), 71–72.

Littwin, S. (1998, December). Olivia Newton-John's personal miracle. *McCall's, 126,* 53–54.

Lo, C. C., A. N. Monge, R. J. Howell, and T. C. Cheng. (2013). The role of mental illness in alcohol abuse and prescription drug misuse: Gender-specific analysis of college students. *Journal of Psychoactive Drugs, 45*(1), 39–47. doi:10.1080/02791072.2013.763561.

Lobel, B. (2010). Playing more than the cancer card. *Performance Research, 15*(2), 29–33. doi: 10.1080/13528165.2010.490426.

Lopez-Guimera, G., M. P. Levine, D. Sanchez-Carracedo, and J. Fauquet. (2010). Influence of mass media on body image and eating disordered attitudes and behaviors in females: A review of effects and processes. *Media Psychology, 13*(4), 387–416. doi:10.1080/15213269.2010.525737.

Louganis, G. (1995, March 6). Book bonus. *People,* 66–74.

Luafik, M. (2012, April 5). Celebrity weight loss: Did these stars get too thin? *Shape*. Retrieved from http://www.shape.com/celebrities/celebrity-photos/celebrity-weight-loss-did-these-stars-get-too-thin.

Lucci, S. (2011). *All my life: A memoir*. New York: HarperCollins.

Luo, W. (2012). Selling cosmetic surgery and beauty ideals: The female body in the web sites of Chinese hospitals. *Women's Studies in Communication, 35*, 68–95. doi: 10.1080/07491409.2012.667055.

Luscombe, B. (2008, January 22). Heath Ledger: Star in distress. *Time*. Retrieved from http://content.time.com/time/arts/article/0,8599,1705981,00.html.

Macatee, R. (2012, November 14). Catherine Zeta-Jones talks bipolar disorder, wants to "help remove any stigma attached" to mental illness. *E! Entertainment Television*. Retrieved from http://www.eonline.com.

MacMillan, C. (2012, February 5). A diabetes dialogue: Paula Deen's diagnosis has us rethinking habits. *RepublicanAmerican*. Retrieved from http://www.rep-am.com/articles/2012/02/28/lifestyle/health/617873.txt.

"Magazines shape culture at women's, minorities' expense." (2012, Winter). Media Report to Women, 40 (1). Retrieved from www.mediareporttowomen.com.

"The Magnificent Mary." (2000, Summer). Role models [Interview]. *Countdown, 21*, 12.

"Mail." (1997, September 29). *People*, p. 4.

Malkin, M. (2000, March 12). Battles against disease are overpoliticized. Retrieved from http://www.townhall.com/columnists/michellemalkin/mm000312.shtml.

Malkin, M. (2014, January 12). Michael Douglas: Wife Catherine Zeta-Jones won't be with him at Golden Globes today. Retrieved from http://www.eonline.com/news/498270/michael-douglas-wife-catherine-zeta-jones-won-t-be-with-him-at-golden-globes-today.

Mandell, A. (2013, May 15). Pitt proud of Jolie's strength, dedication. *USA Today*, 2A.

Mann, D. (2007, July 31). TV's Robin Roberts has breast cancer: Co-anchor of ABC's *Good Morning America* to undergo surgery. *WebMD News*. Retrieved from http://www.webmd.com/breast-cancer/news/20070731/tvs-robin-roberts-has-breast-cancer.

Marcus, M. B. (2009, March 22). Moore's sunny look on life. *USA Today*. Retrieved from http://www.azcentral.com/thingstodo/movies/articles/2009/03/23/20090323moore0323.html.

"Mariah Carey on Twitter: 'Heartbroken'; Others react." (2012, February 11). Retrieved from http://www.cbsnews.com/news/mariah-carey-on-twitter-heartbroken-others-react/.

Marquina, S. (2014, February 3). Giuliana Rancic talks new E! show "Beyond Candid with Giuliana." Retrieved from http://www.ryanseacrest.com/2014/02/03/giuliana-rancic-talks-new-e-show-beyond-candid-with-giuliana/.

Martin, E. M., and T. S. Horn. (2013). The role of athletic identity and passion in predicting burnout in adolescent female athletes. *The Sport Psychologist, 27*, 338–348.

Marwick, A. E. (2013). *Status update: Celebrity, publicity, and branding in the social media age*. New Haven, CT: Yale University Press.

Matelski, M. (1988). *The soap opera evolution: America's enduring romance with daytime drama*. Jefferson, NC: McFarland.

Matelski, M. (1999). *Soap operas worldwide: Cultural and serial realities*. Jefferson, NC: McFarland.

Matsumoto, N. (1992, August 17). Hope in her heart. *People, 38*(7), 74–78.

Mayer, C. (2007, August 16). Why Diana mattered: How Diana transformed Britain. *Time*. Retrieved from http://www.time.com/time/specials/2007/article/0,28804,1650830_1650834_1653460,00.html.

Mayo Clinic. (2014a). Diseases and conditions: Thyroid cancer. Retrieved from http://www.mayoclinic.org/diseases-conditions/thyroid-cancer/basics/definition/con-20043551.

Mayo Clinic. (2014b). Myelodysplastic syndromes. Mayo Foundation for Medical Education and Research. Retrieved from http://www.mayoclinic.org/diseases-conditions/myelodysplastic-syndromes/basics/treatment/con-20027168.

McCallum, J. (2001, August 20). Life after death. *Sports Illustrated, 95*(7), 72–80.

McLeroy, K. R., N. H. Gottlieb, and J. N. Burdine. (1987). The business of health promotion: Ethical issues and professional responsibilities. *Health Education Quarterly, 14*, 91–109.

MDS Foundation. (2014). What is MDS (i.e. what is Myelodsplastic Syndromes?). The MDS Foundation. Retrieved from http://www.mds-foundation.org/what-is-mds/.

Merriam-Webster.com. (2014). Merriam-Webster: An Encyclopedia Britannica company. Merriam-Webster, Incorporated. Retrieved from http://www.merriam-webster.com/.

Mettenburg, J. (2000, June). The Magnificent Mary. *Cfk magazine*. Retrieved from http://www.jdf.org/kids/cfk/rolemodels/2000/marytylermoore.html.

Meyrowitz, J. (1985). *No sense of place: The impact of electronic media on social behavior*. New York: Oxford University Press.

"Michael Jackson." (2011, November 9). *New York Times*. Retrieved from http://topics.nytimes.com/top/reference/timestopics/people/j/michael_jackson/index.html.

"Michael Jackson dead at 50 after cardiac arrest."

(n.d.). CNN. Retrieved from http://www.cnn.com/2009/SHOWBIZ/Music/06/25/michael.jackson/.

"Michael Jackson Dies." (2009, June 25). Retrieved from http://www.tmz.com/2009/06/25/michael-jackson-dies-death-dead-cardiac-arrest/.

"Michael Zaslow speaks out about his fight against Lou Gehrig's disease." (1998, January 20). Retrieved from http://america.net/~gwp/usmz/z-on-als.html.

Miller, H. G. (2005, November/December). Growing up Mary: By taking control of diabetes, Moore tells how she could make it after all. *Saturday Evening Post, 281*, 12.

Mirkinson, J. (2012, June 11). Robin Roberts MDS; "GMA" co-host announces she has bone marrow disease, will undergo transplant (video). *The Huffington Post*. Retrieved from http://www.huffingtonpost.com/2012/06/11/robin-roberts-mds-bone-marrow_n_1586151.html?view=print&comm_ref=false.

ModernMom.com. (2012, November 8). Brooke Burke Inspires Others to Share Their Cancer Stories. Retrieved from http://www.modernmom.com/08027ac4-3b46-11e3-8407-bc764e04a41e.html.

Moe, P. (2012). Revealing rather than concealing disability: The rhetoric of Parkinson's advocate Michael J. Fox. *Rhetoric Review, 31*, 443–460.

Mohammed, S. (2001). Personal communication networks and the effects of an entertainment-education radio soap opera in Tanzania. *Journal of Health Communication, 6*, 137–154. doi: 1081–0730/01.

Moore, M. T. (1995) *After all.* New York: G. B. Putnam's Sons.

Moore, M. T. (2007, Summer). JDRF's most powerful voices: Children's Congress 2007. *Countdown, 28*, 4.

Moore, M. T. (2009). *Growing up again: Life, loves, and oh yeah, diabetes.* New York: St. Martin's Press.

Morton, R. (Ed.). (1997). *Worlds without end.* New York: Museum of Television & Radio.

Moskin, J. (2012, January 17). Chef has diabetes, and some say "I told you so." *New York Times.* Retrieved from http://www.nytimes.com.

Moyer-Gusé, E., A. Chung, and P. Jain. (2011). Identification with characters and discussion of taboo topics after exposure to an entertainment narrative about sexual health. *Journal of Communication, 61*, 387–406. doi: 10.1111/j.1460-2466.2011.01551.x.

Mumford, L. (1995). *Love and ideology in the afternoon: Soap opera, women, and television genre.* Bloomington: Indiana University Press.

Mumford, L. (1997). Taking issue: Social themes in the soaps. In R. Morton (Ed.), *Worlds without end* (pp. 99–110). New York: Museum of Television & Radio.

Murphy, A. G. (2003). The dialectical gaze exploring the subject-object tension in the performances of women who strip. *Journal of Contemporary Ethnography, 32*, 305–335. doi: 10.1177/0891241603032003003.

Murphy, E. (2012, March 22). Whitney Houston died from drowning believed spurred by heart disease, cocaine. *ABC News.* Retrieved from http://abcnews.go.com/Entertainment/whitney-houston-death-report-drowning-heart-disease-cocaine/story?id=15979609

Murphy, S. T., L. B. Frank, J. S. Chatterjee, and L. Baezconde-Garbanati. (2013). Narrative versus nonnarrative: The role of identification, transportation, and emotion in reducing health disparities. *Journal of Communication, 63*, 116–137. doi: 10.1111/jcom.12007.

Murphy Kelly, S. (2012, February 12). Twitter breaks news of Whitney Houston death 27 minutes before press. *Mashable.* Retrieved from http://mashable.com/2012/02/12/whitney-houston-twitter/.

Nariman, H. N. (1993). *Soap operas for social change: Toward a methodology for entertainment-education television.* Westport, CT: Greenwood Press.

Nash, D. (Producer). (2013, January 17). Paula Deen opens up about her diabetes diagnosis. *Today.* Retrieved from http://www.today.com/video/today/46023389#46023389.

National Breast Cancer Foundation. (2012). About breast cancer. National Breast Cancer Foundation, Incorporated. Retrieved from http://www.nationalbreastcancer.org/about-breast-cancer.

National Institute on Drug Abuse. (2014). DrugFacts: Nationwide trends. Retrieved from http://www.drugabuse.gov/publications/drugfacts/nationwide-trends.

Navasky, M., and K. O'Conner. (2010, November 23). Facing death. [*PBS Frontline*]. Boston: Mead Street Films, LLC.

NBC News. (2009, June 25). Nightly report with Brian Williams: Michael Jackson's death report. Retrieved from https://www.youtube.com/watch?v=Q7TflyqRmco.

Nelson, J. (2014, March 21). Amy Robach finds Robin Roberts an inspiration in her cancer fight. *People.* Retrieved from http://www.people.com/people/article/0,,20799106,00.html.

"NFL and the community." (2014, June 3). Retrieved from http://www.nfl.com/community.

Niederdeppe, J. (2008). Beyond knowledge gaps: Examining socioeconomic differences in response to cancer news. *Human Communication Research, 34*, 423–447. doi: 10.1111/j.1468-2958.2008.00327.x.

Niederdeppe, J., H. K. Kim, H. Lundell, F. Fazili, and B. Frazier. (2012). Beyond counterarguing: Simple elaboration, complex integration, and counterelaboration in response to variations in narrative focus and sidedness. *Journal of Communication, 62*, 758–777. doi: 10.11 11/j.1460–2466.2012.01671.x.

Niemiec, R. M., and S. E. Schulenberg. (2011). Understanding death attitudes: The integration of movies, positive psychology, and meaning management. *Death Studies, 35*, 387–407. doi:10.1080/07481187.2010.544517.

Nocera, J. (2009, January 15). Health isn't a private issue when you're a legend. *New York Times*. Retrieved from www.nytimes.com/2009/01/16/business/16nocera.html?_r=1&.

Nolte, S. (2014, March 4). Missed opportunities: Media, celebrities, and BRCA1 screening. Retrieved from http://www.signalsblog.ca/missed-opportunities-meda-celebrities-and-brca1-screening/.

Norris, M. L., K. M. Boydell, L. Pinhas, and D. K. Katzman. (2006). Ana and the Internet: A review of pro-anorexia websites. *International Journal of Eating Disorders, 39*, 443–447. doi: 10.1002/eat.20305.

O'Connor, I. (2001, November 7). Magic put new spin on living with AIDS. *USA Today*, 13C.

O'Gorman, S. (1998). Death and dying in contemporary society: An evaluation of current attitudes and the rituals associated with death and dying and their relevance to recent understandings of health and healing. *Journal of Advanced Nursing, 27*, 1,127–1,135.

O'Keefe, D. J., and J. D. Jensen. (2008). Do loss-framed persuasive messages engender greater message processing than do gain-framed messages? A meta-analytic review. *Communication Studies, 59*, 51–67. doi: 10.1080/10510 970701849388.

O'Keefe, D. J., and J. D. Jensen. (2009). The relative persuasiveness of gain-framed and loss-framed messages for encouraging disease detection behaviors: A meta-analytic review. *Journal of Communication, 59*, 296–316. doi: 10.1111/j.1460–2466.2009.01417.x.

O'Leary, A., M. Kennedy, K. A. Pappas-Deluca, M. Nkete, V. Beck, and C. Galavotti. (2007). Association between exposure to an HIV storyline in "The Bold and the Beautiful" and HIV-related stigma in Botswana. *AIDS Education and Prevention, 19*, 209–217.

O Malley-Keighran, M. P., and M. Coleman. (2013). "I am not a tragedy. I am full of hope": Communication impairment narratives in newspapers. *International Journal of Language & Communication Disorders, 49*, 174–188. doi: 10.1111/1460–6984.12066.

Ong, J. C. (2014). "Witnessing" or "mediating" distant suffering? Ethical questions across moments of text, production, and reception. *Television & New Media, 15*, 179–196. doi: 10.1177/1527476412454687.

Oprah's Next Chapter. (2012, June 17). The Kardashians [Video file]. Retrieved from http://www.oprah.com/own-oprahs-next-chapter/Oprahs-Next-Chapter-The-Kardashian-Family-Part-1.

Oprah's Next Chapter. (2012, June 24). The Kardashians: Part two [Video file]. Retrieved from http://www.oprah.com/own-oprahs-next-chapter/Oprahs-Next-Chapter-The-Kardashian-Family-Part-2.

"Our story: 'Don't give up ... don't ever give up.'" (2013). Jimmy V. Foundation. Retrieved from http://www.jimmyv.org/about-us/our-story/.

Owen, W. (1984). Interpretive themes in relational communication. *Quarterly Journal of Speech, 70*, 274–287.

Ozerky, J. (2012, January 3). Grease under fire. *Time, 179*(4), 56.

Papacharissi, Z. (Ed.). (2011). *A networked self: Identity, community, and culture on social network sites*. New York: Routledge.

"Paula Deen's Food Network shows: No changes to her TV cooking until at least 2013." *Huffington Post*. Retrieved from http://www.huffingtonpost.com/2012/02/07/paula-deen-diabetes-food-network_n_1260827...

Pederson, J. R. (2013). Disruptions of individual and cultural identities: How online stories of job loss and unemployment shift the American Dream. *Narrative Inquiry, 23*, 302–322. doi: 10.1075/ni.23.2.05ped.

Perry, S. (2007, January 23). Keira Knightley sues over anorexia claims. *People*. Retrieved from http://www.people.com/people/article/0,,20009389,00.html.

Petchauer, E. (2012). *Hip-hop culture in college students' lives: Elements, embodiment, and higher edutainment*. New York: Routledge.

Petronio, S. (1991). Communication boundary management: A theoretical model of managing disclosure of private information between marital couples. *Communication Theory, 1*, 311–335. doi:10.1111/j.1468–2885.1991.tb00023.x.

Petronio, S. (2000). *Balancing the secrets of privacy disclosure*. Mahwah, NJ: Erlbaum.

Petronio, S. (2002). *Boundaries of privacy: Dialectics of disclosure*. New York: State University of New York Press.

Petronio, S. (2004). Road to developing Communication Privacy Management Theory: Narrative in progress, please stand by. *Journal of Family Communication, 3*, 193–207.

Petronio, S. (2007). Translational research endeavors and the practices of communication privacy management. *Journal of Applied Communication Research, 35*, 218–222. doi: 10.1080/00909880701422443.

Petronio, S. (2010). Communication privacy management theory: What do we know about family privacy regulation? *Journal of Family*

*Theory & Review, 2,*175–196. doi:10.1111/j.17 56–2589.2010.00052.x.

Petronio, S. (Ed.). (2013). Special issue on Communication Privacy Management Theory and family privacy regulations. *Journal of Family Communication, 13* (1).

Petronio, S., and J. Caughlin. (2006). Communication privacy management: Understanding families. In D. Braithwaite and L. Baxter (Eds.), *Engaging theories in family communication: Multiple perspectives* (pp. 35–49). Thousand Oaks, CA: Sage.

Petronio, S., and S. Kovach. (1997). Managing privacy boundaries: Health providers' perceptions of resident care in Scottish nursing homes. *Journal of Applied Communication Research, 25,* 115–131.

Petronio, S., H. M. Reeder, M. L. Hecht, and T. M. Ros-Mendoza. (1996). Disclosure of sexual abuse by children and adolescents. *Journal of Applied Communication Research, 24,* 181–199.

Petronio, S., and J. Reierson. (2009). Regulating the privacy of confidentiality: Grasping the complexities through communication privacy management theory. In T. Afifi and W. Afifi (Eds.), *Uncertainty, information management, and disclosure decisions* (pp. 365–383). New York: Routledge.

"Philip Seymour Hoffman entered detox for narcotic abuse." (2013, May 31). Retrieved from http://www.tmz.com/2013/05/30/philip-seymour-hoffman-detox-narcotics-heroin-drugs-abuse/.

Phillipov, M. (2013). Resisting health: Extreme food and the culinary abject. *Critical Studies in Media Communication, 30,* 377–390. doi: 10.1080/15295036.2012.755054.

Pisa, K., and S. M. Silverman. (2006, July 4). Keira Knightley dismisses weight criticism. *People.* Retrieved from http://www.people.com/people/article/0,26334,1210070,00.html.

Platt, J. (2013). *2013 Welcome message from the Platts, CC2013 Chair Family* [JDRF blog]. Retrieved from http://cc.jdrf.org/2013/04/29/childrens-congress-2013-welcome-message-from-the-platts-cc2013-chair-family/.

"Prescription drug overdose in the United States: Fact Sheet." (2014). Centers for Disease Prevention and Control. Retrieved from http://www.cdc.gov/homeandrecreational safety/overdose/facts/html.

Press, A. L. (2011). Feminism and media in the post-feminist era: What to make of the "feminist" in feminist media studies. *Feminist Media Studies, 11*(1), 107–113. doi: 10.1080/14680777.2011.537039.

"The Princess and the Pump." (2013, July 8). *Here we go! JDRF's Children's Congress* [Blog]. Retrieved from http://www.theprincessand thepump.com/2013/07/here-we-go-jdrfs-childrens-congress.html.

Prokupecz, S., F. Karimi, N. Turner, and R. Sanchez. (2014, February 5). Source: 4 arrested in connection with drugs in Hoffman's apartment. *CNN.com.* Retrieved from http://www.cnn.com/2014/02/05/show biz/philip-seymour-hoffman-death/CNN's Jason.

Puente, M. (2012, November 13). Catherine Zeta-Jones helps defuse bipolar stigma. *USA Today.* Retrieved from http://www.usatoday.com.

Puente, M., D. Freydkin, and A. Mandell. (2013, May 15). Her mastectomy could change women's lives. *USA Today,* 1–2A.

Radner, G. (1989). *It's always something.* New York: Simon and Schuster.

Ramasubramanian, S., and S. Kornfield. (2012). Japanese anime heroines as role models for U.S. youth: Wishful identification, parasocial interaction, and intercultural entertainment effects. *Journal of International and Intercultural Communication, 5,* 189–207. doi: 10.10 80/17513057.2012.679291.

Randee, D. (2012). *The Today Show*: Giuliana and Bill Rancic: We're having a baby! Retrieved from http://www.greatertalent.com/speaker-news/the-today-show-giuliana-and-bill-rancic-were-having-a-baby/.

Redman, P. (2005). The narrative formation of identity revisited: Narrative construction, agency and the unconscious. *Narrative Inquiry, 15,* 25–44. ISSN: 1387–6740.

Redmon, K. C. (2013, July/August). Soap operas save the world: Melodramas promoting literacy and family planning? Tune in next week. *Pacific Standard,* 26–27.

Reed, L., and P. Saukko (Eds.). (2010). *Governing the female body: Gender, health, and networks of power.* Albany: State University of New York Press.

Reeders, D. (2008). Solutions to stigma. *HIV Australia, 7*(3), 29–49.

Reeve, D. (1999). *Care packages: Letters to Christopher Reeve from strangers and other friends.* New York: Random House.

Reeves, M., and S. Clarke. (2011, April 26). Michael Douglas to Oprah: Wife Catherine Zeta-Jones was "outed" in bipolar struggle. *ABC News.* Retrieved from http://abcnews.go.com/Entertainment/michael-douglas-oprah-catherine-zeta-jones-outed-bipolar/story?id=13456094.

Respers France, L. (2013, July 4). Photos: Celebrity substance abuse confessions. *CNN.com.* Retrieved from http://www.cnn.com/2013/07/04/showbiz/celebrity-news-gossip/substance-abuse-celebs/.

Robach, A. (2013, November 11). ABC News' Amy Robach reveals breast cancer diagnosis.

Retrieved from http://abcnews.go.com/blogs/health/2013/11/11/abc-news-amy-robach-reveals-breast-cancer-diagnosis/.

Roberts, L. (2008, June 16). My Keira HASN'T got an eating disorder—she got her skinny frame from her dad, says her mother. *Daily Mail.* Retrieved from http://www.dailymail.co.uk/tvshowbiz/article-1026596/My-Keira-HASNT-got-eating-disorder—got-skinny-frame-dad-says-mother.html.

Roberts, M. (2013, May 14). "Jolie effect" on breast cancer? BBC. Retrieved from www.bbc.co.uk/news/health-22521844.

Roberts, M. B. (2012, February 26-March 3). Leeza Gibbons: The popular talk-show host finds a new mission after her mother's brave battle with Alzheimer's. *American Profile,* 6–7.

Roberts. R. (2007, August 3). ABC's Robin Roberts: "I have breast cancer." *ABC News.* Retrieved from http://abcnews.go.com/GMA/CancerPreventionAndTreatment/abcs-robin-roberts-breast-cancer/print?id=3430554.

Roberts, R. (2012, June 11). Robin Roberts: I'm going to beat this. *ABC News.* Retrieved from http://abcnews.go.com/Health/robin-roberts-myelodysplastic-syndrome-diagnosis-beat/print?id=16540293.

Roberts, R., and J. Elliott. (2012, January 19). Paula Deen speaks out. [Interview transcript] *Good Morning America.* Retrieved from Regional Business News Database.

Roberts, R., with V. Chambers. (2014). *Everybody's got something: A memoir.* New York: Grand Central.

"Robin Roberts: Biography" (2014). Retrieved from http://www.biography.com/people/robin-roberts-21188247#early-life&awesm=~oEgs7dsp3Lnuos.

Rock, M. (2003). Death, taxes, public opinion, and the midas touch of Mary Tyler Moore. *Medical Anthropology Quarterly, 17,* 200–232.

Rockwell, D., and D. C. Giles. (2009). Being a celebrity: A phenomenology of fame. *Journal of Phenomenological Psychology, 40*(2), 178–210. doi: 10.1163/004726609X12482630041889.

Roderick, M. (2006). Adding insult to injury: Workplace injury in English professional football. *Sociology of Health & Illness, 28* (1), 76–97. doi: 10.1111/j.1467–9566.2005.00483x.

Romo, L. (2012). "Above the influence": How college students communicate about the healthy deviance of alcohol abstinence. *Health Communication, 27,* 672–681. doi:10.1080/10410236.2011.629409.

Rosenbaum, E. H., and I. R. Rosenbaum. (2011, December 31). Attitude! When winning is everything: The will to live. Cancer Supportive Survivorship Care. Retrieved from http:// www.cancersupportivecare.com/attitude.html.

Ross, K. (Ed.). (2012). *The handbook of gender, sex, and media.* Malden, MA: Wiley-Blackwell.

Rothstein, M. (1999). *Genetic secrets: Protecting privacy and confidentiality in the genetic era.* New Haven, CT: Yale University Press.

Rubin, R. (2007, April 26). Cancer steps into limelight. *USA Today,* 4D.

Rutenberg, J. (2011, May 27). The long good-bye. *New York Times.* Retrieved from http://www.nytimes.com/2011/05/29/fashion/farrah-fawcetts-long-goodbye.html?pagewanted=1&_r=1.

Salahi, L. (2011, April 14). Catherine Zeta-Jones sheds light on bipolar II disorder. *ABC News.* Retrieved from http://abcnews.go.com.

Salvatore, D. (2011, November). Robin Roberts: Why this is the prime of her life. *Prevention.* Retrieved from http://www.prevention.com/health/health-concerns/robin-roberts-exclusive-interview-surviving-breast-cancer.

Samuels, A. (2011, May 23). I survived. *Newsweek, 157*(21/22), 62–65.

Sanchez, R. (2014, February 28). Coroner: Philip Seymour Hoffman died of acute mixed drug intoxication. CNN. Retrieved from http://www.cnn.com/2014/02/28/showbiz/philip-seymour-hoffman-autopsy/.

Sanderson, J. (2011). *It's a whole new ballgame: How social media is changing sports.* New York: Hampton Press.

Sanderson, J., and P. H. Cheong. (2010). Tweeting prayers and communicating grief over Michael Jackson online. *Bulletin of Science, Technology & Society, 30,* 328–340. doi: 10.1177/0270467610380010.

Sandvoss, C. (2012). From national hero to liquid star: Identity and discourse in transnational sports consumption. In C. Sandvoss, M. Real, and A. Bernstein (Eds.), *Bodies of discourse: Sports stars, media, and the global public* (pp. 171–192). New York: Peter Lang.

Sandvoss, C., M. Real, and A. Bernstein (Eds.). (2012). *Bodies of discourse: Sports stars, media, and the global public.* New York: Peter Lang.

Saporito, B. (2008, September 15). He won his battle with cancer. So why are millions of Americans still losing theirs? *Time, 172*(11), 36–42.

Satran, J. (2012, October 15). Paula Deen: "I couldn't understand the haters." *The Huffington Post.* Retrieved from http://huffingtonpost.com.

Saukko, P. (2006). Rereading media and eating disorders: Karen Carpenter, Princess Diana, and the healthy female self. *Critical Studies in Media Communication, 23,* 152–169. doi: 10.1080/07393180600714539.

Saunders, A. (2009, November 19). Cancer crusader Stefanie Spielman dies at 42. Retrieved from http://www.dispatch.com/content/stories/local/2009/11/20/stefanie-spielman-loses-cancer-battle.html.

Savage, M. E., and P. R. Spence. (2014). Will you listen? An examination of parasocial interaction and credibility in radio. *Journal of Radio & Audio Media*, *21*, 3–19. doi: 10.1080/19376529.2014.891214.

Scardaville, M. (2003, January 21). Angel among us. *Soap Opera Digest*, *28*(3), 52–53.

Schirato, T. (2013). *Sports discourse*. London: Bloomsbury.

Schlosser, E. (2012). *Fast food nation: The dark side of the all–American meal*. New York: Houghton Mifflin Harcourt.

Schocker, L. (2013, December 31). 13 of the biggest celebrity health battles of 2013. *Huffington Post*. Retrieved from http://www.huffingtonpost.com/2013/12/31/celebrityhealth2013_n_4518887.html?view=print&comm_ref=false.

Schwab, F. (2014, March 3). Peyton Manning cleared after neck exam, will get $20 million and play in 2014. Retrieved from http://sports.yahoo.com/blogs/nfl-shutdown-corner/peyton-manning-cleared-neck-exam-20-million-play-172749413--nfl.html.

Schwartz, A. (2013, September 16). Catherine & Michael: Inside their tragic split. *People, 34–37*.

Schwarz, A. (2011, May 2). Duerson's brain trauma diagnosed. *New York Times*. Retrieved from http://www.nytimes.com/2011/05/03/sports/football/03duerson.html.

Scodari, C. (2004). *Serial monogamy: Soap opera, lifespan, and the gendered politics of fantasy*. Cresskill, NJ: Hampton Press.

Scrambler, G., and A. Hopkins. (1986). "Being epileptic": Coming to terms with stigma. *Sociology of Health & Illness*, *8*(1), 26–43.

Screen Actor's Guild. (2011, September 8). *Mary Tyler Moore honored with 2011 Screen Actor's Guild Life Achievement Award*. Retrieved from http://www.sagaftra.org/press-releases/september-08-2011/mary-tyler-moore-honored-2011-screen-actors-guild-life-achievement-.

Seacrest, R., M. E. Bunim, and J. Murray. (Creators). (2011). Life in the big city. In R. Seacrest, J. Murray, J. Jenkins, G. Goldschein, R. Jay, M. Bidwell, and K. Jenner. (Executive Producers), *Kourtney and Kim take New York*. New York: Bunim/Murray Productions & Ryan Seacrest Productions.

Seaton, E. (2008). Common knowledge: Reflections on narratives in community. *Qualitative Research*, *8*, 293–305. doi: 10.1177/1468794106094067.

Serpe, G. (2012, November 13). Keira Knightley disappointed by droopy "fantasy breasts." Retrieved from http://www.today.com/entertainment/keira-knightley-disappointed-droopy-fantasy-breasts-1C7042433?franchiseSlug=todayentertainmentmain#__utma=…

SFGate. (2013, March 6). Paula Deen encourages you to take a walk in her footsteps and start seeing diabetes in a new light. Retrieved from http://www.sfgate.com/news/article/Paula-Deen-encourages-you-to-take-a-walk-in-her-4333382.php.

Shaffer, V. A., S. Tomek, and L. Hulsey. (2014). The effect of narrative information in a publicly available patient decision aid for early-stage breast cancer. *Health Communication*, *29*, 64–73. doi: 10.1080/10410236.2012.717341.

Shakespeare, W. (1599/2014). Hamlet. In P. Weller (Ed.), *Shakespeare Navigators*. Retrieved from http://shakespeare-navigators.com/hamlet/H31.html.

Sharf, B. (2009). Observations from the outside in: Narratives of illness, healing, and mortality in everyday life. *Journal of Applied Communication Research*, *37*, 132–139.

Sharf, B., L. Harter, J. Yamasaki, and P. Haidet. (2011). Narrative turns epic: Continuing developments in health narrative scholarship. In T. Thompson, R. Parrott, and J. Nussbaum (Eds.), *Handbook of health communication* (2nd ed., pp. 36–52). New York: Routledge.

Shuster, R. (1993, April 29). Courage against all odds is lesson for us all. *USA Today*, 3C.

Sidey, H. (1994, November 14). "The sunset of my life." *Time*, *144*(20), 65.

Silverstein, J. (2014, April 14). Robin Roberts discovered lump while covering 2012 Oscars, she reveals in memoir "Everybody's Got Something." *New York Daily News*. Retrieved from http://www.nydailynews.com/entertainment/tv-movies/robin-roberts-reveals-moment-discovered-lump-article-1.1756287.

Simmons, N. (2012). The tales of *gaijin*: Health privacy perspectives of foreign English teachers in Japan. *Kaleidoscope: A Graduate Journal of Qualitative Communication Research*, *11*, 17–38.

Simpson, R. (2007, January 8). It's itsy bitsy teeny weeny Keira Knightley. *Daily Mail online*. Retrieved from http://www.dailymail.co.uk/tvshowbiz/article-427243/Its-itsy-bitsy-teeny-weeny-Keira-Knightley.html.

"Singer Whitney Houston dies at 48." (2012, February 11). CNN. Retrieved from http://www.cnn.com/2012/02/11/showbiz/whitney-houston-dead/.

Singhal, A., M. Cody, E. Rogers, and M. Sabido. (Eds.). (2004). *Entertainment-education and social change*. Mahwah, NJ: Erlbaum.

Singhal, A., and E. Rogers. (1999). *Entertainment-education: A communication strategy for social change*. Mahwah, NJ: Erlbaum.

Singhal, A., and E. Rogers. (2003). *Combating AIDS: Communication strategies in action*. New Delhi, India: Sage.

Sizemore, R., B. Rott, G. Rancic, and B. Rancic. (Executive producers) (2010a). A Heartbreaking Loss. *Giuliana & Bill.* Style Network Broadcasting.

Sizemore, R., B. Rott, G. Rancic, and B. Rancic. (Executive producers) (2010b). Family Matters. *Giuliana & Bill.* Style Network Broadcasting.

Sizemore, R., B. Rott, G. Rancic, and B. Rancic. (Executive producers) (2010c). Knocked Up? *Giuliana & Bill.* Style Network Broadcasting.

Sizemore, R., B. Rott, G. Rancic, and B. Rancic. (Executive producers) (2010d). Operation Ovulation. *Giuliana & Bill.* Style Network Broadcasting.

Sizemore, R., B. Rott, G. Rancic, and B. Rancic. (Executive producers) (2012a). Holy Baby. *Giuliana & Bill.* Style Network Broadcasting.

Sizemore, R., B. Rott, G. Rancic, and B. Rancic. (Executive producers) (2012b). Meet the Duke. *Giuliana & Bill.* Style Network Broadcasting.

Sizemore, R., B. Rott, G. Rancic, and B. Rancic. (Executive producers) (2012c). Who's Your Nanny? *Giuliana & Bill.* Style Network Broadcasting.

Sizemore, R., B. Rott, G. Rancic, and B. Rancic. (Executive producers) (2013a). Baby on the Loose. *Giuliana & Bill.* Style Network Broadcasting.

Sizemore, R., B. Rott, G. Rancic, and B. Rancic. (Executive producers) (2013b). Duke's Nanny & Pedi. *Giuliana & Bill.* Style Network Broadcasting.

Sizemore, R., B. Rott, G. Rancic, and B. Rancic. (Executive producers) (2013c). Rancic Rewind. *Giuliana & Bill.* Style Network Broadcasting.

Sizemore, R., B. Rott, G. Rancic, and B. Rancic. (Executive producers) (2014a). Home Alone *Giuliana & Bill.* E! Broadcasting.

Sizemore, R., B. Rott, G. Rancic, and B. Rancic. (Executive producers) (2014b). Saving Face. *Giuliana & Bill.* E! Broadcasting.

Sloan, T. (2010). *Changing shoes: Getting older—NOT OLD—with style, humor, and grace.* New York: Gotham Books.

Smart, B. (2005). *The sport star: Modern sport and the cultural economy of sporting celebrity.* London: Sage.

Smith, F. (2014) IMDB mini biography. Retrieved from http://www.imdb.com/name/nm0461136/bio?ref_=nm_ov_bio_sm.

Smith, G. (1993, January 11). As time runs out. *Sports Illustrated, 78*(1), 11–25.

Smith, G. (1993, October 4). "We're going to beat this thing." *Sports Illustrated,* pp. 17–25.

Smith-Chandler, N., and E. Swart. (2014). In their own voices: Methodological considerations in narrative disability research. *Qualitative Health Research, 24,* 420–430. doi: 10.1177/1049732314523841.

Smolowe, J., F. Weinstein, S. Cotliar, M. Green, S. Scully, S. Marquez, et al. (2006, March 27). Dana Reeve brave to the end. *People, 65*(12), 112–116.

Solotaroff, P. (2011, May). Dave Duerson: The ferocious life and tragic death of a Super Bowl star. *Men's Journal.* http://www.mensjournal.com/magazine/dave-duerson-the-ferocious-life-and-tragic-death-of-a-super-bowl-star-20121002#ixzz2wKmlaEkA.

Sood, S., and E. M. Rogers. (2001). Dimensions of parasocial interaction by letter-writers to a popular entertainment-education soap opera in India. *Journal of Broadcasting & Electronic Media, 44,* 386–414.

Spence, L. (2005). *Watching daytime soap operas: The power of pleasure.* Middletown, CT: Wesleyan University Press.

Spencer, A. (2012). Giuliana Rancic: How I got through the tough stuff. CNN. Retrieved from http://www.cnn.com/2012/11/12/living/health-giuliana/.

Spitzack, C. (1993). The spectacle of anorexia nervosa. *Text and Performance Quarterly, 13,* 1–20.

Starpulse.com. (2014). Robin Roberts biography. Retrieved from http://www.starpulse.com/Actresses/Roberts,_Robin/Biography/.

St. Clair, L. (2014, May 28). Loss of appetite: The Food Network loses its way. Retrieved from http://www.sfweekly.com/2014-05-28/culture/network-next-food-network-star/.

Stefanik-Sider, K. (2013). Nature, nurture, or that fast food hamburger: Media framing of diabetes in the *New York Times* from 2000 to 2010. *Health Communication, 28,* 351–358.

Steinfeldt, M., and J. A. Steinfeldt. (2012). Athletic identity and conformity to masculine norms among college football players. *Journal of Applied Sport Psychology, 24,* 115–128.

Stelter, B. (2014, June 11). Paula Deen to host new TV show—online. Retrieved from http://www.kspr.com/life/money/Paula-Deen-to-host-new-TV-show-online/21052342_264…

Stephens, C. (2011). Narrative analysis in health psychology research: Personal, dialogical and social stories of health. *Health Psychology Review, 5,* 62–78. doi: 10.1080/17437199.2010.543385.

Stone, A. (2011). Former first lady Betty Ford dead at 93. *USA Today.* Retrieved from http://www.usatoday.com/news/washington/2011-07-08-betty-ford-obit_n.htm.

Stone, A. (2013, March 2). Celebrity eating disorder confessions: Inspiring or dangerous? Retrieved from http://www.hollywood.com/news/celebrities/55002837/eating-disorder-awareness-recovery-celebrity-spotlight-harmful-katie-couric-lady-gaga.

Stroud, S. R. (2011). *John Dewey and the artful life: Pragmatism, aesthetics, and morality.* University Park: Pennsylvania State University Press.

Stuart, M. (1980). *Both of me*. Garden City, NY: Doubleday.

Stump, S. (2013, November 7). Matt Lauer, Al Roker have prostate exams live on *Today*. Retrieved from http://www.today.com/health/matt-lauer-al-roker-have-prostate-exams-live-today-8C11547011.

Summitt, P., with S. Jenkins. (2013). *Sum it up*. New York: Random House.

Swayze, P., and L. Niemi. (2009). *The time of my life*. New York: Simon & Schuster.

Sweeney, A. (2004). *All the days of my life (so far)*. New York: Kensington.

Syer, J. (1986). *Team spirit: The elusive experience*. London: The Kingwood Press.

Symetra Tour (2014). *Tour player addresses diabetes at JDRF Children's Congress*. Retrieved from http://www.symetratour.com/golf/news/2011/6/tour-player-addresses-diabetes-at-jdrf-children-s-congress.aspx.

"Synopsis." (2014). *Miss Representation*. Retrieved from http://film.missrepresentation.org/synopsis.

Taibi, C. (2014, January 25). Amy Robach's courageous decision. *Huffington Post*. Retrieved from http://www.huffingtonpost.com/2014/01/15/amy-robach-hair_n_4603252.html.

Taibi, C. (2014, April 25).Amazing news for Amy Robach. *Huffington Post*. Retrieved from http://www.huffingtonpost.com/2014/04/25/amy-robach-chemotherapy-session-good-morning-america-breast-cancer_n_5211969.html.

Tan, M. (2008, May 26). Guiding Light star gastric on TV—and in real life. *People*. Retrieved from www.people.com/people/archive/article/0.20204015.00.html.

Tasiemski, T., and B. W. Brewer. (2011). Athletic identity, sport participation, and psychological adjustment in people with spinal cord injury. *Adapted Physical Activity Quarterly, 28*, 233–250.

Tauber, M., S. Cotliar, A. Dennis, J. Jordan, M. Green, and P. Cedenheim. (2013, May 27). "I made a strong choice." *People, 79* (21), 66–72.

Taylor, A., and M. Hutchings. (2012). Using video narratives of women's lived experience of breastfeeding in midwifery education: Exploring its impact on midwives' attitudes to breastfeeding. *Maternal & Child Nutrition, 8*, 88–102. doi: 10.1111/j.1740–8709.2010.00258.x.

Teal, W. (n.d.). Celebrity secrets to losing baby weight. *Parents*. Retrieved from http://www.parents.com/baby/health/lose-baby-weight/celebrity-secrets-losing-baby-weight/.

Teitelbaum, S. H. (2005). *Sports heroes, fallen idols*. Lincoln: University of Nebraska Press.

Tenzek, K. E., A. R. Herrman, A. R. May, B. Feiner, and M. Allen. (2013). Examining the impact of parental disclosure of HIV on children: A meta-analysis. *Western Journal of Communication, 77*, 323–339. doi:10.1080/10570314.2012.719092.

Testa, J. (2013, June 26). Why Food Network dumped Paula Deen: It's about ratings, not racism. Retrieved from http://antennafree.tv/2013/06/26/why-food-network-dumped-paula-deen-its-about-ratings...

Thackeray, R., S. H. Burton, C. Giraud-Carrier, S. Rollins, and C. R. Draper. (2013). Using Twitter for breast cancer prevention: An analysis of breast cancer awareness month. *BioMed Central Journal, 13*, doi:10.1186/1471–2407–13–508. Retrieved from http://www.biomedcentral.com/1471–2407/13/508.

"Thinspiration pictures, Thinspiration photos of real girls, models and celebrities." (n.d.). Retrieved from http://thinspiration-pictures.blogspot.com/.

"This just in." (2014, February 3). Retrieved from http://www.tvguide.com/soaps/guiding-light-star-10094.aspx.

Thompson, T. L. (2009). The applicability of narrative ethics. *Journal of Applied Communication Research, 37*, 188–195.

Tidwell, L. C., and J. B. Walther. (2002). Computer-mediated communication effects on disclosure, impressions, and interpersonal evaluations: Getting to know one another a bit at a time. *Human Communication Research, 28*, 317–348. doi.org/10.1111/j.1468–2958.2002.tb00811.x.

Today Show. (1998, July 8). Profile: Soap opera actor Michael Zaslow battles with Lou Gehrig's disease [Interview transcript].

Tolson, A. (2001). Being yourself: the pursuit of authentic celebrity. *Discourse Studies, 3*(4), 443–457. doi: 10.1177/1461445601003004007.

Trout, J. (2014, March 5). Jennifer Lawrence body-shames you more than you might realize. *Huff Post Women*. Retrieved from http://www.huffingtonpost.com/jenny-trout/jennifer-lawrence-body-shaming_b_4521379.html.

Tuck, L. (2014, May 21). Samantha Harris shares mastectomy selfie from hospital room. Retrieved from http://shine.yahoo.com/healthy-living/samantha-harris-shares-post-mastectomy-selfie-194...

Twitter. (2014a). About. Retrieved from https://about.twitter.com/.

Twitter. (2014b). Brooke Burke-Charvet. Retrieved from https://twitter.com/brookeburke.

Twycross, R. (2007). Patient care: Past, present, and future. *Omega: Journal of Death & Dying, 56*, 7–19. doi:10.2190/OM.56.1.b.

Tyley, J. (2013, November 22). Jennifer Lawrence "refused to lose weight" for Hunger Games.

SciFiNow. Retrieved from http://www.scifi now.co.uk/news/jennifer-lawrence-i-refused-to-lose-weight-for-the-hunger-games/.

Underwood, A. (2012, May). "So many people need hope." *Prevention, 64*(5), 52–62.

U.S. Senate Committee on Homeland Security & Governmental Affairs. (2013). *What is a Senate committee?* Retrieved from http:// www.hsgac.senate.gov/about/whatis.

U. S. Senate Hearing 110–316. (2007, June 19). *The Juvenile Diabetes Research Foundation and the Federal Government: A model public-private partnership accelerating research toward a cure.* Retrieved from http://www.gpo. gov/fdsys/pkg/CHRG-110shrg36614/html/ CHRG-110shrg36614.htm.

U. S. Senate Hearing 111–908 (2009, June 24). *Type 1 diabetes research: Real progress and real hope for a cure.* Retrieved from http://www. gpo.gov/fdsys/pkg/CHRG-111shrg51789/html/ CHRG-111shrg51789.htm.

Vaccariello, L. (2013, May 7). *Reader's Digest* announces "100 most trusted people in America." *Reader's Digest.* Retrieved from http:// www.prnewswire.com/news-releases/readers-digest-announces-100-most-trusted-people-in-america-206435821.html.

Vaccariello, L. (n.d.). Why Robin Roberts is the most trusted woman on television. *Reader's Digest.* Retrieved from http://www.rd.com/ culture/why-robin-roberts-is-the-most-trusted-woman-on-television/.

Valvano, J. (1993, March 4). ESPY Awards speech. Jimmy V. Foundation. Retrieved from http://www.jimmyv.org/about -us/remembering-jim/jimmy-v-espy-awards-speech.

"Valvano remembered as dynamic man." (1999, December 17). *USA Today,* 12C.

Van Dijck, J. (2013). *The culture of connectivity: A critical history of social media.* New York: Oxford University Press.

Van Natta Jr., D. (2013, October 2). Book: NFL crusaded against science. Retrieved from http://espn.go.com/espn/otl/story/_/id9745 797/new-book-denial-says-nfl-used-resources.

Van Vonderen, K. E., and W. Kinnally. (2012). Media effects on body image: Examining media exposure in the broader context of internal and other social factors. *American Communication Journal, 14*(2), 41–57.

Vaughan, P. W., E. M. Rogers, A. Singhal, and R. M. Swalehe. (2000). Entertainment-education and HIV/AIDS prevention: A field experiment in Tanzania. *Journal of Health Communication,* 5, 81–100. doi: 1081–0730/00.

Veatch, R. M. (1980). Voluntary risks to health: The ethical issues. *Journal of the American Medical Association, 243,* 50–55.

Venetis, M. K., K. Greene, K. Magsamen-Conrad, S. C. Banerjee, M. G. Checton, and Z. Bagdasarov. (2012). "You can't tell anyone but…": Exploring the use of privacy rules and revealing behaviors. *Communication Monographs, 79,* 344–365. doi:10.1080/03637751. 2012.697628.

Vitale, D. (1994, April). Unforgettable Jim Valvano. *Reader's Digest,* 78–82.

Vu, H. T., and T. Lee. (2013). Soap operas as a matchmaker: A cultivation analysis of the effects of South Korean TV dramas on Vietnamese women's marital intentions. *Journalism & Mass Communication Quarterly, 90,* 308–330.

Walters, B. (Executive Producer, 2014, May 16). *ABC's Barbara Walters Special, Barbara Walters: Her Story.* ABC News Special.

Wang, M., and A. Singhal. (1992). "Ks Wang," a Chinese television soap opera with a message. *International Communication Gazette, 49,* 177–192.

Weir, B. (n.d). Whitney Houston: Cause of death revealed. *ABC News Video.* Retrieved from http://abcnews.go.com/Entertainment/ whitney-houston-death-report-drowning-heart-disease-cocaine/story?id=15979609.

Weitz, R. (Ed.). (2003). *The politics of women's bodies: Sexuality, appearance, and behavior.* New York: Oxford University Press.

Welch, H. G. (2013, May 18). What Angelina Jolie forgot to mention. CNN. Retrieved from http://www.cnn.com/2013/05/17/opinion/ welch-jolie-mastectomy/index.html.

Wetli, C. (2014, August 12). Robin Williams' suicide illuminating America's failure to deal with mental illness: guest opinion. Retrieved from http://impact.al.com/opinion/print. html?entry=2014/08/robin_williams_suicide_ illumin.ht…

Whannel, G. (2002). *Media sport stars: Masculinities and moralities.* London: Routledge.

Wheeler, M. (2013). *Celebrity politics.* Cambridge, England: Polity.

White, M., and D. Epston. (1990). *Narrative means to therapeutic ends.* New York: W. W. Norton.

"Why Keira Knightley lasted 12 hours on Twitter." (2013, December 30). *The Sydney Morning Herald.* Retrieved from http://www.smh. com.au/lifestyle/celebrity/why-keira-knightley-lasted-12-hours-on-twitter-20131230-302rr.html212–226.

Williams, C. T. (1992). *"It's time for my story": Soap opera sources, structure, and response.* Westport, CT: Praeger.

Wittebols, J. H. (2004). *The soap opera paradigm: Television programming and corporate priorities.* Lanham, MD: Rowman & Littlefield.

Wolf, M., F. Theis, and H. Kordy. (2013). Language use in eating disorder blogs: Psychological implications of social online activity. *Journal of Language & Social Psychology, 32*(2), 1–15. doi: 10.1177/0261927X12474278.

Wolin, R. (2001). *The rhetorical imagination of Kenneth Burke*. Columbia: University of South Carolina Press.

Wolters Kluwer Health. (2014). Patient information: Myeodysplastic syndromes (MDS) in adults (beyond the basics). *UpToDate*. Retrieved from http://www.uptodate.com/contents/myelodysplastic-syndromes-mds-in-adults-beyond-the-basics.

World Health Organization. (2014). Cancer. Retrieved from http://www.who.int/mediacentre/factsheets/fs297/en/.

Wujcik, D. (2009, March). Use celebrities to start the conversation about cancer. *ONS Connect, 24*(3), 5.

Yep, G. A. (2000). Disclosure of HIV infection in interpersonal relationships: A communication boundary management approach. In S. Petronio (Ed.), *Balancing the secret of privacy disclosures* (pp. 83–96). Mahwah, NJ: Erlbaum.

Yoo, S. K., L. R. Smith, and D. Kim. (2013). Communication theories and sport studies. In P. M. Pedersen (Ed.), *Routledge handbook of sport communication* (pp. 8–19). London: Routledge.

Young, N. (2008). Identity trans/formations. In C. S. Beck (Ed.), *Communication yearbook 31* (pp. 224–273). New York: Erlbaum.

YouTube.com. (2014). Brooke Burke-Charvet: Cancer. Me? Retrieved from https://www.youtube.com/all_comments?v=6yvZuWuSIHU.

YouTube.com. (2014, January 31). Amanda Knox interview on GMA Good Morning America with Robin Roberts. Retrieved from https://www.youtube.com/watch?v=n4hafGvxj9o.

Zakarin, J. (2013, April 10). Robin Roberts on her cancer battle, the lowest moments and why "GMA" is no. 1. *Hollywood Reporter*. Retrieved from http://www.hollywoodreporter.com/news/robin-roberts-her-cancer-battle-435868.

Zaslow, M. (1998, January 20). Michael Zaslow speaks out about his fight against Lou Gehrig's disease. *Soap Opera News*, 1–2.

Zaslow, M., and S. Hufford. (2005). *Not that man anymore (A message from Michael)*. New York: iUniverse, Inc.

Zenk Pinter (n.d.) Colleen Zenk Pinter's battle with cancer. Retrieved from http://www.womensday.com/life/entertainment/colleen-zenk-pinters-battle-cancer-64845.

Zimmer, K., with L. Morton. (2011). *I'm just sayin'!: Three deaths, seven husbands, and a CLONE! My life as a daytime diva*. New York: New American Library.

Zizek, S. (1992). *Looking awry: An introduction to Jacque Lacan through popular culture*. Cambridge, MA: MIT Press.

Index

depriving dilemma 76
destigmatization *see* stigma
detached co-owners 57–58, 62–63 *see also* narrative
diabetes: type 1 *see* juvenile diabetes (type 1 diabetes); type 2 64–65 (*see also* Deen, Paula)
dialectic of the gaze 41
The Doctors 6
donor: bone marrow 124, 170, 171–172, 173, 179–181, 183
Doug Flutie, Jr. Foundation for Autism 125
Douglas, Michael 51, 52, 53
Down syndrome 211
Dravecky, Dave 122–123
drug abuse 96–97; classroom conversations 106–107; college students' conversations 105–107; death from 94, 99–100, 108–109; families' conversations 106; fear 109; friends' conversations about 107; Heath Ledger's death and 101, 109; media-related awareness 104–105; Michael Jackson's death and 104, 109; Phillip Seymour Hoffman's death and 104, 109; Whitney Houston's death and 102–103, 109
Drugs.com 94
Duerson, Dave 115–116
Duke, Patty 53, 210
Dunbar, Kate 65
Dyer, Kendall 65
Dynasty 10–11

E! Network: *E! News* 149, 150, 155; *Wild On!* 29, 32–37
early detection *see* screening
eating disorders 80–81, 140; Keira Knightley and 77, 78, 83–85; visual aspects 87–88; websites 81–82; *see also* body image
Ebert, Roger 24
eczema 45
Elizabeth Glaser Pediatric AIDS Foundation 211
Elliott, Missy 23
end of life *see* death and dying
Esiason, Boomer 126–128
Esiason, Gunnar 126–128
Evans, Linda 10–11
Everhart, Angie 24
Everybody's Got Something (Roberts) 167, 170

Fab-U-Wish 150, 159–160
Face to Face with Connie Chung 119–120
Facebook 14–15, 18, 97, 103; Brooke Burke-Charvet 26–27, 28, 30–31, 33–35, 36–37; on Giuliana Rancic's *Today Show* interview 158; Paula Deen 68; Robin Roberts 170; supportive communication 37, 38
face-lift 132–134
Fainaru, S. 115, 116, 117
Fainaru-Wada, M. 115, 116, 117
Farrah Fawcett Foundation 17

Fashion Police 149
Fast Food Nation 74
Fawcett, Farrah 16–17, 78, 97
Field of Dreams 122–123
Fisher, Carrie 53
Fisher, W.R. 12, 13
Flutie, Doug 125
"Follow the Script" 24
Fonda, Jane 81
food: Southern 64–65, 68–69, 70–71; U.S. 64, 74
Food Network 68–69, 74–75
football *see* National Football League
Ford, Betty 11, 188
Forrester, Kristen *(Bold and the Beautiful)* 136
Fox, Michael J. 5, 14, 59, 208–209, 211
Freud, Sigmund 94
front stage 15, 113; *see also* impression management
Fulton, Eileen 136–137

gain-framed message/appeal 154–155
Garland, Judy 94
General Hospital 135
genetics 8, 85
Giuliana & Bill 150, 152, 153–154, 159–160, 161, 163, 165–166
Glamour 155–156, 157–158, 160
Godfrey, Linsey 141–142
Goffman, Erving 9–10, 55, 69, 113
Gold, Tracy 140
Good Morning America: Breast Cancer Awareness Month 178, 203–204; Catherine Zeta-Jones interview 54, 55–56; Mary Tyler Moore interview 190; Robin Roberts 6, 168, 175–176
Goody, Jade 17–18
Goody effect 17–18, 209
Gould, Ellen 193
Graves' disease 23–24
Gring-Pemble, L. M. 17
Growing Up Again (Moore) 186–187, 188, 189, 194
Guiding Light 135, 137, 139–140, 142–143, 144–145, 147

H1N1 virus 169
Hall, Gary, Jr. 192
Hamilton, Scott 123, 124
Hashimoto's disease 23–24
Hayes, Bill 137
Hayes, Susan Seaforth 137
Haythorn, Russell 111
head injury 114–116
health activism *see* public health activism
Health.com 160–161
HIPPA laws 61
HIV/AIDS: Arthur Ashe 117–118, 208; congressional testimony 211; Greg Louganis 118; Magic Johnson 18, 118–121; Rock Hud-